Psy

Exeter

3 Day

ssociated with
hts and devel-
nced overview

ig with those
uding vulner-
l for recovery
s paid to how
'self-healing'

treatment of
s interested in

working with
sor at several
Stockholm hospitals. He is former chairman of the ISPS and has published
extensively on the subject of psychosis.

Psychoses

An integrative perspective

Johan Cullberg

Foreword by Professor Patrick McGorry

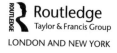

Routledge
Taylor & Francis Group

LONDON AND NEW YORK

The International Society for the Psychological Treatments of the Schizophrenias and Other Psychoses Book Series

Series Editor: Brian Martindale

The ISPS (The International Society for the Psychological Treatments of the Schizophrenias and Other Psychoses) has a history stretching back some 50 years, during which it has witnessed the relentless pursuit of biological explanations for psychosis. The tide is now turning again. There is a welcome international resurgence in interest in a range of psychological factors in psychosis that have considerable explanatory power and also distinct therapeutic possibilities. Governments, professional groups, users and carers are increasingly expecting interventions that involve talking and listening as well as skilled practitioners in the main psychotherapeutic modalities as important components of the care of the seriously mentally ill.

The ISPS is a global society. It is composed of an increasing number of groups of professionals organised at national, regional and more local levels around the world. The society has started a range of activities intended to support professionals, users and carers. Such persons recognise the humanitarian and therapeutic potential of skilled psychological understanding and therapy in the field of psychosis. Our members cover a wide spectrum of interests from psychodynamic, systemic, cognitive and arts therapies to the need-adaptive approaches and to therapeutic institutions. We are most interested in establishing meaningful dialogue with those practitioners and researchers who are more familiar with biological based approaches. Our activities include regular international and national conferences, newsletters and email discussion groups in many countries across the world.

One of these activities is to facilitate the publication of quality books that cover the wide terrain that interests ISPS members and a large number of other mental health professionals, policy makers and implementers. We are delighted that Routledge of the Taylor & Francis Group has seen the importance and potential of such an endeavour and has agreed to publish an ISPS series of books.

We anticipate that some of the books will be controversial and will challenge certain aspects of current practice in some countries. Other books will promote ideas and authors well known in some countries but not familiar to others. Our overall aim is to encourage the dissemination of existing knowledge and ideas, promote healthy debate and encourage more research in a most important field whose secrets almost certainly do not all reside in the neurosciences.

For more information about the ISPS, email isps@isps.org or visit our website www.isps.org

Other titles in the series

Models of Madness: Psychological, Social and Biological Approaches to Schizophrenia
Edited by John Read, Loren R. Mosher & Richard P. Bentall

Evolving Psychosis: Different Stages, Different Treatments
Edited by Jan Olav Johannessen, Brian V. Martindale & Johan Cullberg

First published 2006
by Routledge
27 Church Road, Hove, East Sussex BN3 2FA

Simultaneously published in the USA and Canada
by Routledge
270 Madison Avenue, New York, NY 10016

Routledge is an imprint of the Taylor & Francis Group

Originally published in Swedish as Psykoser: Ett integrerat perspektiv
by Natur och Kultur, 2000, 2004 © Johan Cullberg and
Borkförlaget Natur och Kultur, Sweden

Translation © Johan Cullberg and ISPS

Copyright © 2006 Johan Cullberg

Typeset in Times by RefineCatch Ltd, Bungay, Suffolk
Printed and bound in Great Britain by
TJ International Ltd, Padstow, Cornwall
Paperback cover design by Hybert design

This publication has been produced with paper manufactured to
strict environmental standards and with pulp derived from
sustainable forests.

British Library Cataloguing in Publication Data
A catalogue record for this book is available from the British Library

Library of Congress Cataloging-in-Publication Data
Cullberg, Johan, 1934–
    Psychoses : an integrative perspective / Johan Cullberg.– 1st ed.
       p. cm.
    Includes bibliographical references and index.
    ISBN 1-58391-992-9 (hbk) – ISBN 1-58391-993-7 (pbk) 1. Psychoses. I. Title.
    RC512.C85 2006
    616.89–dc22   2005017913

ISBN10: 1-58391-992-9 (hbk)
ISBN10: 1-58391-993-7 (pbk)

ISBN13: 9-78-1-58391-992-9 (hbk)
ISBN13: 9-78-1-58391-993-7 (pbk)

2006

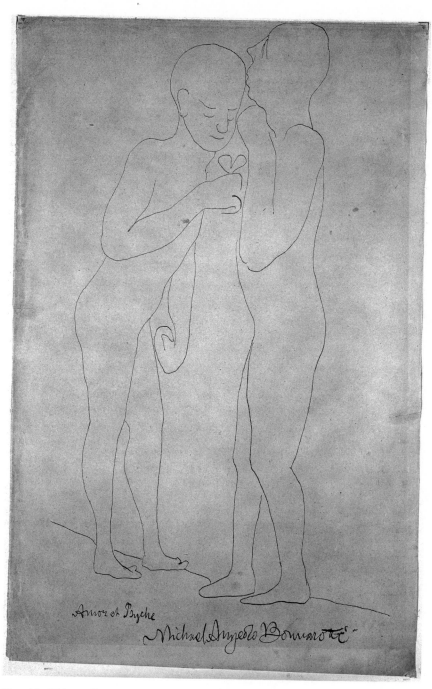

Amor et Psyche

Michael Angelo Buonarotti

Please see over page for explanatory text on this artist, Ernst Josephson . . .

Ernst Josephson (1851–1906) is one of Sweden's most prominent painters. He developed a chronic schizophrenic disorder in 1888 while temporarily living in France. His painting radically changed from a naturalistic romantic style to a naïve directness with visionary force and expressive deformations. A change towards expressionism is often seen in established painters who develop a long-term psychotic disorder. Josephson remained active as an artist, mostly with pen drawings but also with some oil paintings.

This pen drawing is signed 'Michel Angelo Bonnaroti' since Josephson believed that he was in spiritual contact with Michelangelo.

Courtesy of the Swedish National Museum

Contents

Figures and tables

Tables

Foreword

Understanding and treating psychotic disorders, particularly schizophrenia, presents major challenges. Despite significant advances in treatment and liberal reforms to the structure of mental health services, in most parts of the world, including affluent developed countries, the personal experience and quality of life of those affected and their relatives has not improved very much. Indeed the neglect is palpable in North America and other English-speaking countries, and also in the developing world where the fate of people with schizophrenia tends to be idealised. In a general sense, this is due to a failure of societies, health systems and individuals to maintain and extend the humanistic perspective to people with severe mental illnesses. Psychiatry itself has contributed to this problem by lurching from one reductionistic extreme to another. For decades all psychiatric disorders were fully explained on a narrow psychological basis. More recently brain dysfunction and a narrow disease model has taken over. Psychiatry among the medical disciplines truly aspires to an integrative, bio-psycho-social approach, yet this is eschewed in centres for research, elusive in the real world and increasingly lacking in the training of mental health professionals and psychiatrists.

This is why Johan Cullberg's book is so important. It is a seminal scholarly work which draws upon humanistic philosophy, psychoanalysis, lessons from the history of psychiatry, good and bad, the experiences of the sufferer including his brother, his own experiences as a relative of someone with psychosis, neuroscience and epidemiological research, and intervention studies. The result is a rare and precious synthesis of knowledge and experience that should be read by all those responsible for the care of people with psychotic illness. The strength of the book lies not only in pursuing the elusive endeavour to integrate biological and humanistic perspectives (a difficult task!), but also in its ultimate acceptance of the biological basis of the disorder and the need for careful use of drug therapies, while at the same time showing the critical need for humanistic and sophisticated psychological understanding of the patient and his or her predicament, crises and struggle to recover. The book is enriched with wonderfully practical guidelines and innumerable pearls of clinical wisdom distilled from a long and constantly evolving clinical and personal experience. I know of no other textbook on psychosis in the English language which communicates this kind of message. This is why it so pleasing to see Johan Cullberg's hard-won perspective finally becoming accessible to anglophone psychiatry. He is an integrator and a humanitarian and a wonderful ambassador for the values he advocates in the understanding and clinical care of patients and their families.

In his Epilogue, in which he refers to his brother Erland's illness, he closes with the following paragraph. I would like to to highlight it again in the Foreword because I think it contains a basic truth and problem which must be overcome if the care of serious mental illness is to improve in our societies:

> Working in medical care has an almost irresistible tendency to numb practitioners to the realisation that they are treating and tending individuals who are just like themselves. Many claim that they have to dissociate themselves from their feelings if they are to function in the wards, which is plainly not the case. There is more to good care than ethical principles and staff training. It also requires an organisation that accords priority to and accordingly finds room for empathy and humanity without any loss of professional standards. I have seen many places where this has been achieved. It is very much a matter of wanting and being sufficiently courageous to break away from ingrained attitudes. An organisation in which truly humane care is not feasible is a bad organisation. In other words, this has to do with the politics of care in the widest sense.

This is the heart of the matter around which all of the other perspectives, expertise, knowledge and wisdom contained within this book can be layered. It is an essential message for those who provide mental health services. I sincerely hope the work of this very wise, passionate, caring and yet truly modest man, Johan Cullberg, will be widely read in the English-speaking world where its messages urgently need to be absorbed.

Patrick McGorry
Melbourne
1 February 2005

Preface

As a young medical student in the latter half of the 1950s I read a book which describes a psychotherapy carried out with Renée, a schizophrenic girl (Sechehaye 1947). The book had a deep effect on me both because of its authenticity and because Renée was able to recover her health completely. At the same time I came across an American article about research on the ceruloplasmin fraction of the blood protein of schizophrenic patients. When rhesus monkeys were injected with it they reacted with all the signs of catatonic schizophrenia. Today we might ask ourselves what it really was that cured Renée. As it turned out, ceruloplasmin was not the answer to the mystery of schizophrenia. But for me the experiences of reading those studies still represent the vast scope of the area of research into psychosis.

It is easy to forget that psychosis, like schizophrenia, is a phenomenological concept. It can, as yet, only be defined in behavioural terms and as subjective changes in the experiential world. It has not been possible to characterise schizophrenia biologically even if such factors probably play an essential role. In this book I want to show how fruitful and necessary it is to keep the humanistic and biological perspectives alive simultaneously in the understanding of and work with the psychotic condition.

But when it is necessary to act on one's words and to try to uphold an interdisciplinary scientific perspective, one immediately encounters a major problem of a theoretical and practical nature. It is not just a question of separate scientific traditions but also about different and yet indispensable ways of looking at human beings. So we have to work towards a state of holding both areas of knowledge in mind. Both must be examined critically and from their specific conditions. How does the connection between the biomedical and the psychological systems reveal itself? What is the cause and what the effect? At the same time, when does the desire to be strictly scientific become a questionable reduction? If such sciences that are based on experimentally controlled research are the only ones that can be accepted, certain human experiences can easily become devalued and slip through the fingers. On the other hand there is a danger that personal prejudices of professional workers are accepted uncritically.

It has been challenging and exciting to formulate these questions, which I have worked on over many years. Both areas of knowledge are growing fast and sometimes it has felt 'too much' to hold them both together. There is a definite risk that the lacunae will become unacceptably large when only one person is writing a book of this kind and not, as usually happens, a group of writers each representing their own special interest. Nevertheless, I think there lies a point in striving towards offering a comprehensive picture of the psychotic individual as a human being, just as much as thinking about his or her biological aspects. It is precisely where and how the two disciplines come together that the essential problem is contained.

The book is directed mostly towards those professional workers who meet people with a psychotic condition. But I hope that it can also be read without too much previous knowledge by the interested non-professional.

The people whose fates I have described in the vignettes have read and accepted publication with the necessary alterations to, amongst other things, their identity. I thank them for their generosity in sharing their experiences.

Johan Cullberg
Stockholm
December 1999

Preface to the English edition

This book has been written at a time when there is little in the way of contemporary textbooks that have an integrative approach to psychosis. Today our biological and neuropsychological knowledge about the functional disorders of the brain is growing rapidly. In many ways they are guiding lights for medical practice. However psychological understanding and treatments are also expanding their evidence base, especially cognitive behavioural approaches. Psychoanalytically oriented researchers are moving towards neurophysiology and reformulating their theories of aetiological and motivational factors in psychosis. Dynamic psychiatry is now integrating itself as a clinically useful tool alongside the biological, cognitive and epidemiological approaches to psychiatry. This book, I hope, will be one of these integrating voices.

There will always be an epistemological conflict inherent in these efforts to synthesise the natural and humanistic sciences. I have tried to produce a reasonably coherent yet balanced overview of this subject. If this book can help us to develop more productive and humane care for patients with psychosis, its aims will have been fulfilled. I also believe that a better understanding of the psychology of psychosis may contribute to a deeper understanding of ourselves.

I hope the book will prove useful not only to medical students, psychiatrists in training and other mental health professionals, but also to non-professionals with an interest in the subject.

The book has been updated since it was first published in Swedish. The English translation has been partly supported by The International Society for the Psychological Treatments of the Schizophrenias and Other Psychoses (ISPS). I thank the ISPS board for this, and especially Dr Brian Martindale for his unfailing support during this period. I am also very grateful to Dr Michael Layton for his careful and professional checking of the English psychiatric terminology. Finally I thank Dr Philippa Martindale for her linguistic and editorial help.

Johan Cullberg
Stockholm
April 2005

Part I

The psychotic crisis and the schizophrenic disability

Hidden behind his psychotic life, in every schizophrenic a normal psychic life is proceeding. We might add that hidden by everyday behaviour, a schizophrenic life proceeds in every healthy person.

Manfred Bleuler, 1979

Chapter 1

Reason – a thin veil over chaos

Without you there is no me.

E. G. Geijer, 1856

A look at our existential position is hardly encouraging. As specks of dust in an infinite universe we are of no more interest than a single grain of sand on the seashore. We are born and die on time's narrow isthmus in an unfathomable ocean. We struggle, yearn, strive and suffer, gathering knowledge and experience, until it is all over and totally forgotten in a matter of generations.

At the same time there is another part of us on which everything centres, a point where we feel our specific weight and defend our identity, nationality and world view as being self-evident in relation to the different identities, nationalities and world views of others. We assert our existence and the ways in which we consider that the social order should be maintained and improved. In our conscious outlook we make little or no allowance for our own mortality. The risks we perceive have to do with loss of love or property and the possibility of being wronged or put to shame. As a means of preventing such things we construct both conscious and unconscious strategies that hopefully will not be too far out of step with the strategies of others. We aim to build them on what we consider to be a reasonable foundation.

The notion that reason, normalcy and self-esteem are things we can take for granted plays an important part in our adaptation and sense of security. But we are also aware that our rationality is rather fragile. Every night in our dreams, time, space and logic are all suspended. We also daydream to a varying extent, though for many people recalling one's daydreams is more embarrassing than what we dream in our sleep. In our daydreams we are pleasure-seeking, vengeful and engaged in hazy fantasies of power. Although these are our own fantasies and dreams, we find it hard to accept that daydreams express the deeper reaches of our personality. But on looking back at our earliest days, we recognise that our personality has its roots in the fertile soil of childhood to which the daydreams hark back.

We inevitably live in an impossible existential divide – between being just a speck of dust in the universe and simultaneously being its immeasurably important focus. In addition, we live in a psychological divide between respectable reason (our moral code) on the one hand and asocial self-assertion and pleasure seeking on the other. Our lives involve an ongoing dialectical alternation between these two positions and realities. Apart from the occasional impulse to do things that can seem incomprehensible, this alteration leaves little outward trace. Moreover, it is rendered less hazardous by the existence of states of repose and being able to cross bridges to our inner life. If these bridges are absent or break down, finding our way in the world becomes more difficult; our mental health is endangered. In some cases our reaction may amount to a loss of contact with reality – a psychosis.

Regression in the service of the ego

Sigmund Freud (1856–1939) distinguished between *primary process thinking* and *secondary process thinking*. The latter is the rational, logical mode of thinking that we are all trained to develop as an essential instrument for survival as a biological and social being. Secondary process thinking is governed by the reality principle.

Primary process thinking is associated instead with the world of dreams, including daydreams. It is governed by the pleasure principle, with wish fulfilment more or less untrammelled by space, time and persons. Morality and ethics have hardly any say in this omnipotent form of mental functioning.

The possibility of escaping for a time from the strict categories of rational thought and dwelling in its dialectical opposite means a lot for our mental health. The term regression implies that thinking and behaviour are governed to a greater degree by earlier levels of development. A classic psycho-analytic description for this is 'regression in the service of the ego', in contrast to the more destructive and pathological forms of regression that include psychosis. Here are some regressive bridges that span the divide between rational and irrational thought:

- fantasy and play
- creativity
- intimate relationships and sexuality
- religion
- magical rituals and predictions (e.g. horoscopes and astrology)
- intoxication.

Fantasy and play

These vital functions are similar in that they bring together or allow us to find a 'middle ground' between our inner world and the real world. We cannot completely survive in a world of rational order nor can we sustain for long a world of fantasy. The young child, in its fantasy games, animates his 'blanket' into something which allows a transition to take place between play and reality. According to the English psychoanalyst and paediatrician D. W. Winnicott (1971), children create a 'transitional space' between the real mother and the fantasised inner representation of the mother by means of a 'transitional object' – the blanket, cloth or whatever might be favoured. The child engages in a creative act, which allows him or her to deal with the disappointments engendered by its parents and reality. According to Winnicott, the blanket (or the alternative transitional object chosen by the child) represents and *is*, for the two to three year old, an aspect of the mother which allows the child to attain complete control over her. The capacity to use fantasy in play, play which is entirely serious, to transform reality consti- tutes the groundwork for the possibility in later life to create contact with the transitional space. The child will also be able to test out his illusions against reality with the use of his transitional object.

Winnicott wants us to understand that it is through this original tran- sitional space, between reality and illusion, that the adult's creative freedom is born. This is a perspective which has proved fruitful in considering the psychology of creativity. In psychosis the boundary between fantasy or play and reality has been lost.

The intimate relationship

In close conversation as in physical intimacy we venture outside the bound- aries of our selves and reinstate a 'symbiotic' contact with another being.[1] This is something, which the existentialist philosopher Martin Buber calls 'the experience of "you" '. It occurs with intensity, yet at the same time exists outside rationality, within such a symbiotic space.

An active 'you' experience is decisively meaningful in the evolution of our ability to hold on to and function within our experience of a continuous self. This is why unwanted and excessive isolation constitutes a risk for psychic health. One of the most important phenomena in acute psychosis is that the ability to function within the other 'you' category has been temporarily suspended (see Chapter 4 for more).

Sexuality

In today's western world, sexuality is perhaps the factor that has come to provide the most accepted method of reassurance. In its commercialisation it has acquired something like the function of a drug. In the different kinds of sexuality, 'normal' and 'perverse', in reality or fantasy human beings regain contact with an earlier form of pleasure seeking. Through sexuality's connection with procreation it becomes the most potent bridge to our biological-animal selves. Up until the 1960s sexuality was seen as the most dangerous of man's needs and had been held under strict social and psychological control. Man has developed powerful defence mechanisms in relation to his sexuality, repression from consciousness, projection onto others or splitting between an antisocial sexualised part of the self and a socially desirable part.

This kind of splitting mechanism can most easily be seen in certain disturbed personalities. Although outwardly – and possibly in their attitude to themselves – they are experienced as perfectly 'normal', they can secretly behave in a way which is considered from a cultural point of view as unacceptable sexual behaviour. It might concern the priest who indecently abuses children; the politician who regularly consorts with prostitutes and who has a fetish for sado-masochistic rituals; the psychotherapist who has intercourse with his patients; or the farm labourer who engages in bestiality. In such instances the relationship between the moral aspects of these disparate parts of the personality is lax. There is not enough strength in the struggle against acting out to prevent it, even though a part of the personality is presented as acceptable. Many learn to live with foolproof defences against experiencing concern and guilt. Regression does not take place 'in the service of the ego'; rather it happens as an obsession. Although contact with the irrational self is experienced, it is maintained via a destructive and risky splitting of the personality. Those who become aware of their split behaviour or who are dependent on this part of the personality can conduct themselves with the same degree of irrationality as the psychotic. The difference is that psychosis re-establishes the threatened inner continuity by means of the delusion while the mechanism of splitting allows for the maintenance of the self in spite of the contradictory contents.

Religion

A 'you' relation can be experienced outside human relationships in religion or in a mystical union with nature. For those who find in God a person, a 'you', the sense of togetherness can be like that which can occur with their fellow humans or often surpassing that. Religion is also accepted by most people as having a place within the rational community. Today it can be practised either privately or openly.

Religion is expressive of a permanently set vision of the world and an unshakeable ethic. Within this vision a relationship is entered into with something holy which demands complete devotion. Rock solid symbols for good and bad present themselves in stories and traditions carried over many generations, which can be worshipped through pictures and icons. For example, the Christian Holy Communion offers a sublimated strengthening meal that, while expressing an inner communion with mankind, has an unmistakable, symbolic cannibalistic undertone. This act spans the extremes between spirit and nature. The incorporation of the good, which either appears in a metaphorical form as with Protestantism or in the form of transubstantiated body and blood as in Catholicism, psychologically speaking, has the same roots as corresponding rights in earlier cultures where the consumption of a valued body part from an animal or deity offers participation in the equivalent power.

Without entering debates regarding religion, I want to show, with this reasoning, what the essential bridge to our unconscious and deepest personal life is about. Such phenomena as the experiencing of concrete spiritual forces, the hearing of God's voice, belief in Christ as miraculously risen from the dead, in a non-religious context would be considered diagnostic of psychosis with recommendation for medical treatment.

The Swedish author, August Strindberg (1849–1912) went through a deep personal mid-life crisis ('the Inferno crisis') which culminated in the form of a transient delusional state with psychotic ideas of persecution and death threats. Through the studies of religious literature, mainly Emanuel Swedenborg's later writings, he was brought to the understanding that it was really God who wanted to chastise him and by means of terrifying experiences lead him onto the righteous path. Thus he was led back to the Christian vision of life. These psychotic experiences were transformed, in this way, into a religious context that rendered them culturally acceptable.

In the Old Testament (Genesis 22) the story is told of how Abraham, by God's command, is prepared to sacrifice his son, Isaac.

God puts Abraham to the test

And it came to pass after these things, that God did tempt Abraham, and said unto him, Abraham: and he said, Behold, here I am. And he said, Take now thy son, thine only son Isaac, whom thou lovest, and get thee into the land of Moriah; and offer him there for a burnt offering upon one of the mountains which I will tell thee of.

And Abraham rose up early in the morning, and saddled his ass, and took two of his young men with him, and Isaac his son, and clave the wood for the burnt offering, and rose up, and went unto the place of which God had told him.

Then on the third day Abraham lifted up his eyes, and saw the place afar off.

And Abraham said unto his young men, Abide ye here with the ass; and I and the lad will go yonder and worship, and come again to you.

And Abraham took the wood of the burnt offering, and laid it upon Isaac his son; and he took the fire in his hand, and a knife; and they went both of them together.

And Isaac spake unto Abraham his father, and said, My father: and he said, Here am I, my son. And he said, Behold the fire and the wood; but where is the lamb for a burnt offering?

And Abraham said, My son, God will provide himself a lamb for a burnt offering: so they went both of them together.

And they came to the place which God had told him of; and Abraham built an altar there, and laid the wood in order, and bound Isaac his son, and laid him on the altar upon the wood.

And Abraham stretched forth his hand, and took the knife to slay his son.

And the angel of the Lord called unto him out of heaven, and said, Abraham, Abraham: and he said, Here am I.

And he said, Lay not thine hand upon the lad, neither do thou any thing unto him: for now I know that though fearest God, seeing thou hast not withheld thy son, thine only son from me.

And Abraham lifted up his eyes and looked, and behold behind him a ram caught in a thicket by his horns: and Abraham went and took the ram, and offered him up for a burnt offering in the stead of his son.

And Abraham called the name of that place Jehovah-jireh: as it is said to this day, In the mount of the Lord it shall be seen.

(Genesis 22, 1–14)

This story would be considered to be an expression of mental illness today, but within the religious context it contains a quite different meaning. Man has a need through a kind of double bookkeeping to live under the exigencies of reality, something which can be dealt with through the Church and which has been well tried over many centuries. This can be used or abused, as with so many other institutions set up by man. The acutely psychotic individual has lost this dialectic. For such people, they have become the world and much of what occurs in the world is centred on them or is controlled by them.

Magical thinking

The belief that it is possible to control fate and the future by magical methods is closely connected with religion and often merges with religious practice. Magic has always presented itself to people as a method of turning impotence into power and despair into hope. However, there is a fundamental, even if diffuse, difference between religion and magic. In religion a sense of contact with the spiritual and transcendental gives meaning and function to everyday existence. In magic there is the desire to reverse the laws of nature and to make man the master of his fate. In times of crises, horoscopes and astrology, tarot cards and fortune tellers come into their own and otherwise reasonable people consciously allow magical thinking to play an increasing role in their decisions and major choices.

We are all easily given to magical thinking, especially in a crisis. Hence it may be difficult to be sure whether it is a patient's experience that appears irrational to us, even while taking into account their own personal standpoint, which points to a temporarily regressed form of thinking or whether it might be psychotic.

Intoxication

Alcohol and drugs have always been a part of human existence. Intoxication as a way to establish contacts and make a bridge to the world where harsh rationality can be partly lifted is sanctioned in our culture. Just as with religion, it is surrounded by a socially controlled system that can be broken on occasion. Alcohol destroys our inhibitions. We become more friendly and happy, it awakens our sexuality: we approach the Dionysian state. Used in this way it is experienced by many as a reasonably indispensable part of our culture. However, alcohol abuse gradually alters our relationship to reality. Eventually denial becomes the most immediate mechanism of defence followed by rejection from society. Not infrequently it follows that the use of alcohol or drugs and their capacity to mitigate the hard truths of reality can also throw up an otherwise latent psychosis.

Normal vs abnormal thinking

There is a grey area to protect

There are no clear defining rules for what we call 'normal' – and there can't be. What one man calls normal differs from another's concept. The difference in perception between countries and cultures can be even greater. When we consider the conception of what is considered normal it is essentially a question of whether we are speaking statistically or normatively.

A *statistical norm* is to do with a way of being, a quality or representation that is expressed or understood by many individuals. In other words, it is called the average. High intelligence is as abnormal as low intelligence.

In terms of *normative understanding*, on the other hand, normality is expressed by that which is considered acceptable behaviour within a set group. The not-normal, the abnormal or ill are those considered to interfere with the group's ability to maintain the conditions which they value most highly: for example, health, work and social potential. Visions of a religious nature are considered valuable within certain religious cults but are considered of little worth in academic circles and would even merit a psychiatric diagnosis. In the former example the person might become a leader, whereas in the latter he or she risks being branded as strange and would not be taken seriously. Our way of seeing the opposite sex, other social classes or the peculiarities of other races is much influenced by the way we consider what is 'normal'.

Behaviour considered as ill in psychiatric terms should not just consist of that which differs from the statistical norm. It should include suffering or a risk on behalf of the sufferer, or for society. Nor should it have a temporary characteristic such as a plausible and acceptable reasonableness in the face of exterior circumstances. The notion of *crisis*, which oscillates between the psychically normal and the psychiatric, might be used in this case. In concrete situations, a process is implied with a hopeful potential where everyone working together is necessary to ensure the best possible outcome. Even in a severely escalating situation, with marked changes in behaviour which are not normal from a statistical point of view, the crisis perspective is sometimes preferable to perceiving the situation as pathological.

The conception of *the pathological standpoint* has become entwined with factors that lie outside a specific person's understanding and where psychiatric expertise is necessary. Here, a defined meaning may sometimes be lacking in terms of how people in these conditions might be considered. At the same time, the medical standpoint will always be valued as part of a dialectic in dealing with the crisis. (By dialectic I mean, in part, a dialogue relationship but also the relationship between two conceptually opposed attitudes where together they might form a synthetic understanding.)

The conception of crisis does not exclude psychiatric diagnoses. A *diagnosis* is a classification of certain types of behaviour and is not automatically the same thing as a declaration of pathology, although it is often seen to be so. Disturbed behaviour can often be classified as psychotic, depressive or suicidal. Considerations in terms of a crisis do not exclude medical treatment either. In this work, crisis and pathological viewpoints will often overlap.

Summary

We live in a world where it is essential that we are able to orientate ourselves and make sure of our survival, and for this reason we must work together. To maintain such a state it is necessary for us to make use of a logical-empirical way of thinking. At the same time, we all have, in a more or less sublimated form (i.e. expressed in a greater or lesser instinct-driven way) in our waking lives and even more so while dreaming, a primary process thinking that is closely allied to similar experiences which we find within acute psychoses. However, there is an area within our representational world that acts as an imaginary bridge between the outer and inner world. This in-between area, which is also represented in social institutions, is one that we seek out in order to supply a necessary 'regression in the service of the ego'. Even so, sometimes the strength of the bridge does not hold and collapses when the stressful load becomes too great. That which controls the line between our inner and outer world is lost to a more or less pronounced psychotic form of behaviour.

There exists an uncertain boundary, an important grey area between unusual ideas and what we call delusions. An idea that would constitute a delusion if I harboured it does not necessarily mean another should perceive it in this way. Many greater or lesser steps forward in our culture take place through the work of lone thinkers, where both they and others can on occasion question whether they are engaged in some mad venture or whether their work constitutes something of true value.

Chapter 2

Losing contact with reality

Six experiences and six diagnoses

I shall now consider some clinical cases in which patients experienced loss of contact with reality – in some cases completely, in others partially. For some, the loss was short-lived while for others they were never able to completely retrieve their state of health. First I will describe the exterior course of events and then I will carry out a psychiatric analysis and diagnosis (pp. 20–24).

A mental rape

For six months Angela, a single 33-year-old woman, had been manager of a boutique that was part of an international chain of shops. With her staff she had made intensive preparations for that season's sales programme. With only a day's warning, her area manager turned up. Without giving reasons, he complained about her lack of social competence – something that was manifestly unjust according to both Angela and her colleagues. Prior to this visit, there had been no criticism.

Two days later, Angela was called to head office. She was given her notice there and then without any explanation. The boss, a man younger than Angela, was unyielding. Angela was unwilling to lose her dignity and tried to keep her feelings under control. Constraining herself, Angela signed an agreement whereby she was to receive compensation of six months' pay. She confided to friends who persuaded her not to sue the company in order that her reputation should not be undermined within the industry as this might make it harder for her to find employment.

Angela was given a few days to settle her successor into her job. It had already been agreed that she should. She felt 'anaesthetised' but did as she was required with great effort. At night she cried a great deal and talked to her friends on the telephone. Some days later, after a meeting with a lawyer, she began to experience vague death threats from people that she passed on the street. She felt she was being pursued and saw people spying on her from cars. Suddenly everything came clear to her – she felt that her life was being threatened by an international conspiracy. She fled to her parents' home. There her sense of security was further undermined when she heard people speaking in code about her during the weather report. Her parents tried to show her the absurdity of such a fantasy but without success. A few days later, while her panic about being threatened slowly grew, she sought help at an acute psychiatric department. There she was diagnosed as acutely psychotic, placed in an acute ward and treated with antipsychotic medication.

However, the doctor who saw her the following day considered her to be able to function outside the hospital, in spite of her psychosis, with the proviso that she should return to the hospital for frequent visits. The antipsychotic medication was replaced with something to help her to sleep. Angela's persecutory ideas lessened after some weeks and she could now see that her relations and friends had encouraged her to separate her real illness from the 'pursuer' who had actually been after her. During the working through of the crisis a more pronounced sensitivity, feelings of pain and concern over the future emerged. Angela continued for several years in psychotherapy and eventually found employment in a new job where she fared well.

She spoke about her experiences of being dismissed in terms of a mental rape.

On the loss of the good childhood

Beth became acutely ill with auditory hallucinations, fantasies of saving the world and pronounced agitation. She was 30 years old, lived with a partner and worked in a state-operated factory. A year and a half earlier her grandmother had died and a half-brother had succumbed to schizophrenia. These events had caused Beth to become depressed and to seek psychotherapy. On several occasions she considered suicide but restrained herself, primarily because she felt that her sick brother needed her. Several months before she was hospitalised she had sought acute psychiatric help for panic-anxiety attacks and a couple of weeks later she had fantasies that she had been sent to redeem the world by the UN. She heard God's voice and the voice of a famous rock star who cried: 'Persevere Beth!' which supported her in her mission.

The situation was accentuated by a trip abroad. The houses in the city that she visited seemed to her to be somehow like houses from a film set, with the signposts put up to deceive her. She fled her fellow travellers and the city. As a result of her confused behaviour, the police stepped in and sent her home by air ambulance.

Beth was 'put on section' (detained under the mental health law) and given antipsychotic medication, but without success. On one occasion she set fire to her mattress on her ward. A couple of weeks later she was encouraged to join a project for first-time psychotic patients. Yet she still felt as if she was being plotted against and refused her medication. Nonetheless, she showed signs of being able to do some mental work without medication and she was transferred to a special crisis centre. Even so, Beth defended herself furiously against any attempt to critically discuss her feelings.

Beth explained that her dead grandmother, who had been in the Salvation Army, represented something positive and good in her childhood. She had lived with her grandmother between the ages of five and eight on the advice of the social services in order to protect her against negligent treatment at home. She had been living with her single mother who because of her work and her all-consuming love life had been unable to cope with her daughter. Beth described how 'Frequently, in the mornings there was a new man to whom I was to say hello', and who quickly disappeared from the picture. She also described how 'hopelessly in love' she was with her mother and how she tried, without success, to have her love reciprocated during these years. With her grandmother she felt she was noticed and listened to for the first time.

However, Beth's mother remarried and took her daughter back and gave her several half-siblings. She did well at school and at work but 'nothing seemed to interest me'. When her grandmother died it was as if 'the world had lost its contents' and she became ever more depressed with a strong sense of her life being meaningless. 'Life was just empty.'

Six months after being admitted, Beth's psychotic experiences had lessened to a large extent. In her talks she was encouraged to explore what it was that gave reality to her fantasies. The therapist was careful not to appear omniscient. Little by little Beth explored and began to understand her earlier experiences with her mother and understood her sorrow at the loss of her grandmother. Now she encountered a new and important change. During a visit to a convent she met a Catholic nun who reminded her of her grandmother. After this, Beth was able to give up her delusions for good.

In a follow-up discussion four years later Beth was feeling well and was deeply involved with her work. She had had a child with her partner and was experiencing great joy in motherhood. Beth commented on her period of psychosis as having been the most difficult time in her life but she was not sorry that she had undergone it. In many ways she now experienced a greater sensitivity about life than before. She explained that her feelings had more depth and were more intense now: 'It is strange that I have had to have a psychotic episode in order to break through that emotional shell which I had built up over the years.'

Telepathy, thought control and voices in the wind

Carina was 22 years old and attending a private art school when she was first admitted to hospital. She had believed for some time that people on the street were talking about her and even thought that people were making secret television films of her through her neighbour's window. When she watched television she noticed that if she thought about something specific the announcer would alter the channel and Carina believed she could control the announcer with her thoughts. Those who were making the films now began to send her messages by telepathic means. These messages tormented her and claimed that she was a dirty person with perverse thoughts. Eventually they went far enough to send her compulsive thoughts about her having intercourse with dogs. These fantasies felt totally foreign to her character and therefore she felt violently insulted by them. She wondered how many people around her knew about these slanders. Carina withdrew more and more from her friends. She did not join in with school parties but worked in her studio, workdays and holidays alike. When her friends and her mother tried to encourage her to go out, she mostly responded with anger. Nobody had realised just how serious her problems were until she called home from the hospital.

One night when Carina overheard how many people up in the attic were talking about her and criticising her paintings, she went to the police for help. She wanted to identify those who plagued her and those who left her alone. Instead of concerning themselves with her problem the police referred her to the psychiatric clinic where she agreed to be admitted.

It emerged that Carina was an only child. Her parents had divorced when she was 5 years old. During her childhood she had lived with her mother. Her father, who was an academic, had remarried and her contact with him had worsened on the birth of a new child which meant that there was now no place for Carina in his home. Several members of the father's family had been treated for psychiatric illnesses. There had been a period when she was 16 years old when she had become dejected and had spent time pondering the existence of God. She had stopped school but with support from a child psychiatrist had been able to resume after a short while. Carina had always found it easy to make friends, who admired her artistic talent. Teachers too had given her support and she had done well at school on the whole. Apart from a short love affair, which petered out, she had never had a serious boyfriend, although she was considered attractive.

At the clinic Carina was able to feel a certain sympathy for her pursuers. This feeling disappeared quickly once she heard voices that mocked her and forced her to carry out certain meaningless rituals and movements of her body. She dared not take medication and was transferred to a ward where she was compelled to have muscular injections and antipsychotic medication. Disturbing side effects ensued in the form of painful eye movements and an inner sense of unease and restlessness. Although these symptoms could have been relieved she refused to take medication. She was given injections that had a long-term effect. After a couple of months it was possible for Carina to be discharged. Her movements and thinking were slowed down but the voices had disappeared. She did not have the energy to paint and instead took part in the hospital's therapy. The post-hospital care took place in a psychiatric clinic. She refused point-blank to continue with her medication and was slowly able to resume her painting.

Some years later, during preparations for a students' exhibition, she became ill again with delusions and hallucinations. This time her hospitalisation lasted longer. Carina was now able to try out newer antipsychotic medication administered in tablet form and for a considerably longer period than previously. On this occasion she experienced considerable benefits from the medication and was able, yet again, to return to her art.

On developmental regression

David had always been something of an eccentric at school. He had difficulties with sport and was considered to be awkward. His parents worked in a religious community and were open and sociable. His younger siblings found life easier and David was seen as the 'problem child' at home. During puberty he became attached for a while to a small-time criminal gang where hashish was smoked. This was quickly discovered and at the same time David was apprehended for raiding department stores at night. His parents reacted promptly and began to give more time to encouraging other interests in David. He was a pleasant-looking boy and easily likeable. His performance at school was average. At the age of 17 he complained that he could not sleep and his parents found him sitting up at night, sweating with anxiety, on several occasions. He didn't know why he should, but began to wonder whether he was homosexual. He had heard people in town, in queues and on buses, saying that he was but could not remember exactly whom. He was referred to his GP who examined him in full without any positive findings and prescribed something to help him sleep. It was put down to being due to the pressures of schoolwork and a late puberty. It was assumed that he would grow out of it.

David finished school when he was given the chance to start employment at a print works as an errand boy. To begin with his state of mind improved. David seemed happy although his boss complained more and more frequently about his slowness. He did his errand work punctiliously but would sometimes find himself standing by the wayside 'not thinking about anything in particular'. At home there was concern when David began to take less care over his appearance whereas before he had been most particular over his hygiene and about the way he dressed. He smelt of sweat and his parents and siblings had to nag him to wash his hair and change his clothes. David's behaviour changed gradually. He dragged out his mealtimes and could find himself sitting sometimes for as long as half an hour with food in his mouth without swallowing. His father had particular difficulty in tolerating his temperament and the family centred more and more on David's behaviour. They didn't know whether it was a declaration of defiance or a sign of illness. There were no definite indications pointing to 'disturbed thinking'. However he would sit and laugh to himself. When asked what it might be about he would reply with a secretive smile or would say that it was nothing in particular.

When he was 19 years old his parents again sought help and this time he was referred to a psychiatric clinic. It was not necessary to admit him to inpatient care. The family had a series of counselling sessions at home and David worked well with the help of his parents. A thorough medical and psychological investigation did not produce any definite findings. David agreed to try antipsychotic medication in the hope that it might help him. Eventually it was possible to offer him a placement with other young people who had difficulty with their psychological functioning in communal accommodation. He maintained a relationship with a couple of his old friends and started to attend a specially adapted training. Little by little the family were able to reassure themselves that David's life had become meaningful and that he could get on.

Arteriosclerosis and confusion at night

Elizabeth was a 69-year-old widow. Her husband had died four years earlier and her two children lived some distance away. She had always been active in the church and dedicated to work in the community and in the sewing club. In recent years she had had several minor strokes which had little lasting effect save for a weakness in her right leg and a certain loss of memory.

In deteriorating winter conditions Elizabeth slipped on the road and broke her leg. Although there were no complications she was admitted to the surgical ward for safety's sake. On the first night she was frightened and wanted to go home. The night staff managed to persuade her to stay. Around 2 am she found her way to the wastepaper basket where she tried to urinate. When a fellow patient called the night nurse they found Elizabeth in a state of complete confusion. She thought she was at home and imagined that her husband had just gone out. When they tried to help her back to bed she became furious and began to swear. Elizabeth calmed down and slowly became aware that she was in hospital when the nurse turned the light on in her room and brought her a cup of coffee with sugar. After a little she was able to allow herself to lie down and sleep.

The next day Elizabeth had only a vague recollection of the night before. She was quite lucid and her old self again. Elizabeth was soon transferred into a long-term care hospice. Here they gave her a night-light and she had photographs of her husband and children on her bedside table. In this way, she was able to orientate herself whenever she became confused at night. Added to this, she could often be tempted to join in for coffee and a chat. Some years later, Elizabeth had a fatal stroke.

On the other side of 'the doors of perception'

The author of this book was a young medical student in the 1950s. During my course in pharmacology I came across a book by Aldous Huxley (1954), *The Doors of Perception.* It was about the Mexican Indian drug mescaline that was described by Huxley as able, in the most delightful way, to deepen experiences and which was, incidentally, safe and free of addictive property.

After a successful examination in pharmacology I asked my professor if he would like to join me in some research by giving me mescaline. He agreed and one Sunday a couple of weeks later at the professor's country home, I was allowed, together with a fellow student whom I had brought along, 0.4 g of pink mescaline crystals in a little water. The ensuing events were recorded. During the first three hours nothing happened and we began to wonder if the dose had been too small. Coffee was served. When I looked into the coffee dregs I suddenly saw how the colour changed. At the same time the coffee cup turned into a deep well. When my companion shut the door the noise released a clutch of small red snakes which slithered swiftly towards the edge of the cup and down into the well where they mingled with the coffee dregs, and became a confusion of red and blue balls of colour, spreading and bursting, and were replaced by more balls of fire. Every subsequent sound resulted in fascinating new explosions of colour of varying types and form.

It was clear that there had been an effect. However, I was barely able to communicate my experiences. I was convinced that the other two wanted to experiment on me and exploit my vulnerable position. I asked them to leave me for a while. When they returned I was sitting, huddled up and paralysed. I experienced – for the first time in my adult life – a powerful anxiety that only let up when I sat stiff and still and returned whenever I tried to relax. As this was happening, I lost the sense of the passing of time. An overwhelming feeling of timelessness had taken hold. However, if a wisp of cigarette smoke began to flutter in a draught of air, then time could 'start up' for a short while.

I experienced a growing anxiety which increased until in the end it became unendurable. It felt as though I had to give in to it to argue with the professor. I began to rag him and insisted that he had flirted with the prettiest girls on the course and that he had used his position to seduce them. I tried even further to humiliate him and ended up by calling him an immigrant and a dirty old man. The anxiety, which compelled me to throw aggressive vulgarities at a person whom I actually appreciated very much, lessened but returned with renewed strength.

The professor's comments, which struck me as very significant, were that I might find myself troubled by my behaviour later on, but that I did not need to worry for he had been in psychoanalysis and had managed to deal with worse.

Eventually the effects wore off and after about eight hours everything returned to normal for me, even though I assured myself that I would never try mescaline again. I remember my experiences very clearly. Some months later I found myself reading another book by Aldous Huxley. This time it was *Heaven and Hell* published in 1956. Huxley had continued with his experiments and was now in a position to announce that mescaline was by no means an innocent joyride. It could also be a potent force for anxiety.

I came to find psychoanalysis myself later on and was able to discover a deeper understanding for my sudden attacks against my admired professor. The mescaline had loosened my inner censor and for some hours carried into the open things which I was later to meet up with and work through during a long psychoanalysis.

Can we understand the development of psychosis?

Angela

Angela had suffered from depression when she was 20 years old. On the whole she had coped well since then. She was competent and had found herself in a job which she enjoyed. Her notice had come like a thunder bolt. (Later she understood that it had to do with an administrative reorganisation that she had to give in to.) The fact that her boss was a younger man in the same career had not made it any easier and increased the humiliation. She guessed later on that his own insecurity had made him brutal. Her psychosis, which had revealed itself in the form of persecution and anxiety, can be understood in view of the completely unexpected nature of her dismissal. Moreover it had been delivered in an offensive and insensitive way and so the impotence that Angela had experienced was extreme. She slept little at night and had to hold herself under strict control during the daytime.

During her psychosis, which she later described as a waking nightmare with strong overtones of a thriller, the sensation softened by way of a perception that her life was threatened externally. All in all, it is easier to struggle against an exterior threat from which protection can be obtained with help, than to face a total loss of capacity to understand what is going on internally. In this way, psychosis can be seen to represent an adaptive function. A vital factor behind the loss of reality was also the inability to sleep.

The diagnosis, according to the DSM-IV system (see Appendix), is a *brief psychosis with reactive characteristics* (i.e. triggered by stress). Angela's prognosis was very good but she needed psychotherapeutic support to heal her impaired sense of her self.

Beth

Beth's early childhood was filled with disappointing experiences in her relationship to her mother to whom she had been closely attached. She had no clear vision of her father. Presumably she had denied more effectively her need for him and had formed early strategies to compensate for his absence. Her grandmother provided the 'good internal object', which means that the internalised proximity of the grandmother had become essential for Beth's sense of balance in her perception of herself. Certainly it covered over a deep sense of abandonment.

Together with the fact that she had had to leave her grandmother (who lived in another part of the country) in order to return home to her mother and to her new family, Beth developed an inner protective skin which helped her to gain a good but shallow adjustment. This was built on the grandmother's psychological presence for her, something that evaporated when she died. The normal period of mourning for Beth was transformed into an escalating depression with feelings of meaninglessness. Later she experienced anxiety attacks – presentiments about being on the edge of psychosis. Normally her sorrow would have healed, but for some reason this did not occur. We do frequently encounter the fact that those who become psychotic have a low capacity to work through and come out of their depression and its causes.

Instead, Beth became more and more disturbed over a period of some months (though never in such a way that she was able to keep a hold of herself). She began to experience strange situations and allusions at work. Beth was very happy when, in spite of having never been interested in religion, she heard the voice of God that revealed to her that she had been chosen to join the United Nations in a move to redeem the world. It might be imagined that her childhood experience of having been attended to by her grandmother was now, in consequence of an unbearable sense of abandonment, transformed into being attended to by that God whom her grandmother had served.

It is often possible to see that this kind of development in psychosis represents an alternative to suicide: it is a suicide in the literal meaning of the word – a killing of the self. From this point of view psychosis becomes a potential for possible development. But of course not all psychoses can be looked at in this way. Beth's half-brother's illness points to a genetic trait that might have added to her vulnerability to developing psychosis.

The diagnosis is *schizo-affective psychosis*, which means that the symptoms cover the criteria for both affective illness and psychosis. The former manifests in a deep depression and the latter in the shape of hallucinations and prolonged delusions, partly of a grandiose nature. In spite of a tendency to relapse, the progress, as in this case, is favourable in certain cases and can be much helped by psychotherapy. Often it is necessary to prescribe antipsychotic medication and lithium to reduce the risk of relapse.

Carina

Carina's psychosis suggests a somewhat different impression. She had always been a sensitive person and careful to maintain her integrity in relation to boys. However, she had always maintained deep friendships with her girlfriends. Her illness started with a withdrawn state lasting many months, which did not immediately suggest a depressive but rather a ruminative state. The psychosis itself had a more bizarre aspect to it than those earlier encountered. Her fantasies were quite incompatible with her earlier fantasy world and with her specific cultural setting. This indicates that primitive experiences and fantasies had broken into her thinking, for some reason. Carina perceived them as coming from outside – she was unable to see it any other way. Her experiences were frightening and it was impossible for her to share them with others. It is hard to find a clear reason for her becoming ill other than that she must have felt a relatively harsh pressure both from her demanding artistic education and in her need to distance herself from the more adult sexuality practised by her friends. Since she reacted so desperately during a developmental phase that most people of her age come through without too much difficulty, one can surmise that Carina had a vulnerable nature. (The concept of vulnerability is discussed in Chapters 6 and 7.)

A year later Carina became ill again. This time her symptoms lasted over six months. The diagnosis was schizophrenia – a conclusion drawn from both her long-lasting hallucinations and delusions and the fact that they were so bizarre. The second time around she was placed on a more appropriate antipsychotic medication to which she reacted positively.

In retrospect it might have been better to have allowed Carina to receive lower dosages. Her symptoms would have improved without the serious distress from her experience of the side effects, causing her not to want to continue with the prescription.

David

David had always been somewhat eccentric but had not shown any clear symptoms before he was 17 years old. He was easily influenced and not much interested in studying and might easily have been led into more anti-social ways. Through the good work of his parents, this was avoided. The first symptoms were beset with anxieties, due to problems concerning his sense of identity. David believed he was starting to become homosexual and later this was followed by auditory hallucinatory experiences in which people discussed him. There were no concrete indications of homosexuality and his experiences were characterised by delusion. A little later his lack of attention to his appearance, and tendency to laugh without any apparent reason were additional symptoms.

His state was considered hard to shift and medication had an uncertain effect. The diagnosis was *symptomless or simple schizophrenia*. The prognosis in terms of complete return to health is not good but there is a possibility that he might gain, within the limits of his circumstances, a decent quality of life.

Elizabeth

Elizabeth's loss of reality is different. At the time of her hospitalisation she lost her ability during the night to orientate herself in time, place and person. This is a state of *confusion* and only in its appearance can it be likened to psychosis. In the other cases no problems of orientation with mistaken perceptions of time, place and person are evident. These people experienced private inner misperceptions of exterior events; hearing voices coming from the outside world which were not there. A confusional state comes about as a result of an organic dissipation of the capacity to function. In Elizabeth's case it was possible, thanks to her symptoms arising from little embolisms in the brain, to see that she suffered from alterations, due to age, in the brain's blood vessels with the resultant deteriorating flow of blood. This condition is characterised by a lowered threshold at night when the metabolism is lowered and the light level is low resulting in understimulation, disorientation and a cognitive collapse or disintegration. The best form of treatment is to improve the function of the brain in simple ways: by helping her to rediscover her identity, putting the light on and talking to her. Antipsychotic or tranquillising medication often has the effect of worsening confusion.

This is a *delirium* where, in contrast with psychoses, there is a straightforward organic cause. It could also be called an *arteriosclerotic confusion*.

The author

The *toxic-organic psychosis* triggered within the author of this book by mescaline contains as many important distinctions as similarities in relation to these different forms of loss of reality. It is above all the colourful visual hallucination which (as in this case) did not represent anything in particular. These visual perceptions are called *synesthesias*: that is to say, that one kind of perception (for example, hearing) stimulates another perceptual modality (in this case vision). In the literature about mescaline and the closely related drug LSD-25 the different fearful hallucinatory experiences resemble the descriptions given by patients in the grip of the delirium seen in alcohol withdrawal.

Visual hallucinations of this kind do not usually occur in 'functional psychoses', by which we mean those which cannot be understood as resulting from a clearly defined organic cause. In the functional psychoses one may hear of vague images, of visualised inner fantasies or of nightly dream-like waking experiences. Clear visual hallucinations are, on the other hand, usually due to poisoning, drugs or brain damage, especially in the temporal lobe. There are also epileptic seizures that stem from the temporal lobe, which present as a sequence of hallucinated images. These visions tend to be repetitive and stereotypical.

The loss of an inner sense of time is characteristic of the mescaline psychosis and certainly constitutes one of the reasons why mescaline was used to develop religious, mystical states by the Inca people. The similarities with functional psychoses consist in both the tendency to experience delusions and, in the catatonic state, a rigidity which is maintained with tensed muscles, in order to reduce anxiety. A tendency towards impulsive outbursts of disturbed behaviour and primitive thinking are found, as well, in both drug-induced and functional psychosis.

This experience increased my view that it is essential to work with several theories simultaneously in mind when trying to understand a particular psychosis: the biological knowledge regarding mescaline's effects could not alone explain the painful and personal nature of my thoughts during my psychosis. At first, the unsavoury thoughts felt alien to my personality and I believed that they had simply appeared wholly as part of the mescaline. Later, I realised that they were understandable when seen from what emerged from my unconscious during my personal psychoanalysis.

Summary

These six cases illustrate different aspects of loss of psychic reality. Some are easier to understand than others. Whilst the experiences of Angela and Beth could have been gathered from a detective story, Carina described more bizarre delusions. As with David he had behavioural disturbances that were prolonged and even bizarre. The combination of bizarre and long-term psychotic symptoms is characteristic of those psychoses which are known as *schizophrenia*.

Elizabeth's state of mind was a *delirium* due to arteriosclerotic causes, leading to a disturbance of orientation in the realms of time, space and identity. The symptoms are much more directly dependent on organic causes within the brain. The author's mescaline-induced state describes a *toxic delirium* – one that nonetheless had a significant psychic content.

In all these cases an intricate combination between the psychological and social circumstances and the physiological condition of the brain can be detected. It is this combination of perspectives that this book intends to examine more closely in order to provide a map by which the researcher can better orientate himself to the mind of the psychotic individual. We cannot work seriously on these problems if we do not admit the necessity to span the breadth of research into the human mind. This book differs from other psychiatric works in its undertaking of such a broad enterprise.

Maps have to be redrawn from time to time. Many readers will make their own discoveries, which either complement or deviate from what I have to relate in the following chapters. That is the nature of maps.

Chapter 3

The concept of psychosis, delusions and hallucinations

The concept of psychosis

Psychosis is a phenomenological-psychological concept. There is neither a biological definition covering the term, nor is there a specific biological 'marker' for psychosis. Every attempt to find a neurophysiological correlate has been unsuccessful. Through the phenomenology of psychosis, in this chapter we will try to come closer to the psychology of psychosis. (Phenomenological approaches are where attempts are made to describe phenomena and subjective descriptions of experience without using theoretical conceptualisations.)

Without *delusions* one cannot or should not speak in terms of psychosis. Perceptions are often correct in psychosis, but it is the interpretations of the perceptions which are mistaken. This differs from delirium where it is primarily the perceptions that are disturbed. A psychosis can be more or less influenced by the following phenomena, which however cannot be called psychotic in themselves:

- hallucinations
- disturbed behaviour
- confusion or delirium.

Hallucinations

Hallucinations of a visual or auditory nature can occur without a realistic perception of the world being altered. Here, the person has a full insight into his experiences as representing some kind of illness or irrationality. In other words, a hallucination cannot be called psychotic if it does not manifest itself as a delusion.

Disturbed behaviour

Disturbed behaviour occurs in many instances other than psychosis. Moreover, psychotic people exist (for example, with delusional disorder) who do not portray a noticeable degree of disturbed behaviour.

Spirits at a board meeting

A 48-year-old single man who worked for a company that was listed on the stock exchange suffered for many years from spirits that harangued him, wanted to fight him and knock him over. This occurred more and more frequently during board meetings. He would excuse himself and rush off to his own office next to the room where the meeting was held, where the fighting could proceed on the carpet. When this was over he pulled himself together and returned to the meeting without anyone knowing what had occurred. However, his overall anxiety increased and finally he sought psychiatric help. It transpired that the spirits belonged to a wider system of delusions. Three years later he committed suicide.

Confusion or delirium

Confusion or delirium entails the break-up of the person's ability to orientate themselves in time, place and identity. It points to a primary origin in the brain's functioning and usually has to do with potentially reversible organic disturbances (impaired blood supply, hormonal or toxic changes, fever, etc.). The psychotic individual is normally not disorientated even though features of a confused state can occur as a consequence of psychosis.

The concept of psychosis that I use in this book consequently includes a concept of delusion and a vision of reality which clearly deviates from and is not shared by any other. The unusual state of *folie à deux* constitutes an exception, see p. 31. Hallucinations, confusion and disturbances of behaviour can also be features of psychosis, although they are not essential to the concept.

As we have seen, the boundaries between 'rational' and 'irrational' states are unclear: they shift and are culturally determined in every way. This is an extensive grey area. Many live a large part of their lives in these grey zones, and yet are able to manage well in their practical life.

Misinterpretations

The combination of disturbed perceptions and threatening experiences regularly produces misinterpretations. To begin with they allow themselves to be influenced by a capacity for critical thinking but sooner or later become misinterpretations. This was scientifically shown in the 1950s and 1960s in an experiment with sensory deprivation in American universities (Slade 1984: 256–260). Students, of their own free will, were placed in bolstered beds or hung in tanks with water warmed to body temperature making it so comfortable that the body became imperceptible. They were given milk-white glasses and earplugs. The subjects were free to break off the experiment that was designed to last for a long time – eight hours – whenever they wished. At least half of them experienced disturbances of perception, especially of sight and sound. The majority reported fantasies that they were being tricked during the experiment and felt that they were in great danger. For this reason many broke off the experiment before the stipulated time was up.

To walk alone in a forest at night is only a good experience if the person feels himself to be in full control over his fantasies. Another example of the transformation of reality which easily turns into a fearful situation by means of a combination of threat and diminished visual perception is shown in the box.

A desperado armed with a gun was being sought. Reports came in of sightings of the man near a certain coastal area. A group of five military men, led by an experienced sergeant, formed part of the search party. The beach was stony and the sun was strong. They crept forward in line. Suddenly a sound was heard from behind some high stones 30 metres ahead and the sergeant saw, at the same moment, the tip of a gun barrel. Immediately he ordered his men to take cover while he himself led half his men to encircle the stone and in this way the area was stormed. What was discovered was an empty bottle of beer; the mouth of the bottle was gleaming in the sun.[1]

Misinterpretations of reality can also arise within the realm of *hearing* deficits. Older people who suffer increased deafness often believe that others are doing things behind their backs – pulling faces or saying unkind things about them. Deafness is considered an overall more psychically disturbing trauma than blindness and often fuels further misinterpretations.

Even the sense of *touch* can be disturbed with some older people who may experience something creeping on their skin. Together with poor eyesight, loneliness and understimulation these experiences can be interpreted as if insects were crawling on them. The elderly person sees something such as dry skin lying on the skin, scrapes it off and asks the doctor to have it studied under a microscope. Since the skin disturbances continue – and the lack of stimulation remains – the problem endures.

Misinterpretations can occur in old people, together perhaps with premature ageing. With incipient cognitive decline (that is to say, disturbances in logical thinking and memory) they can lose a sense of control over the environment. Mistakes and accidents occur, items are mislaid and appointments forgotten. The person angrily denies these cognitive problems and expects full loyalty from those around them. In cases of road traffic accidents they can deny their part in them. They defend against their forgetfulness by thinking that others have stolen something from them or have moved an object without saying. People around them may not notice that an ageing process lies behind the personality change.

With an *overvalued idea* it is not so much the content that is the cause of the disturbance as the individual's need to cling to the idea. The problem can relate to beliefs about a certain kind of food which might be dangerous to health, the need to keep constant vigilance against the possibility of radioactive rays or the belief about one's huge cultural significance. There are vast areas where we still have little knowledge and it is important to take care not to reach hasty answers – both electrical allergies and telepathy may refer to culturally sanctioned 'paranormal' ideas as well as to irrational delusions. Who is to decide what might be right for others?

Delusions

Paranoia (from the Greek for madness) or *delusions* include a thought content or view of reality that is clearly distinct from a reasonable prevailing view according to observable facts, cultural attitudes, the level of psychological development, and overall circumstances. The delusion must be beyond the reach of influence. In psychiatry, it is necessary to distinguish between the scope, content and degree of bizarreness of the delusions.

Scope

A person can have a delusion that only refers to a small part of reality. However, for the person himself it occupies a large part of their thoughts. It can concern beliefs about having been involved in strange happenings during early childhood, about having been exchanged as a baby and hence finding their adult lives conditioned by these events. The stories become so fantastic and so many other people get drawn into them that they and their lives become divorced from reality, but the person is unable to acknowledge this. It can represent an early stage or be a mild variant of a paranoid psychosis. On the other hand, it seems reasonable that difficult early events might explain later psychological problems. In view of the person's own depiction of the matter it is important in the interests of psychological safety and sensitivity not to invade the person's own beliefs.

The delusions that lead to the psychiatric diagnosis of psychosis are more extensive and are only integrated into social life with difficulty, if at all.

With delusions that become permanent most forms of communal life are impossible.

However, there are people who carry delusional beliefs for years and are unmistakably paranoid but, through a socially protective network or other resources, are not forced to seek help from a doctor. Delusions, which come to the fore during a period of stress or isolation, can eventually resolve without the sufferer ever having recognised his state to be pathological. It can happen, for instance, that the feeling of being poisoned by food can cause complications around eating and a subsequent unhealthy or inadequate diet. It can also feature tenacious and groundless beliefs that all telephone conversations are tapped or that the children are being sexually abused. Usually these ideas are not wholly impossible or bizarre.

Contents

Delusions about others

A common delusion is of feelings of being pursued or spied upon by *groups of angry people*, sometimes involving political organisations such as the CIA or KGB. Many people believed – and some still believe – that after the murder of the Swedish Prime Minister, Olof Palme, in 1986 they were suspected of the murder and were being held under surveillance. For such people misinterpretation of everyday phenomena offer proof that they are being watched: for example, the presence of aircraft in the sky, the fact that cars may drive by slowly, people standing on street corners in a significant way. In the newspapers and on the radio or television references are being made about them. The announcer has a particular way of looking which indicates that the murder she is talking about is the one that the listener or viewer is suspected of. Bugging devices are placed in various strategic places, especially in the psychiatrist's consulting room. Attempts to rationally discuss these beliefs and to show what such surveillance might cost, questions regarding resources and insufficient evidence all fail completely. Yet one can sometimes make contact with a non-psychotic, self-critical part of the patient if his or her trust can be won.

The dividing line between illusions and hallucinations is undefined. Some, as I have mentioned, can relate how they believe themselves to hear people whispering in a dismissive manner as they pass – words such as 'whore', 'shit' and 'idiot'. It is seldom a question of true hallucinations but is rather more likely to consist of *illusions* – that something is actually heard and then interpreted in a specific way. People are thought to grimace in revulsion or to frighten you when you turn around. The registration numbers on cars or company stickers deliver secret messages, as do the labels on cigarette packets lying on the ground.

These experiences can feel like being a part of an experiment or a series of someone else's experiments. Everything is done to frighten you, and to make you give in so that you confess just to prove that you should be put to death. Others want to 'trick' you in different ways. Those who lie behind this persecution may be more or less defined. States of panic can ensue and sometimes suicide is attempted.

Those who live near or are closely dependent on someone who has paranoid thoughts are easily drawn into their paranoid world and so into giving up their ability to think critically. The alternative would be to allow violent angry outbursts to ensue from demands that the absurd ideas must be adhered to. Often it revolves around experiences full of threats and hatred which are felt to issue from all around. Neighbours spy, attempts are made to poison children in school dining halls, and the police listen in on the telephone. A giving up of one's personality to a *folie à deux* is sometimes seen in a partner or child, but relatively soon, the delusions are abandoned if the dependence on the original person is broken.[2]

A delusion can often centre round *a special person* who then takes up the greater part of the deluded person's thoughts. A typical example is a dutiful middle-aged woman who, at work, for many years believes herself to be in a secret relationship with her boss even though they have never referred to it. Over a period of months and years she gathers 'proof' that he shares her feelings and she is able to pick up secret signs from his paperwork or from his behaviour at work. So one day she decides that it is time to come clean. She goes to her boss and declares that now things must be brought into the open, but he, having perhaps never even noticed his colleague, stands amazed. The woman experiences his denial and cowardice as unfathomable when she, as often happens, is referred to a psychiatric clinic. This kind of occurrence is known in German psychiatry as '*Sensitiver Beziehungswahn*' [relational insanity] (Kretschmer 1966).

Delusions about the self

Delusions about body image often lie upon an uncertain dividing line between an overvalued idea and a delusion. The experience of being ugly or of having freakish features when nobody else can see it can sometimes cross the boundaries of delusion. This kind of (usually non-psychotic) preoccupation is called *dysmorphophobia* (for example, see p. 250).

Grandiose delusions refer to heightened significance of the self. From having lived a life untouched by religion, suddenly an assignment comes directly from God to redeem the world from destruction.[3] This anxiety increases if the assignment can only be completed in a specific way such as having to walk between the lines on a pavement or having to maintain, uninterrupted, a certain number in the mind. If you do the wrong thing or forget, the world will be swallowed up. It can be a belief that one is Christ and one must be martyred by throwing oneself off a mountain or by immolating oneself. To be able to control the world or to have telepathic contact with the world's leaders or with well-known personalities, whether living or dead, are other common forms of delusions.

Degree of bizarre thinking

In the early stages of an acute psychosis fantasies can be experienced in a particularly defined way, the perceptions clear and colourful. Hidden meanings can be deciphered from the way things are arranged and one can see how other people have laid the groundwork to confuse you. At later stages, well-known places suddenly become strange, as if someone is secretly creating obstacles perhaps as a test.

If the ideas begin to cross over the boundaries where they cannot be acceptable even within a very fanciful view of reality, it is important to be aware of how the prevailing culture still colours the experiences. An old lady who has been interested in spiritualism and such pursuits for many years could get the idea that she had been hypnotised by strangers without it necessarily being considered deeply pathological. If the same belief takes hold of a young technician it would certainly signify a psychotic alteration in his personality.

Schizophrenic delusions

Experiences indicating that physical integrity (and not just psychic) is transgressed, such as thoughts having been removed from the brain, thoughts or ideas having been placed in the head or that thinking is directly controlled from the outside, are often referred to as *schizophrenic delusions* (see Chapter 11). With experiences of physical manipulation of the mind the sufferer tries to give 'rational' reasons which are as deeply bizarre as the experiences themselves: for example, the conviction that a little metal chip has been inserted into the brain during an operation while asleep. This acts as a radio antenna by means of which others can control and send messages. Or that a little loudspeaker has been placed in a tooth during a visit to a dentist which explains the auditory/vocal hallucinations. The dentist can later find himself persecuted by telephone harassment and other forms of stalking for years.

Protection against radiation

A patient experienced the painful belief that his bed was positioned in the middle of an electrical field which was being controlled by creatures from outer space. He felt discomfort in his whole body and preferred to sleep on the floor elsewhere in his room. In the following weeks he began to experience being bugged by an apparatus set up behind the wallpaper. In his fear, he systematically tore down the wallpaper and cut off the electricity leaving his apartment without light. The contents of his refrigerator rotted and he lived in the ensuing stink, which the carers who eventually entered his home with the help of the police and a locksmith found unbearable.

The need to find some coherence, that is to say, find a meaningful explanation for the strange change which is being experienced internally, outweighs the normal demands of logic and rationality. In psychosis the need for coherence has triumphed and an inner continuity is reinstalled. The price of such coherence is the loss of a shared realistic understanding with others. This does not mean that the logical-rational capacity is lost in other areas of life, which are not directly related to the psychosis. Very bizarre delusions are usually, but not always, accompanied or strengthened by auditory hallucinations.

Brain operation, hypnosis or 'having been a little unwell'?

A 19-year-old student was committed to a psychiatric ward after having developed a condition with hallucinations and anxiety-provoking delusions. After a while he was put on a low dose of antipsychotic medication and the symptoms began to disappear. Three months later I asked him if he could describe his problems. He explained that what had most tortured him was that someone had secretly operated on him, inserting a microchip into his brain. His thoughts could then be controlled electronically. I scratched my head and wondered how such a thing could be possible. The patient thought about it and even began to have doubts. 'No,' he replied, 'it does sound peculiar. It was probably all due to somebody hypnotising me from a distance.'

Even with this response, I looked doubtful. In my experience it was not possible to hypnotise someone who was not aware of being hypnotised. The patient set about thinking this over, again, and after a moment he replied with both a relieved and a small embarrassed smile, that maybe he had just been a little unwell these last months.

COMMENTS

The example illustrates how a person who can give a bizarre schizophrenic explanation – that he is unable to control his thoughts (due to a secret operation on his brain) – can also offer an understanding in terms of a non-bizarre but psychotic fantasy (through hypnosis). He is, at one and the same moment, able to see that these thoughts had appeared in his mind through illness. He is able to do this as he is making good progress towards resuming his health and because the conversation is being carried out in a place which encourages serious reflection about his psychosis.

Delusional psychosis as a waking nightmare

Certain short-lived and longer term psychoses appear to be very similar to the nightmare. The important difference lies in the fact that they are dreamed while awake. The susceptibility for the bizarre and the diminishment of one's critical faculties, the panic-like feeling of being pursued or under the influence of evil forces, the complete aloneness like the premonition of an impending catastrophe, will be familiar to anyone from their own dreams. Many novels about secret agents and science fiction stories have a content that is reminiscent of a paranoid, self-centred world.

Certain less bizarre delusional syndromes can be interpreted in the same way as many dreams. The correctness of the interpretation is only demanded by the patient's response: whether the understanding of the state of mind has increased or not. The interpretation must not be routine – for it to have value the dream interpreter must be experienced and there must be a certain level of co-operation from the patient. In the same way that some night-time dreams feel emptier, dynamically speaking, than others, certain delusions are less interesting or more difficult to understand and to interpret. Those that are rich in symbols appear to be more instilled with feeling and the patient has a more intense relationship with them.

For many patients, above all those who have a good intellectual capacity, pointing out that one experiences their world like a waking nightmare can give them a feeling of being understood. Just as the nightmare's content can never be meaningless, so the acute delusional psychosis describes an inner situation. The person who has an acute psychosis is like the dreamer, his own *dramaturg*, who describes the inner predicament with all available requisites. All fellow performers in the psychosis represent different aspects of the subject's representational world and personal history.

Waiting to be tortured

Eric was a well-built, 40-year-old man who was taken to hospital with the aid of six policemen. He had relapsed into a violent schizo-affective psychosis and was considered to be dangerous. I sat beside him while he demonstrated painful anxiety, waiting tensely. When asked what worried him he replied that he knew that he would be taken into the cell to be tortured shortly and that the hospital was only a front for an organisation controlled by the secret police. When it was guaranteed that this would not happen, I asked him if he could think of any situation in his life where he might have suffered torture. The patient immediately replied that he could. His father had tortured him. Once, when Eric was 11 years old, a person whom his father did not like was coming to visit. Eric, who both admired and feared his father, decided with great agitation to help his father by hiding behind the door to his father's workroom in readiness to beat the visitor over the back with the African assegai that hung on the wall. At first his father was delighted when he heard the plan, but when he realised that Eric was seriously intending to carry it out he became furious and took the spear away from him.

When the patient related the story I was able to confirm that Eric had felt tortured by his humiliation. Eric, in the bewildering circumstances of his being taken into hospital, had found it difficult to distinguish between his actual helplessness and the helplessness he had felt during his childhood. His anxiety faded during the exchange and he was able to begin communicating normally. The fixation belt was released and the conversation continued.

COMMENTS

The acute psychotic delusion was dissolved when the concrete memory was understood as a situation of torture. The patient was able to trust me. The story that Eric told turned out to be only one of many experiences where he had become the butt of his father's practical jokes. Eric experienced them as concrete periods of torture. Later, in addition to medical treatment, he went into a lengthy psychotherapy with me, where, among other events, other psychosis-triggering episodes could be identified.

In order to avoid simplistic conclusions it should be pointed out that psychoses are not dependent on these kinds of experiences but are rooted in both biology and personality.

Hallucinations

Auditory hallucinations

Hallucinations are sense experiences (perceptions) which have no corresponding outer stimulus. All senses, i.e. hearing, vision, smell, taste and touch, can be experienced in a hallucinatory mode. A rule of thumb within psychiatry is that auditory hallucinations are, by a long way, the most frequent within the functional psychoses: that is, psychoses where it has not been possible to find any underlying organic cause. After olfactory hallucination come those of taste and touch. Visual hallucinations more often indicate organic brain damage or a drug-induced influence.

Illusions lie closer to normal experience in that they entail a misinterpretation of an actual outer sense impression. For example, a woman at a noisy cocktail party might think that she can hear the word 'whore' pronounced over and over again with the belief that it is about her. Cars signalling on the road can also be experienced as if they harbour someone who is watching or sending threatening messages.

Hallucinations in healthy people

Many people hear voices or sounds that do not stem from an actual stimulus in the surroundings. More than half the people who have lost someone close to them or a pet that has been around for a major part of their lives react with illusions or hallucinations. When she finds herself alone after her husband's death, a widow might suddenly hear him calling. The dead and buried dog's scratching and whining can be heard as much as the dead child's crying. These experiences come about as a response to certain people's longings; others may feel a terrifying sense of foreboding that they are going mad. The hallucinations and the sense of foreboding are aspects of mourning. In the former the lost one is recreated, in the latter the loss is anticipated in the future. There is a sliding boundary between illusion and hallucination in these cases. The tendency to react in this way also increases if the one who has survived is isolated or has not looked after their physical health, something that often occurs during mourning.

Also, certain *religious mystics* and people with 'the gift of prophecy' can in a lifetime of searching, together with a strong inner tension, hear a Godlike but very concrete voice. In these cases they usually occur after a longer period of social withdrawal and it discharges itself in intense and outwardly directed activity.

The tendency to 'hear voices' and the risk of psychosis

At the end of the 1980s around 400 people in Holland who 'heard voices' met up (Romme and Escher 1989). Most of them were not in psychiatric care but were 'ordinary' people with hallucinatory experiences. This was the beginning of a movement which brought together people with similar experiences in order to support them and to increase knowledge on the hearing of voices.

To repeatedly hear voices without any exterior stimulus in the environment turns out to be something which certain people experience without being or having been psychotic: the apprehension of reality is not even broached and the person knows that the voices do not stem from anyone else. A recent study has observed that around 5 per cent of a non-psychiatric GP population admitted to hearing hallucinated voices talking. Of course, there is a gradual transition between what can be called a thought and a voice. Usually, no doubt, people do not seek out medical treatment and do not consider their experiences as a handicap but rather as a part of their personality. There exist many studies in relation to the character of these voices – whether they are supportive or threatening – or of how they influence people's lives (see Romme and Escher 2000). The dividing line between hearing one's thoughts out loud and having clear auditory hallucinations is vague. Some never have the feeling of an 'inner voice' while others have recurrent experiences of the kind of thoughts which can be heard as voices but which are only seen as a part of their thinking or fantasising. People can report hearing someone talking or whispering to them and not always be certain as to whether it is coming from the inside or the outside. Few people report these experiences to others, either because they have not even thought about it as in any way out of the ordinary or because others might consider them strange.

Many previously psychotic people, who are now free of psychosis clinically speaking, can relate how they almost constantly hear voices. Usually the voices are weak, but sometimes, and especially under conditions of stress, they can be stronger and more disturbing. Voices can be experienced quite adequately as coming from inside with little disturbance. Some, if asked, can tell you about events in their childhood or during their adolescence when they heard voices which are much like the type experienced in psychotic hallucinations. The difference lies in the fact that these earlier voices did not constitute part of a delusion where the person thought about whether they were thoughts of their own or whether they depended on telepathy or some other kind of external influence to their thinking.

A woman described that when she was seven years old and her younger sister told tales about her behind her back, she would lie on her bed and 'thoughts that talked' came to her. Later, she was able on occasion to reassure herself in this way. The first signs of schizophrenia appeared when she was 25 years old, after a long period of antisocial behaviour.

(Levander and Cullberg 1993)

At times people who are not psychotic seek help thinking that the hearing of voices is a sign of mental illness. Naturally, it is important to be able to calm their fears and not to be too hasty with treatment – especially as the antipsychotic medicines often have no effect on voices while they do sedate the personality.

The tendency to hear voices in non-psychotic circumstances can, however, constitute a *vulnerability factor* and thereby increase the risk for developing a psychosis (see Chapters 6 and 7). In a stressful situation the voices can increase in strength and, together with isolation or severe introversion, present an increased opportunity for the messages coming from outside to be misinterpreted as evidence of mystical or persecutory influences. They can start to create a basis for a psychotic development. Then, if the voices do not completely disappear once the acute phase is over, they can be misdiagnosed as a sign of a chronic illness that calls for a higher dose of antipsychosis medication. I have met a number of patients who have had a prior tendency towards this kind of auditory hallucination, and who have not been released from their 'neuroleptic prison' after the stage of acute illness, even though both they themselves and their relatives have complained about it.

Psychotic auditory hallucinations

There is reason to believe that the short-lived, acute auditory hallucinatory state has a different source to the more long-term one, where one or more voices converse or interfere and disturb. The character of the hallucinations is very different. The acute hallucinatory state is often the one that is most clearly tied to the patient's situation in life, making the contents easier to understand. With long-term hallucinatory states, the hallucinations appear more individual, without offering any clear bearing on the actual life situation.

Hallucinations stemming from an acute psychosis often have an 'affective' character. The voices produce critical directives or at times are appreciative, and supportive in nature. 'Shut up!', 'idiot', and other deprecating vulgarities tend to occur. Other auditory hallucinations are less filled with affect. They can occur independently of the actual state of mind of the sufferer and also during remissions from schizophrenic episodes.

Sometimes, many voices communicate with each other: a situation usually referred to as schizophrenic hallucinations. A 20-year-old youth heard how a 30-year-old woman spoke to a complaining 20-year-old, who might have been himself. A nine year old was also involved in the conversation. He was convinced that the nine year old represented himself as a medium, in contact with his childhood.

The voices can be loud or soft, clear or vague, and can interfere with what is going on. They are sometimes described as coming from a radio that is constantly playing, tuned more or less exactly to a station. The voices can be heard as more or less constant ongoing talk or as 'drivel', where specific voices can be made out if one were to listen carefully. Sometimes only a mumble, shriek or call can be heard.

Many patients with long-term difficulties over hallucinations develop their own strategies for subduing the voices so that they do not interfere too much when they are attempting to concentrate on something else. The most frequent strategy is for the sufferers themselves to try to shut up the voices by threatening to shout back if they don't keep quiet. Often people sing, play loud music or clatter about, much to the irritation of neighbours. A professional drummer went for his instrument every time the voices started up. Others try to read a book or say a prayer. It is not unusual for some to use earplugs or to cover their ears. Many continue to hear voices for decades. It is not known how often the voices die away spontaneously or disappear completely, but it is most likely that for the majority the negative and disturbing aspects of the voices diminish in intensity. This is similar to the symptom of ringing or buzzing in the ears, which can be deeply disturbing in the first years, before the sufferer learns to live with the noises. Listened to carefully, they can be heard but they don't interfere with life on the whole. Under conditions of sensitivity or physical difficulties (for example, long-term alcohol or drug abuse), however, they can become stronger.

A study by Cullberg and Nybäck (1992) reveals that these kinds of refractory hallucinations, which are found outside proper psychotic episodes, can go together with an alteration in the brain. It is striking too how much long-term hallucinations remind one of temporary auditory and musical hallucinations, which are sometimes reported after long-term alcohol abuse.

The tendency to hear voices in certain cases goes together with an activation of the motor area for speech in the cerebral cortex (the Broca's area). This has been found in cases of chronic schizophrenic hallucination (McGuire *et al.* 1994). A study with healthy people also shows that the same area is activated when they are encouraged to talk inwardly (Paulesu *et al.* 1993).

Reports of good results in treating disturbing auditory hallucinations with systematic (cognitive) psychotherapy are becoming more frequent. Patients are invited to take command over the voices and to become less dependent on them (see the case of **Chris** in Chapter 16).

Visual hallucinations

Certain psychotic patients describe hallucination-like visual exp[...]
These are mostly fairly vague experiences that have a visual cha[...]

represent extreme misinterpretations of ordinary impressions, that is, illusions. These can have a mystical or frightening aspect. A red switch on the wall begins to shine and appears to be a frightening red eye. The sun can expand and become huge and powerful, something which can turn into a mystical, religious experience. If you try to get a closer understanding of the experience of, for example, a cross in the sky, it is often hard to gather whether it might be a visual hallucination or a strong inner, existentially tinged experience. Some people with schizophrenia can have intense dreams at night and describe how they see different frightening persons or grotesque faces when they awaken.

It can happen that acutely confused people, usually young women, tell of concrete and strong visual hallucinations where the symbolic character is clearly evident. It can be a dramatic story concerning many characters, something akin to a dream that is being retold but where the listener is not quite sure whether they are hearing about an actual hallucination or a dream. Or it might be a very fanciful person who, within a deep regression, allows themselves a creative visualisation of their inner problems. This might be referred to as a *hysterical or dissociative psychosis*.

Organic brain damage or irritant stimuli

Clear visual hallucinations that take place during a waking state are often caused by direct disturbances (poison, brain tumour, etc.) of the brain. They can also appear after long-term alcohol abuse. This is known as *alcoholic hallucinosis*. Pictures appear to move on walls or a troop of dancers enters through the door and disappear again after a short performance. Sometimes these hallucinations, as we have seen, are combined with auditory hallucinations.

Acute *states of poisoning* with benzodiazepine (or barbiturates) are equally likely to produce visual hallucinations. Often they are unpleasant or terrifying: spiders appear and jump onto the bed or nasty animals enter through a crack in the door (see Chapter 13).

With *delirium tremens*, a dreaded state of mind which appears after a long and deep period of alcohol abuse (or tranquilliser abuse), similarly terrifying ʰ ʰⁿllucinations appear. The difference here is that these hallucinations ˢᵗate and so can give rise to reactions of panic. ρen that a patient might throw himself out of . car in order to get away from his pursuers. ucinations are present and sustained in a con- sider the alternative possibility that it might be ρsy which can result in visual hallucinations

Tactile hallucinations

Certain people with a longstanding schizophrenia or with an acute paranoid schizophrenic illness sometimes describe experiencing their body being manipulated, that their organs are being moved about or that they have been injected with dangerous substances (not medication). They do not always have to be actual hallucinations of touch but can appear like a delusion. The ways these experiences are described differ greatly.

Older people can quite often have a sensation that an insect or something else is creeping over their skin (see p. 28). Sometimes this kind of belief becomes reinforced and the experience turns into a hallucination as the person does not allow himself to yield to reasoning.

Olfactory hallucinations and hallucinations of taste

The interpretation of the sense of smell is very much dependent on the psychological situation. This becomes clearer if one thinks of the similarity between, for example, some culturally highly valued smells of cheese and the equally strong negative smell of unwashed feet and excreta. Many acutely psychotic people believe they smell gas or putrefaction: hallucinations that they seldom describe of their own free will. Similarly, food can taste as if it has been poisoned, 'sharp' or rotten. Whether we are dealing with delusions or true hallucinations can be a matter of degree and varies from person to person. The appearance of hallucinations of smell or taste need not point to a bad prognosis. Unpleasant, disgusting olfactory hallucinations can also imply that there is a depressive aspect to the psychosis (see Chapter 10).

Summary

There is as uncertain a dividing line between misinterpretations and delusions as there is between illusions and hallucinations. A hallucination without a delusion (for example, where voices are heard which the person knows to be due to his own thoughts) cannot be called psychotic but must instead indicate a disturbance of perception. Such disturbances of perception can be experienced within different senses. They point to factors suggestive of the development of psychosis if the person has been in a state of stress. Clear visual hallucinations seldom appear except with brain damage and poisoning. They can be confused with psychotically coloured visual fantasies in creative patients and are known as dissociative conditions.

Chapter 4

The ego, the self and psychosis

In this chapter I discuss some theoretical models that describe the development of the self and its dynamic context. A model is a working tool and of
use only insofar as it fulfils its function of increasing our understanding.
When it no longer does so it must be revised or exchanged. We must have
good enough theories and models of the mind if we want to set out to
understand what happens to the personality before, during and after a
psychosis. In this book I shall be using psychodynamic and cognitive theories of the ego and the development of the self. I do not know any other
theory of personality with the same complexity that has the same clinical
relevance.

The ego and the self

The ego is the organising principle for 'the mental apparatus' that
integrates the person's experiences and memories in the face of the demands
of the environment and of somatic impulses. One of the ego's most important functions is to ensure that the experience of the self has continuity and
consistency. Since the notion of the ego is a theoretical construct, a model,
the ego cannot be experienced (see Chapter 17).

The self represents the conscious and unconscious experience of the
person. Consciousness can be seen as a continuum where a clear thought
process can exist alongside diffuse, often contradictory ideas and feelings.
It is an essential part of psychoanalytic theory that the self and the notion
of the ego are not interchangeable.

To a great extent, the self is built out of *representations of the object* and
object relations.[1] It contains an inner system of reference which is built up
out of experiences of life and of representations of the most important
close relationships, which are activated through the experiences of the person's own self. This *inner system of reference*, which superficially can be
likened to the programming of a computer, will link the genetic biological
constitution and lay the foundations for the way the individual handles life
combined with the conscious and unconscious processes that he or she

develops. There are several important theoretical systems describing the psychodynamic aspect of the self. I will confine myself to Otto Kernberg's (1980) synthesis of ego and object relations psychology and with Daniel Stern's (1985) theories concerning the development of the self.

The early installation of representations of important objects in the immediate environment is called the *process of internalisation*. Conscious and unconscious representations of the object remain within the self. The representations of the person's own qualities are also preserved within the self as *representations of the self*. These conceptions of the self make up a large part of the inner world.

With *acute psychosis* the ego's ability to maintain the experience of a continuity and consistency within the self has broken down. The person reacts to this breakdown (discontinuity) in his experience of himself with an acute panic and tries to sort out the new, incomprehensible situation by reinterpreting the outer world to create a new coherence. The attempt to bridge and repair will take place with the help of unconscious regressive ideas, which thus have delusional and often threatening qualities. However, it creates an interim continuity in the self. The cost for the new consistency is a break in the ability to keep a realistic relationship with the environment.

In *long-term psychosis*, the fantasised conceptions have become more organised. The person has adjusted himself or herself to the threat that might be contained in the delusional content, and lives in a prolonged state of emergency. The ego's integrating function has been dislocated in favour of the inner world and the surrounding world is seen filtered through the inner world. Primary process thinking is less contradicted by the reality principle and this is manifest in long-term psychiatric illness (see Chapter 16).

The self–object differentiation

The infant develops a sense of self soon after it is born. This self will become more differentiated and stabilised during the following years. The increased stability gained from the ability to distinguish the self from the outside world constitutes the basis for a sound orientation within the real world. Different events of an inner, biological, social and psychological nature (interaction with the environment) will influence the actual ability to differentiate between the self and the world around. Dynamically, the definition of psychosis is in terms of a disorder in the self–object differentiation. This is not to say that psychosis is 'caused' by early disturbances of development.

Object constancy

The small child has simultaneously different experiences, or 'inner representations', of the same object (for example, the parent) depending on whether the parent gratifies or frustrates, is reassuring or threatening. This is referred to as a 'split' or dual conception in the child's object (parental) representations. A similar duality appears in representations of the self: the child has a group of positive, loving representations of itself. These are separated from the negative self-representations (where there is hunger, anger, envy or a sense of unworthiness). Slowly, the child learns that the two inconsistent groups of good and bad object representations belong together with one and the same object, just as the good and bad representations of the self describe different aspects of the person himself. This work of 'reconciliation' between the good and the bad representations is, on the whole, accomplished by the age of three years. The child has now reached an *object constancy*. It has begun to experience a 'realistic' ambivalent vision of itself as bearer of both good and bad intentions and is able to see, in relation to other people, the possibilities of their having good as well as bad or contrary attitudes.

These ambivalent views are very dominant and, in extreme cases, can begin to control our fantasy world: we can criticise others (or ourselves) for good or bad without paying too much notice to the details or to what might be realistic in our judgements. However, in principle, this inclination to project our outer ideas and needs onto the world is universal and is adjustable for those who have reached a well-grounded object constancy.

If the individual's inner representations of the surrounding world are overwhelmingly disturbing – insecure and frustrating development is not protected by a stable and well-functioning self – it means that the possibility of learning from reality becomes uncertain. The ego develops a difficulty in clearly differentiating outer reality from the warning signals sent by the world that is governed by the object representations. The representations of the surrounding world can give rise to a wide-ranging and early distrust. A tendency to confuse fantasy and reality remains and this tendency is strengthened by frustration and threat. This is the situation with certain personality disorders.

About 'the schizoid and the depressive position'

According to Melanie Klein's theories, the early object relations development takes place by means of a *'paranoid-schizoid position'* at the age of five to six months. The important objects are not yet held together by an object constancy but are still divided into good and bad aspects. Between seven and nine months, the infant has reached a preliminary object constancy which allows it to reach a mutual relationship of a 'you' character. The child has entered into a *'depressive position'* which implies that it cannot easily split off its bad ideas (Klein 1988).

This specific Kleinian terminology can seem bizarre for a reader who comes across it for the first time and will need a deeper explanation than supplied in this book. However, it does hold a strong position within psychoanalytic thinking and clarifies many of the clinical and structural connections between depression and psychosis (Jackson 1994).

Object constancy implies that the conflicting cognitive representations of the parent and the different affects which accompany them become more easily held together in a single conception of the parent. During the period where the representation of, for instance, the maternal gestalt is not fully consistent but divided into different representations, unbridled, hateful and murderous feelings can be directed against the inner representations of the frustrating 'bad mother'. As fortune would have it, the 'good mother' does not succumb but survives and reasserts herself. During the depressive position, the murderous impulses are as likely to strike the good mother as the bad one, since they are now experienced as being directed at one and the same person. The child is therefore forced, in its concern for its vision of the good mother, to control its attacks.

The depressive position, which should not be confused with depression in its clinical sense, describes an early 'concern' (in Winnicott's terminology) offered by the child when it begins to understand the risk that it might destroy the good with its bad and hating feelings. The ability to reattain the depressive position is necessary for all future relationships. At the same time, it becomes the basis of a conscience and demands a certain maturity within the ego. If this capacity fails, the child will fall back into an earlier and more primitive stage of development, the paranoid-schizoid position. In this position, the contrast between the inner and outer representations of reality are not distinguished as there is a 'split' between the good and bad representations of the same object.

By analogy, during a depression which has come about through a loss of a deeply important object, either of a symbolic or concrete kind, one can see how the adult begins to function regressively and to develop a psychotic splitting, usually via a paranoid experience of the world (see Chapter 10 regarding affective psychoses). In this theory, depression is seen as a developmentally 'higher' form of thinking than psychosis, since it assumes an object constancy, which is lacking in psychosis.

The tendency to splitting in adult personality disorders

As stated, the development towards stable and supportive object constancy is disturbed in certain cases of personality disorders. This tendency is characteristic in *borderline personalities*, who present a reduced ability to tolerate anxiety in the face of both idealisation and denigration of both themselves and of others and a tendency towards self-destructive behaviour. On the other hand, the risk of psychosis in these people is not usually particularly high since, more often than not, they have a functioning capacity for self–object differentiation.

The inclination towards splitting has *three main causes*. In the first case, the person in question can have been conditioned in early childhood by long-term and/or repeated *traumas* such as ill-treatment, sexual abuse, changing carers, and an overall lack of security in their home lives. This means that the psychological and developmental work of 'reconciliation' between the good and bad representations has become too complicated.

A second possibility concerns an early destructive interrelationship between *the parents or carer and the child*, where the child's needs have systematically been misunderstood or neglected. The result is a contradictory sense of the self, which struggles with the difficulty of developing an object constancy. The capacity to make a reasonable judgement about other people's attitudes is reduced.

The third ground is *genetic*. We know that a tendency towards personal sensitivity to hurt is often seen in certain families. But a genetic sensitivity can relate to good treatment as well as bad. Those who grow up in a sympathetic home and who are given time to develop their sensitivity in a positive way are certainly less likely to risk developing a personality disorder. Where a child with difficulties in separating from its parents is not forced to develop independence too quickly, such sensitivity can develop creativity. The opposite situation leads to a higher risk of a split occurring within those who are not supported during their development. We still have very little knowledge about these issues.

People who develop a psychosis show signs of a striking split in their object and self-representations. Such a split will usually not remain in the personality after the psychotic state. Thus it differs from the enduring state of the borderline disorder split. In acute psychosis we see a combination of the lack of object differentiation and the lack of object constancy. It can concern a young man who complains that his mother wishes to divest him of his worth by having him admitted to hospital, or of a daughter who complains of her father's incest (this need not have taken place concretely – rather, it may be an expression of the daughter's unconscious fantasy world which is now free of repression).

This function of splitting of the good and bad aspects of the parent, which every psychotherapist knows about from their work with borderline psychotic personalities, has contributed to fostering a picture of the 'schizophrenogenic mother' as the cause of schizophrenia. However, more recent research indicates the inadequacy of this theory. Instead it reveals that it is the personality disorders which predispose to psychosis that are often the result of neglect and abuse in early childhood (see Chapters 6 and 7).

Projection and projective identification

Projection is a psychological defence mechanism that everybody makes use of in a stressful situation but it is especially characteristic of people who are on the edge of psychosis. Projection means that a negatively loaded unconscious thought is placed in the outside world, instead of being experienced as part of the self. Through this mechanism, it becomes unnecessary to take responsibility for the feelings that are awakened by the unwanted thought. The unacceptable character of the projected thoughts means that they are often experienced as threats or as insinuations, such as he is a homosexual or a paedophile.

In *projective identification* two interwoven sequences occur. First, the person will unconsciously reject unacceptable desires and fantasies and project them into another person or object. Then, following the projection, the person unconsciously identifies with the projected aspects of himself/herself now located in the other person who may well be then experienced (through the identification) as trying to control him or her as they are believed to be projecting back the unacceptable. The situation described may be further complicated if the negative nature of the mental contents is unconsciously accepted by the other, leading to guilty feelings in the other. In these ways the phantasied control can become actualised. In psychotic personalities, projective identification is strengthened by means of their tendency to use splitting mechanisms, leading to another person being experienced as totally bad and evil. These situations where projective identification is operating can be difficult for professionals to identify and there is a risk of denial and re-projection into the patient of painful and unwelcome attributes rather than containment.

Acute psychosis as suspension of a 'you' relationship

Acute psychosis implies a linguistic relationship with the world which can be characterised as the sufferer not being able to relate in the second person: that is, in a 'you' relationship (Buber 1962). This 'you' relationship, built on being able to experience oneself in a trusting relationship with the other, is lacking or denied. Instead, the psychotic person lives in a third-person relationship. He or she is alone in his or her universe and is threatened by closeness and afraid of being tempted into a trusting relationship which is thought of as a trap. In order to find security and a sense of meaningfulness, he or she must meet her world according to the criteria that have developed in his or her confined state. There is a logic within this world that can easily be disregarded if notice is not taken of the way he or she experiences their condition.

The mistrust of other people's intentions and fear of accepting help is similar to the feelings of somebody wandering around, disguised, in an alien territory. It is helpful to see this when discussing the psychotic person's 'lack of insight' and lack of willingness to co-operate in the world. It is necessary to allow things to take their time in terms of new events and experiences before trust can begin to develop. When trust grows, the psychosis gives way. For this reason, the care environment together with its personnel's psychological knowledge and ability are of the utmost importance in the treatment of psychosis.

Summary

Acute psychoses imply a dislocation from the experience of the continuity of the self. The self tries to keep the anxiety-filled situation under control and to repair it, through creating a new state of consistency and continuity. This takes place by means of fantasies of a regressive nature and where things are held together by means of the primitive and the irrational – known as a delusion.

An acute psychosis points to the ego's loss of ability to differentiate between certain aspect of the inner and the outer world. The centre of the self lies nearer to the inner world with its magical devices and primary process thinking, where causality, time and place have become negotiable quantities. At the same time, second-person relationships are abolished.

Chapter 5

Phases of acute psychosis

A crisis model

Why describe acute psychosis according to different phases? The simplest answer is that thinking in terms of phases makes it easier to orientate oneself when, as a clinician, a difficult and upsetting situation must be confronted and it is necessary to understand what is being experienced. There is a similarity between a psychotic process and the phases of shock in a traumatic crisis, reaction, adaptation and reorientation. Thinking about phases is also important in the work of helping the patient to recognise early signs that he or she is about to relapse. It is possible, thereby, to get a closer understanding of the fact that a certain symptom can have a different meaning in relation to the phase in which it appears. Finally, those who are treating the patient and the patient's relatives become more capable of seeing the acute psychosis as, in principle, an understandable difficulty in the life of a vulnerable person. It gives a more realistic sense of hope to the work ahead.

Understanding phases within this crisis model is most helpful in the piecing together of events. In some rare cases it can be difficult to discern the separate phases. The progress in some psychoses is so hidden that thinking in terms of crisis does not appear relevant.

The classical model of a crisis is characterised by escalation, turning point, and recovery. This model makes it possible to identify and understand situations which one might otherwise have seen as primarily pathological and hence obscure. Instead, psychosis occurs as a form of failed adaptive strategy within the personality in an otherwise confused and chaotic state of affairs. The acute psychosis is usually a reaction to having to carry too heavy a mental burden when a degree of confusion between the self and the surrounding world occurs. Difficulties stemming from abuse interact with differing degrees of genetic/biological vulnerability resulting in psychosis. A threatening dislocation of continuity within the sense of the self becomes manifest by the attempt to find some meaningful consistency using regressive, magical thinking. The ego's capacity to test reality and its integrative function breaks down. Measured in terms of 'common sense' the external stresses need not be overwhelming. From the individual's point of view, it is normally easier to understand the provocation that has induced the first outbreak of psychosis. This psychotic alteration of the self, by means of different adaptive procedures, can eventually turn into a healing process where the ego resumes its integrating function.

As with a non-psychotic, traumatic crisis, different phases can be distinguished with a certain regularity. Here I will describe a *model* for an acute psychotic crisis. In reality, as stated, phases can either succeed each other more quickly, some phases can appear to be bypassed, or the process can be locked into a particular phase, etc. To my knowledge, Klaus Conrad (1958) has been the first to point out different phases in psychosis in a study interviewing 117 individuals with schizophrenia in the German army. The first phase, which can carry on for several years, he calls the *trema phase* (trema refers to an actor's stage fright, which occurs before he walks onto the stage). This anxiety-filled depressive experience can, according to Conrad, be likened to the inner pressure which is awakened in those who 'know', but not from others, that they have murdered someone. Such a person's reality and world view have totally altered. There is a distance between him and others, which creates an escalating reduction of openness and capacity for closeness. This 'trema phase' is better expressed in its modern term: the *prodromal phase*.

Prodromal phase

This phase, which particularly characterises those psychoses we term schizophrenic, can only be identified with certainty if followed by a psychotic episode. It can continue for weeks, months, or sometimes years. Often the state becomes acute through lack of sleep, isolation or physical exhaustion. The difficulties in life begin to feel all the more alienating and obscure. Difficulties arise when *everyday events defy interpretation*: Why doesn't the post arrive on time? Why do I exist? Why am I walking on this particular street?

The natural sense of security gained from living in a community wavers. The thoughtful person can experience increasing difficulties in differentiating between what belongs to his or her inner world and what constitutes the outside world; what might be a fantasy and delusion and what might be fact and reality. Thinking is closer to *primary process thinking*, which is more dreamlike in its nature but still not taken over by unconscious desires or threats. At the same time, *defensiveness* arises in that a withdrawn state is preferred and the sufferer isolates himself from the company of others. This combination of inner intensity and outer withdrawal can, when confronted by the surrounding world – relatives or friends – release strong and, to those around them, bewildering *outbursts of fury*.

Typically, in the prodromal phase, the capacity to function in work or study diminishes. Many people report a feeling that their thinking has become vague and laborious, that they have completely lost their ability to concentrate. Sometimes, these feelings are increased by the experience of having a complete blockage in their thought processes.

Many people have experienced functioning on a similar level for shorter or longer periods without becoming psychotic. The situation can be altered through positive exterior events and relationships, through psychotherapy or spontaneously. However, it may persist, apparently driven by a deeper psychotic process which we have little understanding of, and consequently little capacity to control. We certainly do not know either how we should differentiate prodromal symptoms from other psychic crises or disorders. As yet, no one has been able to give a valid diagnostic description of the differences. Heightened perceptual experiences such as sharper colours and louder noises can herald a psychotic illness. Descriptions of trance-like states such as short periods of withdrawal from thinking are also important in the diagnosis (Chapman 1966). If these kinds of perceptual disorders occur in a person who has shown a psychic deterioration in functioning and where a relative has suffered a psychosis, the risk for a psychotic illness is high (Yung and McGorry 1996).

Pre-psychosis

For around half of all psychoses, instead of a prodromal phase, only a pre-psychosis stage occurs. This indicates a closeness to a pathological experiential world and means that the threshold to psychosis is about to be crossed. Often there will be a quick deterioration into an overt psychosis but it may continue for several weeks. The world around is experienced as *altered* and all the more *threatening*: angry people are encountered with sharp, searching eyes in the stairway; there is less and less coherence to what people are saying when these people find themselves in groups; and they detect important and frightening attitudes in others and events. Am I performing in a theatrical event which others are directing and which I have not been told about? One imagines that others are *whispering and jeering*. Suddenly one feels that one's *thoughts have a voice* and that they can be heard loudly – perhaps others' thoughts too – causing even greater terror, and one wonders if one is about to go mad. A warning of an *approaching catastrophe* causes *rising anxiety*. Whether the catastrophe is occurring in the world or within the self is never clear.

For some, the need for sleep begins to diminish (usually sleep disturbances will have been occurring for some time) and instead the sufferer may wander around the house at night, *playing music at a very high volume* as this seems to lessen anxiety. *Mealtimes are no longer adhered to* and food brought by carers remains untouched in the fridge. A world totally taken up with fantasies alternates with moments of critical frustration, desperation and, perhaps, suicidal impulses. Evidence of *increased speed of thoughts* can be seen even though it may not result from a manic illness. The person can turn the day around, sleeping too little, devising unrealistic plans or make irresponsible decisions: for example, making contact with superiors in order to chastise them. The high level of inner tension can easily result in explosions of anger when other people are around. Helpful relatives become the recipients of *furious criticism and even physical attacks*. People can find themselves ending up as the object of malicious fantasies and can be sought out as the enemy, without them understanding why. All energy is now taken up by the desire to survive within this altered universe.

Psychosis – early phase

Conrad's picturesque label of the '*Copernican revolution*' illustrates how a person suddenly goes through a change where his perception of the world is turned 'inside out'. From having been a neglected, peripheral person without any power to make an impression on the world that person suddenly becomes its centre. If the delusions and hallucinations that existed during the pre-psychotic phase were strange and frightening experiences they now become the centre of the person's world. Everything that happens in the world is directed at altering his perceptions, at destroying his psyche, and at rendering him impotent.

Now the psychosis can really be seen to have taken control. The impression is that the world has become more clear-cut but in a totally subjective way. Suddenly situations, previously hidden, reveal themselves clearly. It is now quite obvious that he is dealing with a gang operating with the help of laser rays. They enter and steal material from the computer or transmit electrical charges into the person's bed which control his thoughts. The voices that are heard become less difficult to understand when he discovers that people sitting in the neighbour's house are sending them over by hypnotic means.

These extreme sensations of not being in control of one's thinking can, in this way, gain meaning where they might not otherwise have been understood. Now, all at once, we gain access to an internal rationale. The patient believes he can more clearly discern different *messages* as a threat or a danger through the television as if they were being sent directly to him. Newspapers are also full of signs that the patient believes he can now recognise and decipher for the first time. Paradoxically, observing the situation from outside, it can sometimes appear that the anxiety appears less acute in this phase where the obscure and frightening events start to take on an order and clarity. The *threat* that is believed to be there is no less frightening than that which would be experienced in a real situation of being pressurised by or sent death threats by the Mafia, for example. *The enemy is identified* and can be fought off or kept in check. Now the front door can be barricaded, electric wires can be torn out of the wall, and the television can be taped over or thrown out of the window. The blinds are not drawn up in the morning, the poisoned food is left untouched and the tapping messages coming through the radiators can be repulsed by hitting back at them in a threatening manner.

Some can sense the horror of having *their thoughts sucked out of their heads*, or of how *other people's thoughts*, through telepathic means, brain operations during sleep, or quite simply through radio waves, are *inserted into their brain* in the form of obscene pictures, rude suggestions, and contemptuous insinuations or through meaningless talk or babble. They feel they are held under hypnotic or telepathic control by those who live nearby or by powerful international gangs. Neighbours or children that they meet in the stairway are felt to have been posted there to spy on every step they take. Consequently they are subjected to angry glares or furious criticism.

An *archaic primitive world* has now come to the fore for interpretation. There is a force for the bad, which has to be fought off by all possible means. *Directives or distinct orders* are issued to think *specific thoughts or to carry out certain actions* such as removing one's clothes and walking naked in the streets even if it is winter outside. If these directives are countered *the whole world will be destroyed*, and this will be one's own doing. If others try to stop the person it is essential for him or her to use every means possible to fight them and to drag themselves free in order to carry out the necessary action. Loneliness is deep and the mistrust towards other people total, but it is compensated for by the experience of the person believing themselves to have a *unique insight and of being at the centre of existence*. The frustration of others will not alter his or her mind. For the sufferer, the situation is life threatening both to others and to themselves.

This new order of understanding is repeatedly confirmed through special signs, for example, car registration numbers that have particularly significant letter and number combinations, revealing a clear message thanks to their special insight. ACD means Anti-Christ Doomsday, a clear message that soon a world catastrophe will occur. TMP signifies Temporary Motorised Police, who control one's activities. The interpretations appear with lightening speed, clear and are wholly logical from the point of view of the sufferer. The way that cars drive around, stop or start just as one arrives is read and thus reveals how the opposition is playing out their strategy. *Auditory hallucinations* can become even more dominating. It can be the same voice which returns repeatedly, it can be an irritable and contemptuous commentary accompanying one's activities, or it might be different indecipherable voices which are easy or difficult to make out. Some sufferers only have occasional experiences of hearing voices during their psychosis.

If an element of confusion increases, the sufferer in his terror can suddenly *become violent* in this phase. Violent behaviour is seen from the point of view of the psychotic person as self-protective. For example, he might throw himself at a driver whose driving is misinterpreted to be part of the conspiracy that threatens the sufferer. By this time, the surrounding world has usually reacted and tried to get the person to seek help. If the offer for help had occurred or been accepted earlier it might have saved much pain, but by this stage it is often fruitless. Instead, there is a medical examination and often the police are brought in, forcing the sufferer to be taken to a psychiatric clinic for compulsory treatment.

The fear of opening up to or 'taking in' something from the outside world is usually massive, even if the people in question care, are well intentioned, and want to help. The mistrust is not lessened by those in the environment when, in their concern and fear, they attempt to help by giving a conflicting or double-binding message or have difficulty in remaining with the situation. Often the sufferer protests against the medication which, correctly(!), is experienced as an attempt to control his or her mind. The attitude of the helpers is felt to be threatening and a proof of harassment and persecution. To accept hospitalisation could be taken as meaning that one clearly will never get out again and one will be kept there in a hopeless state. The sense of being an outsider is now experienced at its worst.

The feared alternative to possessing this deep understanding of the world's conspiracies is to be mad. Hidden behind the psychotic's mental world is a healthy side where the sufferer can sense the threatening possibility of finding themselves in a horrifying bubble which everyone else feels the need to burst. What is one to do then with one's violent inner chaos? This outcome (of releasing the violent chaos behind the delusional protective front that everyone else wants to remove) is fought against energetically – *a way of refusing to go along with the demands of relatives and doctors*. In the language of psychiatry this refusal is usually termed *'lack of insight into the illness'*.

Psychosis – late phase

A common problem in the late phase of psychosis is that the antipsychotic medication has been prescribed in too high a dose and so the patient experiences side effects. Admittedly, the hallucinations seem to have gone but the patient's behaviour is slow and withdrawn, which is easily interpreted as an expression of the continuation of the illness. Instead of lowering the medication, it may become increased. The result is a higher degree of passivity or 'compliance', which now suggests an indication that the increased medication was justified. This catch-22 situation still occurs all too often in psychiatric care with the consequence that the healing process is slowed down. Moreover, it results in undesirable and unnecessary suffering. The patient and relatives are under great pressure to do as the doctor advises, even if intuitively they feel that the medication should be reduced or removed.

The passing of the psychosis and the assumption of a more normal form of thinking often takes a fluctuating course. Weeks or months can pass before the acute psychosis begins to give way. It is noticeable that the *'islands of sanity'* appear more frequently. The 'Copernican turn' can swing back and forth. Delusions, as with hallucinations, play a lesser and lesser role and their meaning and background begin to be questioned. Even then the temporary improvement often seems to disappear and the *psychotic experience is as strong as ever*. However, the fact that it had been possible to control it at all is a good sign that it will begin to yield steadily.

With a psychotic episode that has been triggered by an experience of loss, or which stems from a difficult conflict in the patient's life which has resulted in the psychotic denial of reality, the depressive contents of the crisis will be able to return afterwards. The experience of having been psychotic makes it more difficult to work through the depression. There are people who after they have recovered say that the psychosis was easier to live with than the ensuing reality. One has to face one's ill-judged behaviour and one notices that those near to one are fearful of making contact. During the psychosis it was possible to fight the dangers believed to be stemming from outside. Afterwards, it is necessary to take responsibility for what has happened as coming from oneself. This can induce a tendency to remain in an *apathetic state, in between psychosis and depression.*

Occasionally, a person protests against the loss of the delusions because they have represented the most important experience in his or her life. In cases of psychoses tinged with affect, especially with religious-mystical experiences, unforgettable traces of blissfulness and inspiration remain, where nothing that follows can compare. Religious literature illustrates the uncertain borderline separating what might be seen as psychosis and what might be considered religious revelations. Huge demands are made on the carer's tact and humility in the face of their desire to confront the truth. Can the person's experience be integrated with the post-psychotic reality without denying their spiritual significance?

Post-psychotic phase – new orientation

In certain psychoses the return to health does not take place completely. It is one of psychiatry's greatest challenges to prevent or minimise the deficits which are characteristic of schizophrenia. Usually the reality principle has reasserted itself in its controlling function in the ego, but often there remain 'shadows' of the psychosis. The sense of the self has usually been shaken to the core. Sometimes, perhaps in the early morning or at specific moments, a thought breaks through suggesting that maybe the delusions represented the truth and that the present represents nothing but a false state. But such thoughts disappear just as fast. Perhaps they are still stored somewhere ready to reappear years later?[1]

The experience of having been mad, that the control over one's logical thinking can be lost, is experienced as painful and distressing. Many patients, maybe even the majority, are wont to hide this phase or deny the psychosis and they react with irritation if it is talked about. This represents a negative prognostic sign and means that the healing process is occurring only on the surface. It might mean a series of relapses has to occur before the patient admits that it has been a psychosis, so that work can lead to self-understanding and towards diminishing the risk for a further relapse.

Painful memories of the time around the relapse and the admission to hospital reappear for a long time. Feelings of *shame* are mixed with *relief* that the psychosis is over, but the problems in life remain. The big question is whether the bridges to the surrounding world have been burned.

Summary

Over time, a *prodromal phase* is seen in the first instance with certain psychoses, which lasts some weeks but sometimes continues for years. It is often characterised by a depression filled with anxiety. A noticeable disintegration of functioning with regard to study or work and/or relationships often occurs during this period. Some can also experience strong visual and auditory illusions. The prodromal phase intensifies during the *pre-psychosis phase*, which features traces of delusional and hallucinatory experiences.

The pre-psychosis phase and early psychotic phase is often stormy but sometimes it is relatively controlled on the surface, even if the underlying tension is intense. A 'Copernican revolution' has occurred where everything of importance that happens in the outside world is connected with the person himself or herself who develops a quite new and extreme centrality. Frequently the last vestiges of self-control disappear around the time of a compulsory admission to hospital – with an ensuing increase in symptoms.

In the *late psychotic phase*, 'islands of sanity' are noted. At the same time, the depressive component is often on the increase as the events that occurred at the beginning of the illness and during hospitalisation return to the mind all too forcefully.

The *post-psychotic reorientation phase* occurs when one sees oneself as a fully functioning person able to return to life in the community coupled with an acceptance of one's illness. If the patient gains insight into his psychosis and works through his experiences without denying them, it increases the possibility of preventing a psychotic relapse. This demands insight and informed support where hope for a realistic future can develop.

Chapter 6

Neurobiological vulnerability factors

[. . .] The room's only window faces something else: The Wild Market Square,
ground that seethes, a wide trembling surface, at times crowded and at times deserted.
What I carry within me is materialised there, all terrors, all expectations.
All the inconceivable that will nevertheless happen.
I have low beaches, if death rises six inches I shall be flooded.

T. Tranströmer, *Carillon* 1983

From a model of illness to a stress-vulnerability model

When psychiatry has tried to explain schizophrenia and other psychotic conditions it has been conceptualised predominantly as a medical illness. A simple and clear cause has been sought: brain damage, a diseased gene, a damaging mother.

The discovery of the bacteria treponema pallidum in 1905 revealed that the syphilitic's dreaded general paralysis of the insane was due to a disease of the brain. Later came the successful effects of the early treatment with salvarsan, followed by penicillin. Since general paralysis of the insane had been thought to be a mental disorder professionals wondered if schizophrenia might also turn out to be an organically determined disorder.

A model of illness can be formed according to medical, sociological, psychoanalytical, magical or other explanatory theories. The cause of the illness and the specific method of treatment are congruent with the core of one's particular theoretical standpoint or world view. The struggles over which school is the 'correct' one have been bitter and ultimately the patients have been the losers.

In the mid-1970s the American psychiatrist Joseph Zubin formulated what is known as the 'stress-vulnerability model', which unites different scientific schools of knowledge and makes it both possible and necessary to foster development towards a combined form of treatment (Zubin and Spring 1977). The thinking behind the model is that people have a differing vulnerability towards the development of psychosis. The illness is triggered by a variety of factors, which are mainly psychosocial in nature. A person with a low degree of vulnerability needs a high level of stress in order to become manifestly ill, while the person who has a high degree of vulnerability succumbs to illness with only a small amount of frustration from outside. Figure 6.1 gives a schematic picture.

The stress-vulnerability model is useful in relation to many illnesses both of a psychic and somatic kind. Diabetes mellitus is often triggered by a physical or psychic frustration in a specifically vulnerable person. In the case of psychotic illnesses our thinking is more complex, but the concept of stress and vulnerability is similar. The onset of psychosis together with rehabilitation and the future prognosis are to a high degree dependent on interactions with the environment and social circumstances.

In this chapter and in Chapter 7, I illustrate different vulnerability factors of both a biological and psychological nature and how they interact with protective factors. Factors that function as triggers of stress are discussed in Chapter 8. Interactionistic aspects are highlighted in Chapter 16.

Our research-based knowledge chiefly concerns the group defined as schizophrenic psychoses. The neurobiological researches cited have chiefly

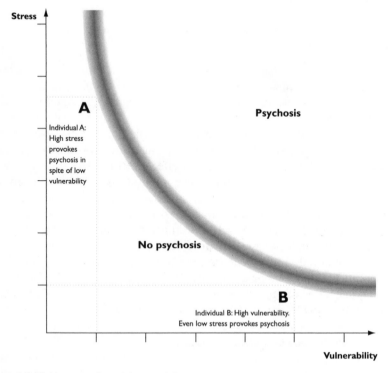

Figure 6.1 The stress-vulnerability model.

been carried out with a narrow definition of schizophrenia that came into use with DSM-III at the beginning of the 1980s, which was an attempt to discern the group with the worst prognosis. The vulnerability theory also concerns the non-schizophrenic psychoses, even if the importance and nature of the underlying factors probably differs.

Today, two main groups of biological underlying factors are described: genetic and pre/perinatal disturbances to the development of the brain. Both can contribute to vulnerability; that is, there might be both genetic and neurodevelopmental forms of schizophrenia – or possibly some form of contribution from both factors. These matters are discussed intensively in international research. I also want to highlight that what today are looked upon as agreed truths may tomorrow be shown to be of no value. The results of research on the brain and schizophrenia are contradictory and suffer a great deal from lack of meaningful diagnostic and good theoretical models. On the whole, the same is the case for psychodynamic knowledge about psychotic conditions.

Genetic vulnerability factors

The spectrum of schizophrenia

The risk of developing a schizophrenic psychosis is usually considered to be about 1 per cent, independent of race or area of birth. This constitutes a simplification of the reality. It has been shown that the risk is 2.4 times as large for those who are born in a large city, in this case, Copenhagen (Mortensen *et al.* 1999).

The sibling of someone with schizophrenia has a risk, according to different studies, of 7 to 10 per cent of developing the illness, and the likelihood of a parent with schizophrenia having a child with the illness is a little over 9 to 12 per cent.

Monozygotic (single-egged) twins, by definition, have the same inherited potential. Different studies suggest a concordance of 15 to 60 per cent: that is to say, if one of them has the illness then that percentage of the second twin develops the illness. Dizygotic (two-egged) twins have the same genetic heritage as ordinary siblings. In the case of dizygotic twins, the risk variation is given as between 4 and 27 per cent, dependent, among other things, on the diagnostic criteria being used.

Is a schizophrenic spectrum inherited?

Adoption studies have also been used to investigate the contribution of non-genetic factors. Comparisons have been made between the rates of illness in adopted children of a parent with schizophrenia and in those whose parents were both psychiatrically well. In a large Danish–American adoption study, undertaken over several decades, research has been made into discovering how often psychiatric illness occurs at an adult stage of the adopted children's lives (Cannon and Mednick 1993). If narrow diagnostic criteria of illness, such as those for chronic schizophrenia, are used, the contribution of an inherited component was reduced. With wider diagnostic criteria – where the occurrence of so-called schizotypal personalities were included in a 'schizophrenic spectrum' – the inherited component proved significant.

For a long time it has been recognised that those with a schizotypal personality have an increased risk of developing schizophrenia. The term schizotypal implies the tendency towards an inward-looking private system of thoughts and ideas. There is also an inclination towards magical thinking and 'superstition' in this group. Where these features are prominent, pervasive and limit psychosocial function, the condition is called schizotypal personality disorder (see Chapter 11 for further discussion).

It is possible that there exists a continuity relating schizotypal thinking – schizotypal personality disorder – with schizophrenia. That which is inherited is not the illness schizophrenia as such, but rather a tendency to a certain type of thinking ('latent schizophrenia'). This thinking can be a risk factor for schizophrenia (Kety *et al.* 1994). It has also been discovered that this kind of 'schizotypal thought disorder' – such as loose associations, incoherent (distorted) thoughts, neologisms (making up new words) and private ways of using words – happens more often within a family of a schizophrenic individual than in others. Even among biological relatives to schizophrenic adoptive children this kind of thinking has been shown to occur more often than amongst non-schizophrenic adoptive children's biological relatives. It shows that there are genetic elements and that it is not just nurturing and early experience which lie behind thought structures (Kinney *et al.* 1997).

However, at the same time it is necessary to offer a warning in the face of a hypothesis concerning pre-schizophrenic thinking. The schizotypal factor is not well defined. We do not know for sure which factors in those with schizotypal personality disorder increase the risk for development of psychosis. It is easy to use this hypothesis to discern that a sensitivity for symbolisation, which might equally be a source of creativity, becomes pathological. There exists a psychiatric terminology that we can easily find ourselves using for behaviour we do not really understand and which differs from psychiatric symptoms. For example, when analysing the speech of psychotic patients, the instruments that we have are rough and ready attempts to find logical-semantic mistakes or divergent uses of words and grammar. Presumably, if the same instrument were used to analyse well-known poems, it would point to an overriding sign of pathology in the poet. The reasoning can, however, be of clinical use if it is understood that speech habits can be more relaxed for some people while for others they are more formal, and that this can be for the good or not. If a relaxed use of speech constitutes a factor for increased vulnerability to psychosis, it can at the same time form part of the creativity that requires a thought process which is full of fantasy. The Danish psychiatrist Bent Rosenbaum (2000) has suggested studying semiotics (the science of signs in language) specific to schizophrenic thought disorders (see Chapter 15 for further discussion).

Concerning the family as protection against negative hereditary factors

The Finnish psychiatrist Pekka Tienari's large study of adoption (1991) has endorsed the higher risk for developing schizophrenia and in schizophrenic borderline states[1] in adopted children with a schizophrenic biological mother compared with adopted children, who have a healthy biological mother.[2] In these cases, however, it has also been found that the children who become ill have more often been raised in adoptive families which show disorders in communication within the family. This implies that a good and protective family environment can work against the forces of genetic hereditary influences that predispose to illness.

For this theoretical and practically important interpretation to be meaningful, it is vital to be able to show that the family dynamics have been disturbed before the child's psychic illness has become manifest. Otherwise the more obvious interpretation cannot be rejected: namely, that the child who shows signs of psychiatric illness influences the family's communication to such a degree that the family's functioning is negatively influenced. There is a risk, for that reason, of confusing the cause with the effect. (Other research has shown that perhaps a third to half of the children who develop schizophrenia have been functioning at a low level for some time before the illness has presented, which in itself must have created problems for the parents.) The follow-up research has not yet been completed, but the Tienari study strongly supports the hypothesis that there are protective psychosocial factors within the well-functioning families that counter inherited vulnerability. This does not mean that the disturbing effects which the child's mental disorder has on the family can be dismissed (Wahlberg et al. 1997).

This research has been carried out in a population with an identified high genetic loading, by focusing on children of biologically schizophrenic mothers. Those studies say nothing about the development of schizophrenia in children where early brain injury or neurodevelopmental disorders appear to predominate over and above the genetic risks for a later development of schizophrenia.[3]

One gene or many genes?

What is the genetic defect in schizophrenia? Several different theories, which are not mutually exclusive, have been suggested:

1   The classic view is that there is one abnormal gene, which is responsible for a stage in the metabolism of a transmitter or receptor in the brain. A metabolic product that increases with stress could, then, induce psychosis. A theoretical model (which is ultimately not realistic) is adrenochrome, a hallucinogenic breakdown product of epinephrine that could accumulate with stress and thus produce psychosis.

2   Genes that lie behind the kind of personality factors which increase the risk for psychosis, for example, schizotypal personality.

3   Polymorphisms (minor mutations) in genes responsible for the neurodevelopment of the brain

4   Changes in genes (maternal/foetal or both) that negatively influence gestational or placental function may increase the vulnerability of the child for developing schizophrenia. The reason for this may be that the neuronal development of the brain is affected.

Huge resources have been dedicated to mapping man's genome (overall gene sequence). Researchers have begun to abandon the idea that it might be possible to find a specific gene that explains schizophrenia and other psychoses. Numerous 'linkage' studies have identified regions (loci) on various different chromosomes (5 and 7 to name but two) that appear to be linked to schizophrenia. However, they have not been reproduced in different populations.

The belief that there is one cause for schizophrenia appears naive in the face of clinical experience regarding the remarkable differences amongst patients with schizophrenia and in the range of exterior (both physical and psychic) factors influencing them.[4] Today, most researchers think that many genes, perhaps 15 to 20 or more in different combinations, may interact and thus, in a complex manner, constitute vulnerability to psychotic illness.

The question remains as to whether these putative genes individually confer risk for psychosis or whether we must change our way of thinking, focusing on interactions between different factors. We can ask ourselves if the risk relates to a lack of (genetic and non-genetic) ego-strengthening personality factors, where the personality in the face of certain stressors is no longer protected against psychotic reactions. The strange thing is not that certain people become psychotic under stress; it is rather more a question why human beings do not react more often with psychosis when we think about the complex work that the ego has to do in keeping a balance between the inner and the outer world. The integrating function of the ego must have strong genetic underpinnings in order to survive. (Chapter 17 explores this subject further.)

The dopamine hypothesis

What is known as the dopamine hypothesis has dominated research into the biology of schizophrenia for a long time. It is based on the knowledge that dopamine, one of the many substances which facilitate neural transmission between the synapses of nerve cells, is blocked by treatment with classical antipsychotic medication known as neuroleptics. These transmitters have their main effect in the basal ganglia of the brain; that is, the nerve centres situated towards the centre of the brain. These centres control the automatic regulation of thought, feelings and motor functioning.

During the last decades it has been suggested that vulnerability implies an inherited tendency to produce a greater concentration of dopamine or a difference in dopamine receptors. This would explain the advances stemming from treatment with dopamine-blocking neuroleptic drugs. We also know that schizophrenia-like psychosis can be triggered by longstanding amphetamine use. The molecule in amphetamine, which is structurally similar to dopamine, stimulates the dopamine receptors into releasing dopamine. A person with a high concentration of dopamine receptors of a particular kind within certain areas of the brain would be considered to have a greater vulnerability for psychosis. However, it has been possible to show that an increase of dopamine receptors does not occur in cases of untreated schizophrenic states. However, they do increase as a result of treatment with neuroleptic medication, something which should guide the use of these substances (Farde *et al.* 1990). (Users help groups have called this effect 'the neuroleptic trap'.)

We also know today that many other neurotransmitters are implicated in the understanding of any given brain activity including schizophrenia spectrum disorders. Hence the original dopamine hypothesis should be open to question on the basis of oversimplification (Henly 1990; Farde 1997).

Types of personality and vulnerability for psychosis

A recent study has shown that the concentration of dopamine D2-receptors in the brains of healthy subjects is lower if they have a 'detached' personality (Farde *et al.* 1997). This is to say, the less dopamine receptors that exist, the more likely the person in question is to avoid deep or close contact with others. If the tendency towards inwardness and withdrawal in schizophrenics is a sign of this kind of deficit, it would explain why treatment with neuroleptics has the effect of worsening negative schizophrenic symptoms: neuroleptics restrain the release of dopamine and thus further reduce its levels.

Genetic research has been more focused on the understanding of the schizotypal personality, which stresses the tendency towards thought disorder and strange or magical thinking. However, it should not be a surprise if schizoid personality disorder, that is, the tendency towards internality and low degree of socialisation, also reawakens interest. Does the schizoid personality structure have causes other than a genetic one? How much is it due to the environment in the earliest years of growth? Experiments on animals illustrate how the young are dependent on the mother's caring attitude (grooming) during a specific period of development in order to achieve a functioning dopamine system in the frontal lobe (Schwartz and Goldman-Rakic 1990). The dopamine system appears to contribute greatly to motivational behaviour of different kinds. Chapter 7, concerning psychodynamic vulnerability factors, illustrates how constitutional factors can influence the development of the self dynamically.

Manfred Bleuler (1984) describes contradictions within the personality that can be provoked in certain situations within young or older people and function as a trigger towards psychosis. Sometimes a heightened sensitivity for experiential impressions or for existential/metaphysical questions can, when combined with schizoid introversion, create difficulties in working through the problems that provoked the psychosis. With others, a combination of strong instinctual drives together with an inhibited personality causes such deep conflicts that the possibility of finding a non-psychotic solution may be greatly reduced. Those who are attracted to the border areas of fantasy but who find no creative expression for this might be seen as being at risk.

Affective vulnerability

Apart from the vulnerability for psychosis there is the affective vulnerability, which has an even stronger genetic root. It concerns an inclination to swing periodically between the extremes of pleasure and pain. Some swing only towards the depressive side, others can swing between both a manic and a depressive state (bipolar illness), whereas others – though fewer – only find themselves experiencing manic or hypomanic (that is to say a not fully developed mania) states. With many people, in these extreme states, paranoid or schizophrenia-like psychotic symptoms are seen. Affective, schizo-affective or cycloid psychoses are dependent on how the symptoms are formed. In my experience, a dominating aspect of people with a first-episode psychotic is that they have affective traits in their psychosis (see Chapter 10). This is not just an academic question, since these people have a better prognosis than other psychotic states. In certain cases an affective illness may act as a stressor that is in itself a trigger for psychosis. Alternatively, a psychosis can also lead to a depressive episode (see Chapter 8).

The prevalence of affective disorder (including unexplained suicide) in the first-degree relatives of those with bipolar affective or schizo-affective disorder has been estimated to be 20 per cent. A full 10 per cent have had or will have the same type of symptom as the ill relative. Even here adoption studies stress (apart from psychological influences) that there are essential genetic factors. It has also been shown that relatives of people with bipolar (manic-depressive) syndrome have a greater creativity, professional success and higher education than those related to patients with purely depressive problems (Coryell *et al.* 1989). It is important not just to see a genetic factor here as the decisive threat for illness. It is more a question of how the vulnerable person can deal with it and if the vulnerability increases through physical developmental damage or psychological difficulties. As we said earlier, the genes need a supportive environment.

Neurodevelopmental disorders

The hypofrontality theory

In a classic study, the Swedish neurophysiologists Ingvar and Franzén (1974) have shown that a group of chronic schizophrenic individuals have lowered metabolic activity in the prefrontal brain region in comparison with healthy subjects. The study has been repeated many times with varying results.

A theory stating that 'hypofrontality' should be characteristic of schizophrenia has, however, won a certain popularity even though it has been open to more and more questioning. Hypofrontality should mean the loss of complex frontal lobe functioning such as judgement, motivation and ethical judgement. It could also imply that signals which normally stem from the frontal lobe and are transmitted down to the basal ganglia are reduced. In the basal ganglia different executive functions are prepared as well as affects and complex patterns of coping. Because of hypofrontality, basal ganglia are no longer open to the restraint and control as the prefrontal cortex is less dominating. They therefore function in a more primitive, less restricted way. This theoretical model has tried to capture schizophrenia's so-called 'deficit' symptoms (passivity, inwardness) as well as the 'positive' symptoms (hallucinations, delusions, and disorders of thought, speech and behaviour) in the increased subcortical activities (see also Chapter 15).

However, it is unlikely that this theory of hypofrontality can represent a complete explanation of schizophrenia. Hypofrontality can also be triggered by the subduing effects of antipsychotic medication. PET studies[5] show that it is not possible either to tell the difference between the reduced functioning in the frontal lobe which is seen in depression and that which appears in schizophrenia. In other words, could hypofrontality of the brain be explained as a non-specific expression of lowered brain activity – as a result of depression, schizophrenia or neuroleptics – just as well as it (hypofrontality) could be an explanation for these conditions?

Today, interest is also taken in other centres such as the amygdala as well as the hippocampus, parahippocampus and thalamus. These areas are important for strategic thinking, learning, short-term memory, and connecting emotions with appropriate emotional behaviour. According to a brain injury theory, which is dominant in the USA, schizophrenia is seen as being dependent on prenatal neuronal development disorders in the brain (Weinberger 1995). How much is genetic and how much is dependent on factors related to intrauterine lack of nourishment or the possibility of the influence of a virus is not known (Figure 6.2).

A meta-analysis[6] from 40 studies where the brain of both schizophrenic and normal control cases were studied with a magnetic camera technique (MRI)[7] showed a significant reduction especially in the right temporal lobe volume (amygdala/hippocampus complex) and an increase in the volume of the lateral ventricles (Lawrie and Abukmeil 1998). It was mainly the grey matter that appeared to be reduced and the finding was primarily observed in men.

However, it is important to keep in mind that these results refer to statistical means. Even among people with schizophrenia there are many with normal values, just as within the control subjects there are many whose anatomy deviates just as much but who do not develop an illness.

One study strengthens the contention around a (non-genetically deter-

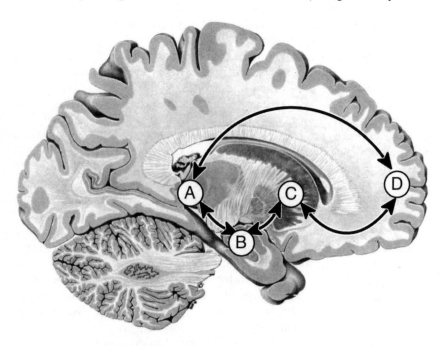

Figure 6.2 A schematic picture of connections and centres in the brain actual in schizophrenia. A represents thalamus, B amygdala and hippocampus, C nucleus caudatus-putamen-globus pallidus, D prefrontal cortex. After Masterman and Cummings (1997).

mined?) deviation or inhibition in the development of the brain in a group of schizophrenic patients (Suddath *et al.* 1990). An MRI scan was conducted with a group of discordant (where only one of the siblings had schizophrenia) monozygotic (one-egged) twins. In 14 out of 15 cases the researchers were able to identify the sibling who had schizophrenia through the MRI pictures showing that they had larger lateral ventricles and a smaller hippocampal volume compared to the healthy sibling. One can speculate as to whether the explanation for this might possibly have been that the brain development in one of the twins had been disturbed, for example, because of less access to nourishment from the placenta resulting in an increased vulnerability.

The findings of abnormal brain structures are more pronounced in men. Since schizophrenia occurs more often in men than women, while women have a greater amount of non-schizophrenic psychoses, it suggests that there are different causes which lie behind but which overlap each other (Castle and Murray 1991). It has also been suggested that oestrogen in women helps to protect against schizophrenia (Häfner *et al.* 1998).

Early abnormalities in childhood development

In an English follow-up study by Jones *et al.* (1994) of all 5362 children born on specific days in 1946 it was possible to identify 30 individuals who have been diagnosed with schizophrenia as adults. When researching into children's care centres, school reports, etc., it was found that these children had a delayed psychomotor development compared with those who did not develop schizophrenia: they took longer to walk, had more difficulties in learning to talk and lower school performance. They also had a tendency to play by themselves. During the routine examination at 4 years of age, their mothers were also judged to have a lower capacity to understand or handle their children in comparison to other mothers.

A new study of Finnish children born in the 1950s who later developed schizophrenia, compared with those who did not, shows a difference only in respect of practical school subjects such as sport, drawing and carpentry where those who developed schizophrenia did not perform so well (Cannon *et al.* 1999). The performances in other subjects showed no difference. On the other hand, attendance broke down more often before secondary school. Boys featured more prominently amongst those who had a lower performance at school. There was no difference between the sexes in respect of their performance in the practical subjects.

How should one interpret this data? Those who have a great deal of experience with patients with schizophrenia know that many of them have not had a low school performance or been physically less able, and that a substantial number have had manifestly wide personal resources. However, one group, predominantly male, has this kind of long-term perhaps lifelong difficulty before they become ill, which may be linked to neurodevelopmental disorders before or at birth. This is supported by studies of monozygotic twins who are discordant for schizophrenia (Torrey *et al.* 1994). In one-third of the discordant children who later developed schizophrenia, their development began to deviate by the age of 5 years. Has the mother's placenta functioned differently for these children?

Pathology in the structure of cells

Knowledge regarding the nature of the neural damage is still scant. Many studies show that such damage, which might result from traumatic destruction of neural tissue or lack of oxygen at birth, is not a major cause. In such cases one would find a growth of connective tissue in the brain, something which has not been reported. The findings instead point more to an inhibition or disturbance of brain development during the foetal stage.

The enlargement of ventricles reflects the lack of tissue in the medial part of the temporal lobe where subcortical centres such as the hippocampus, amygdala and pallidum reside. Any progressive damage as mentioned by Kraepelin, has not been demonstrated in most of the studies (Jaskiw *et al.* 1994). However, it is possible that a subgroup does have such variations (Knoll *et al.* 1998). One can imagine one subgroup with damage early in the brain's development and another small group with a progressive neuronal degeneration who may only present clinically after the first psychotic episode. It would explain the few patients who develop deeper psychotic illnesses that defy all attempts at treatment.

There are several reports suggesting that schizophrenic patients have a lack of cortical tissue in the hippocampus, which is part of the temporal lobe and has important connections with the frontal lobe and amygdala (Jakob and Beckmann 1986; Arnold *et al.* 1991). Such research is often done on those who have undergone lobotomy and on chronically debilitated older patients and consequently this research's application to others is questionable.

Pregnancy and birth complications as risk factors

With regard to obstetric risk factors (the complications of labour such as instrumental delivery, birth asphyxia), some studies identify one, two and sometimes three significant risk factors; however, these are seldom confirmed in other studies. This can be due to the method used but can also be seen as a reflection of the heterogeneity of the group of individuals with schizophrenia.

Several studies claim that if the mother becomes ill with influenza during the second trimester (the middle period of pregnancy) the risk of the child developing schizophrenia is increased (Mednick *et al.* 1988). This presumably would be caused by early damage to the brain through viral infection.

The increased risk is no doubt significant but in practice small and also, potentially, connected to other problems that the mother might have.

For some time it has been known that children who are born during the winter months have a higher risk of developing a schizophrenic illness (Dalén 1978). This could be interpreted as the child's increased vulnerability to infection being greater during this period when the mother's nourishing function is less efficient. Further evidence for the association of winter births with schizophrenia has been reported in a large Danish study (Mortensen et al. 1991; see Figure 6.3).

Children who were conceived in the Netherlands during the period of extreme starvation at the end of Would War II in 1945 were up to three times as likely to develop a schizophrenic illness along with other disorders on the schizophrenic spectrum (Hoek et al. 1998). Another study investigated the impact of the stress that the Dutch people lived under during the German invasion (Van Os and Selten 1998). It shows that a high degree of psychological stress during pregnancy also causes damage to the child in utero, perhaps through neuro-endocrine mechanisms.

During the Finnish winter war many men were killed on the battlefield. A comparison was made between the later frequency of schizophrenia in the children who had not yet been born at the time that the death of the father was reported and in those who had just been born. The risk to the child was greater in the former case, especially during the second trimester of pregnancy, and suggests significant psychosomatic reactions within the pregnant mother (Huttunen and Niskanen 1978).

The so-called Jerusalem study (Fish et al. 1992) shows that birth

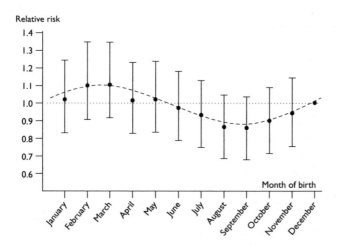

Figure 6.3 The birth month and relative risk for the later development of schizophrenia in the child. The vertical lines give a 95 per cent confidence interval. December is the base month (after Mortensen et al. 1991).

weight was lower in schizophrenic patients in comparison with patients with affective disorders. This finding of a low birth weight, especially when occurring together with prematurity, re-emerges in studies of schizophrenia. Whether they imply that the intrauterine period has been unfavourable with disordered physical (including the brain's) development or whether it depends on other factors, for example, increased stress which can change endocrine activity during delivery is not always clear.

With epidemiological methods and time series analyses it has also been shown that the risk for schizophrenic illness is higher in the case of socially underprivileged classes such as second generation immigrants from developing countries (Warner 1994). This increased risk may be due to a combination of poor perinatal care in these groups and mothers who, due to an earlier lack of sufficient nourishment and vitamin D, develop unfavourable pelvic conditions. The greater degree of mental stress for these deprived groups also needs to be taken into consideration. Can the reduced frequency of schizophrenia that some report in many areas of the western world result from better prenatal, perinatal and neonatal care together with improved welfare? At the same time, it would seem that an increase in the survival of many prematurely born children may contribute to the opposite outcome. Pronounced prematurity is one of the more certain risk factors in schizophrenia.

In a large epidemiological study by Dalman *et al.* (1999) of children born in Sweden between 1973 and 1978, a national register of illness has been combined with a register of birth injuries. Of these children 238 had at some point been diagnosed with schizophrenia according to ICD-9; that is to say, with somewhat wider criteria than DSM-IV. Since the people being studied could not be more than 22 years old, it is only possible to draw conclusions with regard to early onset psychosis. According to their underlying theoretical and practical model, three relatively independent mechanisms for injury were identified:

1   Evidence of intrauterine undernourishment through disorder in the function of the placenta, for instance, pre-eclampsia.[8] Here the risk is more than doubled. Children who have suffered this complication developed schizophrenia twice as frequently as expected. Undernourishment was seen more often in boys.

2   Immaturity was indicated by prematurity. Delivery before week 33 was associated with a 2.5 times higher risk.

3   The Apgar score was chosen as an indicator of lack of oxygen during the delivery. This is measured immediately after birth and then at 5 and 10 minutes. The risk of schizophrenia was non-significantly increased by high stress during delivery.

It should be added that at least one of these perinatal problems occurred in about 20 per cent of the children who later developed schizophrenia. This may be compared to a frequency of about half of that in a normal population. In the future we will probably find new risk factors. A theoretically interesting possibility is infantile jaundice (kernicterus) which, in a case control study was shown to be significantly increased (Dalman and Cullberg 1999). An area of important future research lies in linking different types of obstetric complications in with specific alterations in the structure of the brain.

Even if pregnancy and birth complications increase the risk for schizophrenia, the overall risk that these children will develop schizophrenia later on is still low. Complications around pregnancy and delivery are common but only 1 out of 250 with such complications develops schizophrenia during their lifetime.

The phospholipid hypothesis

At the same time as the dopamine hypothesis began to be challenged, the phospholipid hypothesis started to arouse interest (Horrobin 1999). This connects with the notion of neurodevelopmental disorders. Phospholipids are the foundation of all neural membranes through which signals need to pass. A phospholipid contains essential fatty acids that must be obtained in the diet. It has been found that in schizophrenic patients (as well as in those with dyslexia) there is an increase in the loss of these important fats, perhaps due to an altered metabolism of phospholipids. If this loss is not compensated for by dietary supplementation, then the development of the neuronal system may be disturbed.

Those who put forward this theory link the discovery of disturbed CNS neural development with a genetically determined increase in the loss of fatty acids in neurones. Furthermore, if the synthesis of phospholipids is disturbed in foetal development or because of reduced breastfeeding, the underlying genetic predisposition, can become a clinical problem. Known risk factors such as stress and viral infections reduce the body's capacity to synthesise phospholipids. Several studies show how those who develop schizophrenia have had a shorter period of breastfeeding than others (something which in itself makes one wonder whether there might also be important psychological differences in early development). Breast milk contains more essential fatty acids than formula in bottle feeding. It is still too early to be decisive about this theory. It derives its strength from knowledge about biochemical conditions. Clinical correlation is still weak.

Are brain damage findings specific to schizophrenia?

A comparative meta-analytic study (Elkis et al. 1995) has been carried out between patients with affective illnesses and with schizophrenia regarding the prevalence of enlarged ventricles and signs of atrophy (reduction in neural tissue) of the cerebral cortex. The findings are that both groups of illness are statistically associated with certain brain alterations in comparison with normal people. This suggests that those brain alterations which have been found in schizophrenia are not specific for that disease. Rather, they indicate an overall heightened risk factor for mental illness.

Summary

If you take into consideration the overwhelming quantity of research into schizophrenia, brain changes and genetic factors that has been carried out over the last one hundred years, it is striking both how contradictory the findings are and how few specific findings, if any. There are many reasons for this. The clinical delineation (i.e. diagnosis) of schizophrenia is unsatisfactory. Schizophrenia is not a simple disease: rather, it can be seen as a set of reactions to an earlier vulnerability with many causes. Furthermore, there is very little research into non-schizophrenic psychoses; most research has been carried out in the chronically ill.

The genetic component is probably the most essential biological dimension underlying schizophrenic vulnerability. It appears to be a manifestly polygenic inheritance. A clearer inheritance can be seen if the diagnostic criteria are broadened to include the schizophrenia spectrum disorders. The available data indicate that the genetic factors for schizophrenia may lead to a tendency towards schizotypal thinking.

Another dimension that could be genetically determined, but which also presumably functions independently and increases the effect of genetic vulnerability, is early disturbance in the development of the brain. Interest has been shown in the fact that there is a reduction in brain tissue in perhaps a third of chronic schizophrenic patients, and more in men than women. Potential causes of this kind of damage include lack of adequate nutrition, developmental disorders during pregnancy and shortage of oxygen at birth, though these factors only help explain a small proportion of the total illness burden.

Research within the next decade will certainly produce essential new knowledge about pertinent biological factors, but it is unlikely that neurobiological research will be able to give us a comprehensive explanation for 'the enigma of schizophrenia' which some hope for. Rather it must be looked for in an interdisciplinary approach.

Chapter 7

Psychodynamic vulnerability factors

Psychodynamic vulnerability factors are those particular to a given individual's internal world. They are often contradictory psychological issues that threaten the individual because they pose difficulties in finding the strategies necessary for dealing with a problematic situation, a crisis, overstimulation, or other stresses. The contents of such experiences become so threatening or incomprehensible that the ego loses its ability to function and to integrate.

— schizophrenics

Early trauma and problems in growing up

There is a dearth of scientific knowledge about the influence of childhood circumstances and early experiences on the development of psychosis or schizophrenia. It is more clearly understood how negative experiences during childhood can create or increase the tendency for personality disorders of different kinds. Negative childhood experiences and personality disturbances can function as psychological vulnerability factors for psychosis.

According to the psychoanalytic object relations theory, the ego acquires its structure through the inner representations of our earliest carers, which takes place by means of processes of identification of different kinds. Those children who suffer early lack of security and serious interference in their early relationships develop weaker ego structures, which can be the cause of personality disorders. In a study by Beck and van der Kolk (1987) of 26 chronically psychotic women in a hospital in the USA, half of them recalled incestuous experiences during childhood. Even if the truth of the reports cannot be proven, they indicate that experiences of incest, just as with other abuse during childhood, can constitute a serious vulnerability factor for different kinds of psychic illness.

Experimental studies in mammals can contribute to understanding the importance of the attachment phase. If the relationship with the mother is severed at an early date, the breach will become manifest in serious disorders of the animal's behaviour later in life. It has not been possible to corroborate the excessively reductionistic theory that dominated the 1940s and 1950s psychoanalytic literature which argued that schizophrenia was caused by the disruption of an early mother–child relationship.

A lack of sensitive understanding, of closeness and of faulty interpretations of the child's communication and needs were recurrently cited as factors. Such situations certainly add to the development of personality disorders. In order to develop schizophrenia a combination of vulnerability factors may have to be present such as a particular biological constitution (i.e. genetic and neurodevelopment factors), in combination with early deficiencies in care or abuse which is sufficiently traumatic that it damages the development of the self (Kraemer *et al.* 1984; Siegel 1999; Meuser *et al.* 2002).

Systematic research in these areas remains poor and our knowledge rests mostly on anecdotal data. A review states that the number of schizophrenic patients who have grown up under traumatic circumstances are over-represented (Read 1997). Among this group are included those who have experienced sexual or physical abuse as children or who have experienced serious neglect at an early age. The reason why this has not been noted in earlier literature, according to the writer, is the tendency not to ask about these problems when taking the past history of patients.

The descriptions that schizophrenic patients give of their parents are coloured by their split inner representations. This one-sided picture of a bad mother or father can easily awaken identificatory notions in the person who reads or hears about these parents. For many years parents have found themselves being regarded as the scapegoats for their child's illness.

Infants are constitutionally very different from one another in their developmental level in terms of maturity and sensitivity to stimulus. Thus, it is necessary to be careful when making judgements about how parenting problems contribute to later psychosis. Sensitive children demand more from their parents, who are also often acutely frustrated in their dealings with the child. The only certain fact that we know is that most parents who have a child with a serious physical or psychic illness have a tendency to react with irrational self-reproach and feelings of guilt.

Many (most?) schizophrenic patients, in my experience, have not suffered particularly severe neglect. On the other hand, certain biologically sensitive children have been in special need of a close bond and a more lasting attachment period to their parents. A large part of the ego is genetically determined but important aspects are also formed by way of the earliest internalised object relations.[1] With regard to people with affective psychoses (see Chapter 10) an early trauma is more often the case. Many have noted that people with psychosis have had more psychosocial difficulties during the later part of their development (adolescence and early adulthood), compared to others. These difficulties should be included with the other vulnerability factors already described.

An interview study was carried out by Sonja Levander and the author. We studied eight people with well-controlled DSM-III[2] schizophrenia, who had recovered after intensive and long-term dynamic psychotherapy. Their hospital records were also studied and we interviewed their therapists. There was no indication that they had experienced traumatic stress during their early infancy (Cullberg and Levander 1991). On the other hand, all of them had had very stressful experiences during preschool age or before their puberty. A marked number of patients also had relatives who had been under psychiatric care. We interpreted these findings as evidence of individuals with a genetic vulnerability, who had been under stress from the external world during their development. Later, in late adolescence or early adulthood, they had reacted with psychosis when undergoing a particular stress. During their interviews they were able to describe fully how they had been on the way to becoming stuck in an inflexible state akin to personality disorder, a situation which was altered by the breakthrough of the psychosis. The psychotherapeutic working through, which sometimes continued long after the inception of the psychosis, seemed to have been a decisive factor in curtailing the development of the illness. Some had affective components in their illness; a factor that often indicates that dynamic psychotherapy will be constructive.

Theories of vulnerability and personality development – neuropsychodynamic

The American psychoanalyst James Grotstein, who is well informed in neurobiological issues, has developed a theory regarding children who have a biologically high vulnerability that will confer an increased risk of psychosis (Grotstein 1995). I will give the main points of his theory with some small additions. Grotstein's view is that certain children are born with a reduced level of protective capacities ('filters') when it comes to external stimuli. Hypothetically speaking, it can be due to a genetically orientated higher sensibility or to early developmental disorders resulting from damage to certain brain centres. These are the causes of cognitive micro-defects, which involve the capacity to solve certain types of problem or to think in certain ways. This kind of child may then be placed in an environment that does not cater to its specifically strong needs to be 'held' and 'contained'.[3]

Neuropsychological research supports the theory that the brain is not such a self-determined organ as had been previously thought. Its biological development is quite dependent on adequate external stimuli during critical periods. The infant has the subjective experience from early on of very strong psychological discomfort or painful sensations in connection with stimuli of different kinds (hunger, heat, cold, colic, loneliness). The child is not yet able to tell the difference clearly between stimuli coming from the exterior and those which are from inside. The building of stable inner representations of the surrounding world is made very difficult if the infant is overwhelmed with painful experiences. The unconscious becomes filled with 'demons' (see Chapter 4). There is an excessive early overloading of negative self and object representations. The difficulty in dealing with and interpreting stimuli correctly is exacerbated and the ability to symbolise and to differentiate between abstract and concrete becomes open to error. With this overload there is a lowering of the potential for establishing a well-functioning 'area of transition' between fantasy and reality which young children usually have as a bridge between their image of the mother and the surrounding world (see Chapter 1). These bridges are called transitional objects and phenomena and take the form of blankets, bedtime rituals, hide-and-seek games, and the like.

For those children who have low stimulus thresholds of a physiological kind the transitional areas can be developed, but they risk becoming stuck in these states. The protective buffer against the surrounding world also functions as a barrier against it. Their games turn into compulsive attempts to control, which can disturb family life. Rituals become more and more prolonged and emotional outbursts painful, when the parent no longer wants to go along with the rituals. Activities appropriate to their age become delayed.

The dynamically compensatory strategies that the child unconsciously takes up in order to increase his ability to cope (and perhaps 'survive') takes place, according to Grotstein, in terms of a development of a vicarious 'false' self. He speaks about a 'Faustian pact'[4] where the child 'chooses'[5] safety instead of authenticity. This false self is characterised by concrete thinking and shallow relationships so as not to disturb the deeper layers, where the 'demons' are lurking. It means that situations that might otherwise risk feelings of mourning and loss are barely felt and pushed away. For the authentic buried self these experiences of loss would in fact be experienced as catastrophic and akin to death (annihilation). The false self takes over and forms a personality that shields against the outside world. Relationships, which in a more adult world might lead to attachment and dependency, are avoided by withdrawal. If the impulse towards dependency is much too powerful, for example, an impulse to form an attachment of a regressive type such as that of infant with a mother figure, there may arise aggressive attacks when these impulses are frustrated. Since the authentic self is split off from the conscious self, those deeper more threatening feelings that are provoked can be experienced as coming from the world outside. Negative 'angry' aspects of the self are projected into the environment and form feelings of persecution or other delusions.

Grotstein's theory gives us a model that helps to understand how biological factors can influence the development of the self and how psychodynamic states interact with neurophysiological circumstances. It also shows why certain experiences and events can have a psychotic outcome just as the development of the self and delusions can go together with early biological development. The so-called need–fear conflict between the deep need for warmth and the equally powerful fear of closeness characterises the state of mind of the schizophrenic. The model is a dynamic (interactive) one. Whether it will retain its usefulness only the future will tell.

Personality disorders

In the previous chapter we have seen how *schizotypal* personality characteristics can indicate a potential for schizophrenic development. In this context it would be appropriate to remind ourselves of the psychoanalyst Otto Kernberg's dynamic theory about the organisation of the personality on three levels with different sorts and degrees of disorders manifest in descriptions and experiences of the self (Kernberg 1984). In DSM and ICD diagnostics a similar grouping has been made with more phenomenological criteria (see Appendix). Here I will summarise Kernberg's classification:

1   *The neurotic personality organisation* features clear boundaries between the self and the world, that is to say identity is relatively well defined. The ego is strong and flexible with repression as the dominating defence mechanism. Reality testing is efficient and the ability to relate is relatively good. Included are anti-aggressive, dependent, obsessive-compulsive and avoidant personality disorders. Psychotic regression is not necessarily expected to occur. Even so, one can find acute psychosis in an especially vulnerable person (see the case of Eve, p. 79). The prognosis is usually good.

2   *The borderline personality organisation* is determined by a diffusion of identity. The defensive mechanisms are made up of splitting between idealisation and contempt, love and hate. The ability to make relationships is disturbed. The ego is weakened and there is difficulty in sublimating instinctual wishes and controlling anxiety. Impulsive behaviour is common. Narcissistic, histrionic and emotionally unstable (borderline) personality disorders are included within this category. Reality testing is good. There are certain borderline type personalities who have a tendency to react with schizophrenic-like psychoses when presented with exterior frustration (see the case of John, p. 81).

3   *The psychotic personality organisation* is one where the borders between the ego and the surrounding world have partly been dissolved. One could describe it by saying that there is permeability between the inner and the outer world. The defence mechanisms are more primitive, including splitting, denial and projective identification through to clear-cut projections. Reality testing readily breaks down and the ability to

make relationships is limited. Here we include the schizotypal, paranoid and schizoid personality disorders. The first two disorders are seen as risk factors for psychosis more often than the schizoid.

Personality disorders and psychosis

The examples that I cite below are not chosen systematically. They represent personality types that, according to my experience, present a risk for break-down into psychosis. Usually their defence mechanisms are enough to stem anxiety when in conflict. In some situations, however, their defences do not adequately protect the personality and a psychotic collapse of the ego function takes place. Often this is diagnosed as an acute, brief psychosis, affective psychosis or schizophreniform psychosis.

A personality trait that can act as a risk factor for psychosis is *immaturity*. Today this is not considered to be a personality disorder, and is not included in the current classifications. According to my experience, it lies between the borderline and the neurotic organisation of the personality. The adult's immaturity reveals itself in a 'childish' way of being. One finds a repeated gullibility and tendency to 'see' good parental figures with persons who show clear signs of being the opposite. The immature person's background not infrequently shows a combination of early and long-term periods of mistreatment or of having witnessed mistreatment or sexual abuse together with an emotional tie to abandoning parents. The inner representations (images) of the adult world are filled with angry and frightening threats leading to a need to protect themselves against leaving the child's world. Violence and sexuality are, for these people, closely connected and full of anxiety, but they unconsciously find themselves drawn to both poles just as moths seek out flames. This can sometimes take place in a sublimated form such as finding a way to a caring activity, wanting to save an abused partner or entering into an extreme religious movement. Others get taken over by a pimp, prostitute themselves or find themselves in a repetitiously abusive situation.

When the contrast becomes too strong between the denied difficulties in reality and the inner need for security, catastrophic reactions and chaos occur, sometimes ending in psychosis. If the immaturity is linked with a *low intellectual capacity* or cognitive impairment then the prognosis is worse, and the potential for working through in treatment and rehabilitation is diminished.

Similar problems lie within personality disorders of *a hysterical or histrionic nature*. These people have an intense fantasy life and a strong need to express their emotions. They may also present an attractive and 'exciting' outer image, which contrasts with an inner world dominated by early, repressed conflicts. They often find themselves in crisis situations due to their attractiveness and because they are often curious. When reality becomes hard to face, their intense fantasy life may take over in a concrete psychotic way.

Many of these personalities also have borderline traits. Regressive psychotic states are common. Feelings of guilt, of being an outcast, create a situation where retrieving themselves from regression becomes more difficult, especially if they are not supported by psychotherapy. Sometimes people have marked dramatic psychosis-like symptoms that are not in fact truly psychotic (see the case of Nina, p. 125).

Obsessive-compulsive personalities usually have such a severely ritualised life that outer or inner frustrations only serve to increase the ritualised, compulsive behaviour. In these cases the genetic aspect is an important factor. Here it is clear to see how in combination with immaturity the risk is increased. Conflicts surrounding sexuality or aggression can cause the rigid personality to break down instead of reacting with a compulsive defence.

On the fear of having children

Eve, a 35-year-old senior civil servant, lost her child at birth. She had, for reasons which were unclear, been against her pregnancy but agreed to it when her husband insisted, declaring that he would otherwise leave her. Eve, who had no other children, lived a protected life as an adult, with a great stress on the aesthetic. She had given much time and effort to controlling and planning her life with care. Some weeks after the birth she went into a chaotic psychosis that was followed by powerful depressive feelings, where she blamed herself for the death of her child, preoccupied that she had not loved it.

In our psychotherapeutic work it transpired that when she was only 2 years old Eve's parents had adopted a 1-year-old child with brain damage, which had resulted in disturbed behaviour. The little boy concretely broke up Eve's safe world with his aggressive and destructive behaviour and she came to harbour an intense hatred for him, which she had been unable to show openly until her psychotherapy. She had firmly decided not to have a child until she was ready. After her psychosis she went through a deep suicidal depressive crisis. When it had subsided, after a combination of psychotherapy and antidepressive medication, she decided with her husband that she would become pregnant again. This pregnancy she experienced with a deep sense of pleasure and birth and postpartum period occurred without difficulty.

COMMENTS

The characteristics of Eve's personality with its ordered, controlled and aesthetic sense had been reinforced as a reaction to her early childhood trauma. The need to be able to love a baby conflicted directly with her early feelings of hatred. Through her husband's 'blackmail' of her for his love she had become pregnant. The belief that she had caused the child's death through murderous fantasies became overwhelming and her sense of guilt seemed unresolvable.

Narcissistic personality

People with deep narcissistic problems carry a split between a conscious and a threatening unconscious self-image. This conscious picture of the self is grandiose and maintained and nourished by ideas of being successful, being admired by important people, or by sexual conquests. This view of the self hides and balances a denied and split off early picture of the self filled with frustration and fury. Not infrequently these people enter into deeply depressive states in the later part of their middle age or during their old age. Either a series of misfortunes or violations occur or age invades, with its inevitable humiliations and losses. These rupture the protective grandiosity and the grandiose picture of the self without time enough to compensate and recover equilibrium. People with a defined narcissistic personality may end up being quite lonely during their later years, when the friendships have not been kept up and relatives can no longer deal with the narcissist's neglectful and egocentric way of living. Old age becomes filled with bitterness and contempt, which is directed as much outwardly as inwardly towards themselves.

The compressed, split off, early hatred can no longer be held in check. Instead, it finds its way in, flooding the personality with self-contempt, which can be horrifying in its merciless grimness and swift development. Sudden and violent bids for suicide occur. Alternatively, a psychosis can develop, where aggression is projected onto the outside world, which is in turn then experienced as persecutory and life threatening and must be fought against with violence or avoided. The person can end up violently taking his own life or can enter into a paranoid psychosis or state of bewilderment where he might commit some violent act. Not infrequently this too can end in suicide. These developments are well known within forensic psychiatry. We see them as an aftermath to scandals, for example, within the higher executive world, misfortunes in business or in the criminal underworld. But even with more ordinary disappointments in love, say, a paranoid psychosis can develop with jealousy which is maintained and nourished by the interpretation of different signs and symbols in a psychotic way.

The specialist in eighteenth-century French literature

John was a 40-year-old self-educated man who specialised in eight-eenth-century French literature. He was homosexual and thanks to a timely inheritance from his mother he was able to make long journeys to the continent, where he met up with friends and mingled in literary circles. When the inheritance was used up, John returned to Sweden.

He could hardly maintain a living on his very specialised literary essays. In John's own view, his talents were unique. He only wanted to talk to people who were not too far beneath his own level and so his circle of friends became sparse. He was seen as a gifted eccentric and was offered an early pension because of his narcissistic personality disorder. His mother died, to whom John was very attached, triggering a depression in her son.

At the same time, he was blackmailed by a gang of teenagers because of his homosexuality. The police were unresponsive. His anxiety escalated and it became difficult for him to sleep. John began to see persecutors on every street corner and was convinced that he would be murdered. He tried to get himself admitted to the psychiatric clinic but was sent away because there was no room for him. A day later he became confused and in the evening he dared not go out without first arming himself with a sheath knife. When he saw a car follow him and stop at a red light, he jumped out, flung open the driver's door and plunged the knife into the driver. The man died instantly. John did not fight off the police who arrested him, rather he was relieved.

He was committed to a forensic psychiatric ward in a secure institution and treated for many years with high doses of neuroleptics because of an incorrect diagnosis of schizophrenia. When I met John after eight years he was handicapped by side-effect symptoms in the form of compulsive muscular spasms around the mouth. (These spasms are called tardive dyskinesia, a late onset side effect of neuroleptic medication.) He remained detained because of the risk of impulsive acts but could have been eventually released to live independently.

COMMENTS

This case illustrates how treatment with neuroleptics can be misused. No differentiation had been made between John's short-term, stress-triggered psychosis and his long-term personality disorder which was mistaken for schizophrenia. It also illustrates the risk of not paying heed to early signals of psychosis. Neuroleptic medication is often an effective treatment for schizophrenia but may be counterproductive with other mental disorders. The grandiose self-image of this man who was very gifted indeed was mistaken for a schizophrenic grandiosity, which invariably carries more bizarre traits.

Is alexithymia a vulnerability factor for psychosis?

The American psychiatrist Peter Sifneos (1973) described a condition where patients displayed clear difficulties in putting affects and feelings into words, and in distinguishing verbally the differences between feelings such as anger, sorrow, anxiety, joy, etc. These people avoid situations that could lead to conflict or distress. Sifneos discovered this problem in many people with psychosomatic difficulties and called this state *alexithymia* (Greek for lacking the words for feelings). The same observation had been made earlier by a French psychoanalyst and was called *pensée opératoire*. If such a person experiences a negative or threatening feeling, it cannot be symbolised in the form of words or thought with which to work it through. Instead it is expressed physiologically in psychosomatic activity. They do not themselves seem to be aware of the handicap. This becomes more obvious once one has worked with such a person for a while. Their capacity to work together within a therapeutic relationship and to make use of traditional psychotherapy is limited.

The reason for discussing this notion here is that I have been able to see in a number of cases of schizophrenia how alexithymia has been a factor in the triggering of psychotic episodes. Even during periods free from psychosis marked numbers of patients with the tendency to react psychotically have pronounced difficulties with defining let alone verbalising their feelings.

A gifted 30-year-old man, who had been free from symptoms after a schizophrenic illness over a period of a year, described having had a relapse into delusions a couple of evenings earlier. When asked how this had come about, it transpired that his wife had asked him some questions while he was preparing for his exam. She had been stressed by her own family problems and wanted his advice. The patient was busy and felt he was a little stupid for not being able to reply so he suggested she ask someone else. His wife took no notice and continued to ask him questions. At the same moment he started to think that the neighbours were talking about him through the wall and to believe that people were eavesdropping and spying on him. The experience continued for half an hour, with the forceful intensity of his earlier psychosis. However, this time he was able to control himself as he was consciously aware that this could be a psychotic symptom. At a subsequent appointment there was no sign of psychosis.

When I asked him again to describe his feelings when his wife had disturbed and embarrassed him, he was not able to put words to them. 'She must ask ... she knows that I love her ... she didn't have anyone else to ask ...' At my question as to whether he had, in spite of his love for his wife, felt himself to be irritated, he could not understand why this might be the case. At the same time he began to wonder whether there was a bugging apparatus hidden in my office. His anxiety intensified painfully but decreased when the subject of conversation was dropped.

This case and other similar cases point to the fact that alexithymia can constitute one of the factors that lies behind an increased risk of relapse in the face of affective reactions from others in the home[6] (see the later section on expressed emotion).

Family structure and schizophrenia

Research into family structure in schizophrenia (by which I mean a prolonged psychosis), shows that problems in communication and disturbed relationships more often occur in a family with a schizophrenic child than in other families (Alanen 1968; Goldstein 1992). This might be expected as a result of the genetic relationship between personality disorders and schizophrenia. Often the parent with a personality disorder has been singled out as the cause of the child's illness, whereas in reality the association may be because of shared genetic vulnerability.

It has also not been sufficiently acknowledged how much an ill child can influence his family, contributing to the stress. Here too the relationship between cause and effect is often misinterpreted. In the past parents of the schizophrenic individual have more or less been outcasts and blamed for the illness by the psychiatric team. However, now things have changed and in the last decade parents have no longer been scapegoated. Not many would today blame them for the child's illness. Attitudes have changed to such an extent that it is sometimes difficult meaningfully to discuss the effects that family dynamics might have on the development of illness. If one sticks to a vulnerability theory it is necessary, all the same, to pay heed to the family's pattern of communication as it is of central relevance in terms of positive or negative ongoing stresses.

It is possible to distinguish between different types of home atmosphere in the life of schizophrenic patients. One group has had a *fairly unremarkable (in terms of dysfunction)* home life with a family who care and who maintain a sense of integrity. This kind of background is usual in the kind of person with schizophrenia whose illness has had a barely perceptible inception and who eventually proves difficult to treat.

Another type of family appears on the outside to be well integrated and socially progressive. Looked at more closely, *serious* difficulties in *communication* are revealed. The parents might be incapable of showing warmth and, consequently, the frustration within the family is intense but hidden. The demands and expectations on the children are often quite unreasonable and there is a low tolerance for those children who differ or who fail to live up to expectations. Traits of personality disorders are evident in one or both parents in these families, which suggests that they may be carrying vulnerability factors.

A third and smaller group consists of *those children who have had concrete problems during their upbringing*. They might have grown up with a single, personality disordered parent, have suffered abuse of some kind or have been sent away during critical periods in their growth. Their carers may have changed many times, etc. The Danish study of adoption (Cannon and Mednick 1993) found more early separations (from a schizophrenic parent) amongst high risk children who later developed the illness, compared with children who did not fall ill.

For a sensitive child, the possibilities of building up a stable personality and image of the self are diminished in the kind of setting described in the latter two groups. It is also common that a personality disorder of a borderline or antisocial nature will develop in adaptation or as a form of defence. This kind of 'adaptation' becomes at the same time an additional vulnerability factor, since for these disturbed people there is an increased risk of finding themselves in socially distressing situations.

Expressed emotion (EE)

During the 1970s British psychiatrists were able to show that the psychological atmosphere in home life was just as important as the medication in diminishing the risk for relapse in people with schizophrenia (Vaughn and Leff 1976). In families with a *high level of critical comments and hostility* relapses occurred more frequently. The same was true for families with an overinvolvement with the patient, where the patient's feelings were not left alone. These were identified as high expressed emotion (HEE) environments in contrast with low expressed emotion (LEE) environments. The latter were characterised by a higher degree of integrity within the family. If the patient lived at home and was 'exposed' to an HEE environment for more than about 35 hours a week, the risk of relapse into psychosis was high. In LEE environments relapse was less common and the prognosis was much improved, even without medication. These findings are compatible with the stress-vulnerability concept. It would be reasonable to think that high expressed emotion could act as a trigger factor in people becoming ill for the first time, even if for practical and ethical reasons it was not possible to carry out an experimental study (Figure 7.1).

These findings are now well established and special educational programmes have been developed with the aim of helping families to change their way of communicating from HEE to LEE. It can also be shown that where mental health facilities (such as patient wards, residential accommodation) have high EE, they have reduced recovery rates for patients with psychosis. Here, an HEE environment may well be, in part, a consequence of the mixture of manic, brain-damaged or severe personality disordered patients (see Chapter 21).

A comprehensive neurodynamic model of psychotic vulnerability

The risk of developing psychosis and especially schizophrenic psychosis should be seen as multidimensional, where neurobiological, psychodynamic and social factors work together and strengthen or alternatively counteract each other. The difference between the forms of the psychosis lies in the relative contribution of these underlying factors. We can differentiate between three principally different dimensions of vulnerability (see Figure 7.2).

1   *A genetic personality factor*: in psychodynamic terms a 'thin-skinned' personality or permeable self with uncertain boundaries between the inner and outer world.
2   *Neurodevelopmental disorders*: these result in cognitive disorders that

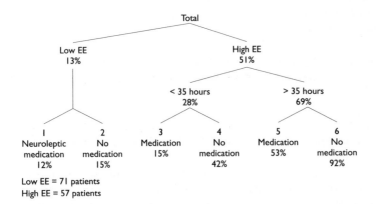

Low EE = 71 patients
High EE = 57 patients

Figure 7.1 Relapse rates at nine months in patients with schizophrenia according to the level of expressed emotion and use of antipsychotic medication. The frequency of relapse is lower in families with low EE (irrespective of medication) than patients on neuroleptics and with high EE (Vaughn and Leff 1976).

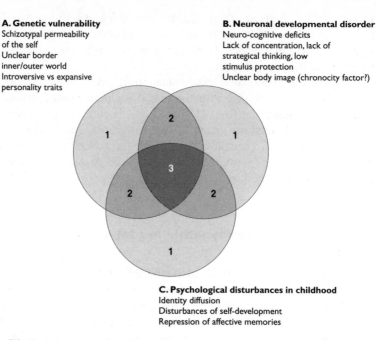

A. Genetic vulnerability
Schizotypal permeability
of the self
Unclear border
inner/outer world
Introversive vs expansive
personality traits

B. Neuronal developmental disorder
Neuro-cognitive deficits
Lack of concentration, lack of
strategical thinking, low
stimulus protection
Unclear body image (chronocity factor?)

C. Psychological disturbances in childhood
Identity diffusion
Disturbances of self-development
Repression of affective memories

Figure 7.2 Hypothetical vulnerability dimensions that increase vulnerability the more factors appear together: I = no or low risk for psychosis, 2 = low risk, 3 = high risk.

are not noticeable in the early stages of life. They both increase the risk of psychosis and make the potential for improvement more problematic. These disorders include difficulties in articulating speech, the ability to express feelings and to symbolise. Moreover, difficulties can occur with awareness, memory function may be poor and the stimulus threshold might be low.

3   *Disorders that affect the healthy development of the ego* and development of the personality where early traumatic experiences and negative object representations work against the personality's ability to build up adaptive characteristics.

The circles in Figure 7.2 overlap in parts. The degree of overlap indicates the hypothetical degree of risk where one is low risk and three is high risk for the development of psychosis.

The ego's integrative task supports an inner continuity of the self, even when personality problems or a cognitive deficit creates difficulties. If the person, through the exigencies of life, ends up at a point where their ego no longer manages to cope with ongoing events, the ego's integrating capacity ceases – something which may have been deteriorating by degree over many years or which can break through more abruptly.

The continuity of the self, the experience of identity, coherence and meaning, are interrupted in the pre-psychotic phase. When the process of disintegration threatens to take over, the self begins to seek out reparative possibilities. The possibility of creating a new meaning and coherence presents itself as more important than whether the meaning and coherence correspond to reality. The ego has partly abdicated its integrative function and the self chooses from the unconscious representational world in what way the difficulty should be repaired or replaced. When the new, regressively coloured understanding intrudes in the form of a psychotic delusion, it functions as a reparative element. Seen from this point of view, psychosis constitutes an attempt to solve an unresolvable dilemma.

Chapter 8

Factors that trigger psychosis

You are a garden into which a bomb once fell and did not explode, during a war that happened before you can remember. It came down at night. It screamed, but there were so many screams. It was heard, but it was forgotten. It buried itself. It was searched for but it was given up. So much else had been buried alive.

Other bombs fell near it and exploded. You grew older. It slept among the roots of your trees, which fell around it like nets around a fish that supposedly had long become extinct. In you the rain fell. In your earth the water found the dark egg with its little wings and inquired, but receiving no answer made camp beside it as beside the lightless stones. The ants came to decorate it with their tunnels. In time the grubs slept, leaning against it, and hatched out, hard and iridescent, and climbed away. You grew older, learning from the days and nights.

The tines of forks struck at it from above, and probed, in ignorance. You suffered. You suffer. You renew yourself. Friends gather and are made to feel at home. Babies are left, in their carriages, in your quiet shade. Children play on your grass and lovers lie there in the summer evenings. You grow older, with your seasons. You have become a haven. And one day when a child has been playing in you all afternoon, the pressure of a root or the nose of a mouse or the sleepless hunger of rust will be enough, suddenly, to obliterate all those years of peace, leaving in your place nothing but a crater rapidly filling with time. Then in vain will they look for your reason.

W. S. Merwin, A Garden, 1970

Psychological stress and vulnerability

When an individual presents with an acute psychosis one often finds an identifiable stressor that predated the psychosis and turns out to be a significant trigger factor (Rabkin 1980; Bebbington *et al.* 1993). A Finnish study into acutely psychotic patients found that there was a marked association with a recent loss (Räkköläinen 1977). Amongst 30 consecutive Swedish patients, who had suffered psychosis for the first time,

Table 8.1 First episode of psychosis and identifiable stressful trigger

	Clearly triggered by stress	Uncertain stress	No clear stress
Schizophrenia	8	4	5
Other psychoses	9	2	2
Total	17	6	5

two-thirds had undergone a definitive life event before they fell ill (Cullberg 2002). But there were also those who had become ill slowly, where one might say that every stressful occurrence had contributed to the deterioration. In five cases of schizophrenia where no clear triggering factor could be found, four of the patients had had an extremely traumatic childhood (see Table 8.1).

Experiences that may not appear to be traumatic for one individual can be highly traumatic for another. The notion of vulnerability implies that the person who becomes psychotically ill has a constitutionally thinner 'mental skin'. There may be many reasons for this: for example, some may have had a 'special' childhood, which need not necessarily be traumatic or 'bad' but rather might be considered as a cultural or peculiar distinctiveness which revealed itself within the parental home. Sometimes very specific intellectual gifts or uncommon artistic or religious interests may be found in one or both of the parents. An isolated childhood may have created a precocious child who found it difficult to forge friendships. Sometimes the parents' divorce – today a statistically normal phenomenon but from the point of view of a young child not at all 'normal' – lies as an incomprehensible event with many unresolved loyalty conflicts. Contact with the mother or father may have become infrequent resulting in a compensatory overdependence on the other parent.

All this may lead to a psychological vulnerability. It can manifest itself in unsuccessful attempts to leave home or in unhappy relationships with the opposite sex. It can be provoked by the expectations of self-assertion at work or by the shock created with the arrival of a firstborn child. High vulnerability suggests an increased sensitivity resulting from earlier and possibly repressed traumas. In such cases it is even more difficult for those around to understand why the psychosis has occurred. This is because the individual has reacted unconsciously to a level of stress that others accept as normal, as a result or earlier memories of abuse, violence or loss.

The psychotic relapse seems to become entrenched, reinforcing the tendency to react with psychosis at the instigation of a new frustration. For each recurrence the outer 'cause' becomes all the less remarkable to the perceiver, especially for the person who does not know the patient's inner world and its particular contents very well. This increasing vulnerability does not differ from other psychologically triggered disturbances such as anxiety, depression or self-harm and suicide.

Stress or crisis?

Today it is usual to use the word stress to cover frustrations that can trigger a psychotic reaction (see Figure 8.1). Since a stressor, as the notion's begetter Hans Selye originally understood it, is something that instigates the body's physiological, normal adaptive stress reaction, I consider that the notion of stress is best used for such frustrations which are primarily understood from

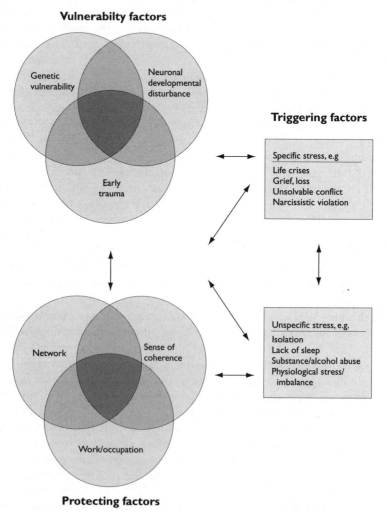

Figure 8.1 Triggering factors, vulnerability factors and protecting factors.

the point of view of physiology: inability to sleep, overwork, disruption of daily routine, somatic illness, etc. They are termed non-specific stressors[1] below.

However, it is also very important that such experiences which tie in with an inner interpretative process and which are specific to the individual who undergoes them are included in the possible triggering factors for psychosis. Here we enter into the individual's specific qualities, preconscious or unconscious processes where we need to be helped by dynamic interpretations. This produces a certain degree of scientific 'unreliability'. Such unreliability does not legitimate the attitude commonly seen in psychiatric research that these processes are non-existent. On the other hand, in individual cases we need to be especially self-critical in checking over our assumptions and interpretations. This group of specific subjective stressors is called crisis and conflict situations. Often non-specific stressors such as lack of sleep or somatic illness lower the threshold for specific crisis and conflict situations that become so subjectively pervasive that they function as triggers for psychosis. The triggering factors interact with vulnerability factors just as they also interact with both the individual's and the environment's protective factors in a complex way that is outlined in Table 8.1.

Non-specific stressors that trigger psychosis

Lack of sleep

Everyone who is unable to sleep will start to lose his or her sense of reality after a certain time. Perhaps after two or three days perception will become uncertain or hallucinatory, as will the experience of the self. The interpretation of the surrounding world alters radically and this may result in delusional misinterpretation. Prior to a psychotic episode most people experience difficulties with sleep. Lack of sleep is probably the one factor that can be counted as definitively contributory towards the onset of psychosis. Thus it is a priority to help a person with an acute psychosis to regain healthy sleep patterns.

Isolation

In the 1950s a systematic attempt was made to minimise the sensory inflow in subjects: 'sensory deprivation' at several universities in the USA. For example, subjects were suspended in a vat of water held at body temperature in a greyish light and in complete silence (see Chapter 3 for further details). Within a period of five to eight hours it was found that they experienced delusions and/or hallucinations. Confinement in prisons can produce similar reactions; in the German literature this reaction is known as 'Zuchthausknall'. Even loneliness in a city or in an alien culture can, in certain cases, cause psychosis because of the lack of reality testing with its fantasy-correcting conversations. Paranoid states have been described as being more frequent among immigrants than with others. The increased isolation of old age, together with lowered cognitive ability, also reduces the threshold for psychosis. This is not an infrequent event with deaf people. Deafness is the physical handicap that most often provokes paranoid reactions.

The withdrawal from society into an isolated state in many people constitutes an early symptom of psychosis. The threshold for psychosis is lowered by the lack of reality testing that comes with reduced social contact. It seems likely that the incidence of psychosis could be reduced if this kind of isolation were to be addressed. Presumably such interruption of psychotic processes happens more often than we are aware of.

Somatic disturbances or dysfunction

Endocrine imbalance is another common factor in the lowering of the threshold for psychosis. Vulnerable women tend to cross the border for psychosis during a premenstrual phase. The postpartum psychoses have endocrine and psychological causes, either of which may predominate.

Certain hormonal illnesses can contribute to the development of psychosis: for example, Cushing's disease with overproduction of adrenocortical hormones or thyrotoxicosis with overproduction of the thyroid gland hormone. Treatment with corticosteriods or the pituitary hormones ACTH and LH may precipitate psychosis.

Other somatic illnesses can also act as a trigger for psychosis. Intracranial pathology such as cerebrovascular disease or tumours may trigger psychosis, especially if the temporal lobe is affected. They may also have an overall effect of lowering the threshold to psychosis. Systemic illnesses such as lupus erythematosus are sometimes accompanied by transient psychotic periods, as are sudden disturbances of electrolyte balance. The combination of gastroenteritis, often seen in travellers, psychological stress and perhaps the misuse of alcohol can trigger an acute psychosis. The group of acute confusional states that form the subgroup of organic psychoses classified as 'delirium' are looked at more closely in Chapter 13.

The influence of alcohol, drugs and poison

In some individuals, a period of heavy misuse of alcohol can trigger a schizophrenic-like psychotic state, which may persist for quite some time. In rare cases, a chronic auditory hallucinosis is thought to result from brain damage caused by heavy drinking. Hallucinogenic drugs directly influence the receptor systems. In certain cases they induce a more slowly developing psychosis as in the case of amphetamines. In some cannabis users a psychosis is triggered after only a day's relapse into abuse. There are also medical drugs such as atropine that lower the threshold for psychosis just as they can produce hallucinosis. Even SSRI antidepressants can bring out psychotic symptoms in individuals with a vulnerability to psychosis, especially in a depressed, temporarily non-psychotic schizophrenic patient. The treatment of malaria with chloroquine has also been shown to be liable to trigger psychosis on rare occasions.

A combination of a toxic reaction together with stress occurs fairly frequently in post-operative psychosis (acute confusional states), which may in part result from intoxication with narcotics where the degree of confusion is proportionate to the dose of narcotics used. During the early years of heart-lung operations, post-operative confusion was reported in 30 to 40 per cent of cases. They usually presented with paranoid reactions or visual hallucinations, often of a terrifying nature, which may fluctuate and last from a few hours to a few days.[2]

Other causes

Not infrequently, overwork is a triggering factor in affective psychoses. There are many possible mechanisms: for example, reversal of the sleep–wake cycle in night workers or neglect of family members resulting in feelings of guilt or low self-esteem.

Extreme affects

Powerful episodes of depression or mania can in themselves be a non-specific stress factor that contributes towards an affective psychosis. If there is a vulnerability to schizophrenia as well, a schizo-affective psychosis can develop. Clinical experiences show that depression not only acts as a non-specific stressor but can also result in a specific form of psychosis which is understandable psychologically and dynamically.

Specific triggering situations of crisis and conflict

Developmental and transitional crises[3]

If the psychosocial environment is complicated or changes for the worse, adapting to the new situation can lead to temporary or permanent difficulties. Most people will react with anxiety, depression or psychosomatic symptoms. For some, the reaction can deepen into a psychosis that is not usually malignant but which may develop into a long-term psychosis. Puberty and possibly the menopause are especially risky times. In both cases, the psychological experience of an alteration in the body, the new role in life and the hormonal changes are all important.

Even transitional crises that are not complicated by physical problems can trigger psychosis. The number of first-time sufferers of schizophrenic psychoses increases after the ages of 18 to 20 and reaches its height at 24 years in men and 25 years in women. During this period the adult's expectations intensify. The decisions as to whether to leave the parental home or to stay, to move in with a partner or not, to meet up with one's own and the world's sexual expectations and demands, to be conscripted or to venture out into the employment market are all problematic. They must be attended to but may stir up deeply threatening emotions for many people.

Postponed maturity or psychic illness?

At present we have no means of distinguishing benign delayed maturity from the prodromal phase of a psychotic illness. There are some suggestive features nonetheless:

- in the late teens or early twenties a deteriorating performance at school or work, or an inexplicable failure to achieve the level which would have previously been expected
- disturbance in social interactions or a subjective feeling of alienation from others
- a history of psychosis in close relatives (especially first degree).

The situation can be turned round by an individual who, perhaps unwittingly, turns out to function like a pilot and can steer the person out of dangerous waters. Naturally, other possibilities for a 'moratorium' can occur.[4] We do not know how often this happens in everyday life, outside the awareness of psychiatrists. However, it almost certainly happens more often than we are aware of. We are only engaged with those individuals who are not able to manage without professional help. Suddenly an opportunity can turn up in the form of work or an activity that feels worth trying. Perhaps the time has come for a talent to find its way into the open, offering a channel for making relationships with others. In my experience, religious or political/anarchist groups which may be frowned upon within intellectual circles have come to the rescue of young people uncertain over their identity and with a predisposition to psychosis. However, it should not be forgotten that there are also cult societies that exploit needy young people without due consideration.

Paranoid and affective psychoses reach their peak incidence between 30 and 40 years of age. Loneliness and isolation can result from the different kinds of disappointment and difficulties seen during this phase of life, especially around relationships and child rearing. This in turn can increase the risk of a psychotic episode. Many have given up on their 'optimism capital' during their twenties. For those who are withdrawn or manifest a schizotypal personality, demands made for openness and involvement cause anxiety and feelings of resentment, which are not diminished by the arrival of children. Exactly which factors are involved may, of course, be difficult to determine in specific cases. Sometimes it is hard to find any reasonable explanation for the breakthrough of psychosis.

Often the whole family may be going through a crisis and the member with the highest degree of vulnerability develops a psychosis. The family crisis may precede the psychosis or follow it. Burdensome factors affect them all: for example, the parental marriage may be coming apart, even though it appears stable from the outside. The threat of unemployment can cloud the whole family. Important changes in the family routine often precede the illness. This suggests that the family's protective function has been diminished, especially if one of its members has been particularly adversely affected.

Loss and separation

Our personalities are made up of our inner depiction of ourselves (our internal representations), of our own physical bodily being and of those people who are or have been near to us. The spoken and unspoken ideas with which we have grown up and which we have incorporated – our inner representations of relationships and meaning – are the bricks or, better, the mortar of meaning. All these aspects, which can be thought of as our 'self', give us our inner experience of continuity and consistency (see Chapter 4 for further elaboration).

If vital parts of our 'selves' are damaged, which is something that happens when we lose a representative of the mental world upon which we are deeply dependent and with which we are psychically entwined, something occurs which could be likened to a mental amputation. It might be an infant dying at birth or a partner dying after a long marriage, but it could also be a young woman losing her womb in an operation. The loss or damage may bring about a traumatic crisis. An intense period of mourning begins. However, if the person has been able to prepare themselves well, usually a process of self-healing takes place. The inability to function is eventually replaced by increased strength, which is characteristic of the healed scar. Sometimes the healing process is more complicated and attended by painful subjective suffering.

In some cases the damage is very deep seated – the symbolic representation in our experiential world is vital (something which does not need to reflect what one can 'objectively' describe as a major exterior event). Here the self can lose the ability to give meaning to what has happened or make room for events in a meaningful consistency. The reparative process has, to a greater or lesser extent, come to be mediated by the primary process[5] functions by means of new, regressive, magical reparative ways of seeing things. With an early vulnerability, this regression can become expressed in a psychosis. The ego's ability to control the formation of meaning has been stretched to the point of breakdown.

Guilt for triumphing over the father

Eric had grown up in an upper middle class home replete with his father's bizarre approach to child rearing. He was closely tied to his mother who had secretly attempted to protect him. He was now a 40-year-old man in a responsible technical/intellectual job, but from the age of 20 had had many attacks of schizo-affective psychoses with both depressive and manic periods. A close relative suffered from bipolar psychosis. I treated Eric with lithium and at the same time with insight-orientated psychotherapy.

At this time, the father developed rapidly progressing Alzheimer's dementia. Since his wife was no longer able to look after him at home a place in a care home was arranged. After a short while he died of a brain haemorrhage. Eric travelled to see his mother to help her with the funeral. A week before he had begun to experience difficulty in sleeping and increased agitation. At his mother's home he was invited to sleep in his father's bed, which was in the same room as his mother's. His mother also gave him his father's bunch of keys as a way of indicating to him that he might like to take over. Eric developed an acute anxiety and could not sleep. In the morning, he began to feel that a spy network was following him. However, Eric had called me as he was able to see for himself that he was about to relapse. He was able to make it back to his own home, but with a fully developed manic psychosis he was immediately taken into hospital voluntarily.

COMMENTS

Eric had a deeply ambivalent relationship to his father. His father's death awoke in him guilt about his old death wishes against his father. The guilt was strengthened by his 'Oedipal triumph', which lay in the fact that unconsciously the mother had symbolically lured him into replacing his father by offering him his father's bed and keys. This conflict was not something he was able to work through, but instead he reacted with a psychosis, prompted by his vulnerability. Eric found psychotherapy helpful in two ways. It deepened his understanding of this and similar events which had brought about his illness. It also helped him work through the underlying conflicts. (Eric's psychotic thinking is also described in Chapter 3, p. 34.)

The case of Beth (Chapter 2, p. 13) offers a further example. This case also illustrates the development of an affective psychosis after a death that appears to have an especially heightened symbolic significance. However, a death can also trigger a schizophrenic psychosis.

When a grandfather dies

Stephen was a 27-year-old law student. He was preparing for his final examinations when his paternal grandfather, who was getting on in years, died a couple of months before the examination was to take place. His grandfather had meant much to Stephen as his parents had divorced when he was 10 years old and his grandfather had partly taken over the role of father to him.

Stephen's childhood had been filled with his mother's depression, suicide threats and periodic alcohol abuse. He had always, like a good son, stood loyally by her side when others criticised her for neglecting him. On one occasion, when he was about 10 years old, he came home to find the house empty. The bedroom and bathroom were covered in blood. His mother had been taken to hospital after cutting herself severely in an attempt to take her own life.

Stephen remembered having been able to control his feelings for many years in the belief that feelings were not for him, but after his grandfather died he became inconsolably miserable. He failed his final examinations and some weeks later developed delusions that he had been the subject of an experiment on the course. He also experienced intense auditory (and at times even visual) hallucinations, which continued for more than six months.

COMMENTS

Some time before his grandfather's death Stephen had already begun to worry whether it was worth continuing his studies. This was a sign of how his controlled personality was beginning to break down in prodromal symptoms. The death of his grandfather made Stephen re-experience his earlier painful memories with his mother. He had never before talked about them or verbalised his feelings of loneliness as a child. With psychotherapy and low dose antipsychotic medication, he was eventually able to resume his studies. However, a couple of years later he relapsed and had to continue with medication.

'Irresolvable' conflicts

In principle, there are conflicting situations that on a conscious level are thought to be impossible to resolve. Vital needs are set against each other and every choice is felt to bring with it an unacceptably destructive outcome. Psychosis can ensue. Afterwards, psychotherapeutic support may be helpful in dealing with the disappointment that an ideal answer cannot always be found and that prioritising one solution may mean neglecting another priority.

'To kill your father or your child'

Karen, aged 30, lived at home with her ailing parents. She had not continued with her education as she had to take care of them. Her father had epilepsy which was hard to treat. This followed a brain haemorrhage and he also had high blood pressure. Her mother suffered from an auto-immune arthritis illness. The family were active members in a religious community. The nearest neighbour was a married homeowner who was also active in the religious community. This man began a secret affair with Karen which eventually resulted in her pregnancy. Karen experienced the positive results of the pregnancy test as a catastrophe and she told no one. She dearly wanted to get married and to have children. Abortion was equal to child murder. On the other hand, the thought of going ahead with the pregnancy meant that her parents must be told. She knew that her father might have a fit if distressed and that this would constitute a threat to his life. Thus she was met with a choice between killing the child she carried or killing her father. She could not sleep and after some days became acutely confused and was admitted to a psychiatric clinic. After a few weeks a spontaneous abortion was found to be in progress. At the same time the psychosis gave way. In Karen's discussion with the social worker, she decided that her parents should receive help from social services as she was thinking about applying for a study grant and leaving home.

Major depression

To be able to tolerate a depression and to deal with it implies that the psychological capacity to do so can be developed. Dynamically, it appears that certain people function analogously with the Kleinian understanding of the schizoid and the depressive position (see Chapter 4), where the depressive capacity is insufficient and a split in the experience of reality takes place instead. The depressive hatred towards the inner representations of the self is projected outwards into the world around, leading to the belief that it is other people who pursue and hate you. Reality therefore becomes most distorted with delusions and other often paranoid psychotic experiences. A deep depression, as with a manic state, seems to function as a strong non-specific stressor for some and can trigger an acute psychotic reaction.

Narcissistic injury

People with high personal prestige may gamble their reputation with one throw of a dice. This can lead to a position that turns their project upside down and may challenge their status and honour. Such sudden reversals might include failed final examinations, a scandal, a particularly bad investment, or a disappointment at work. Sometimes it can happen to someone who has a narcissistic personality, as described in the previous chapter. Often, it concerns gifted successful people who have built up a prestigious image that is now destroyed.

The natural and healthy solution is for the person to lick their wounds and, after some mourning, to start again, this time with less grand illusions and benefiting from the experience. Suicide is another solution. This is not infrequent in these kinds of cases where a powerful super-ego maintains control. Such a suicide may come suddenly without any obvious warning, 'like lightning from a clear sky'. The financier Ivar Kreuger's suicide after the crash in 1932 presents such an example. The third possibility is 'a 'murder of the self' in a more symbolically understood sense. This consists of a swiftly developing psychosis, where the violation and self-hatred contained in the experience of the painful event can be diminished by means of projecting the person's own hatred against themselves onto the world outside. The evil outer persecutors now replace the inner 'persecutor', with its self-hatred. A new explanation and survival strategy is offered for the time being or for a longer period within a paranoid state. The price of such an easing of the situation is social exclusion as a result of the development of a paranoid psychosis. The process of isolation has, more often than not, already paved the way for a psychotic breakdown. People with narcissistic personality problems often have a tendency to paranoid reactions, which usually pass very quickly when the balance is replaced with appropriate strategies. If the failure is too major and the effects too overwhelming, the suspicious attitude can deepen into psychosis. Often simultaneous burdens such as family problems, erotic entanglements, abusive tendencies, etc. may accelerate the process.

The grandiose project breaks down

During his mid-forties the Swedish writer, August Strindberg (1849–1912), experienced a deep crisis in his life, known as his 'Inferno crisis'.[6] This was triggered by marital breakdown and the loss of custody of his children. He had also encountered a writer's block. He could not repair himself without 'shedding my shell like a crayfish'. Strindberg had lost his leading position in the world of literature in his home country and, in addition, he was being sued for blasphemy. He moved to Berlin where he entered into a new but unhappy marriage.

A grandiose idea grew within him whereby he would revolutionise the whole world of science through alchemy and that later he would set about manufacturing gold. With this in mind, he left his new marriage and children and in 1894 settled in Paris with high expectations regarding the great triumph which was to come. When this project slowly but surely failed, the depressive experiences and psychosomatic difficulties increased. In July 1896 Strindberg suffered a paranoid psychosis with delusions of a non-bizarre kind that could not be explained simply by consumption of alcohol and absinthe. His hallucinations are not recorded but he believed himself to be pursued by an international gold Mafia and gangs of art dealers. In a panic, he fled both Paris and his experiments to create gold. Strindberg never came to terms with his scientific failure, but through his religious studies turned instead to Emanuel Swedenborg's (1688–1772) theories about the existence of God who sent out Spirits to punish and instruct. In this manner, Strindberg could reinterpret his delusions of persecution in terms of religion. He believed that God, in his love for Strindberg, wanted to put him on trial. With this creative safe conduit back to his childhood Christianity, Strindberg conceived for himself a manageable explanation for his persecution. In principle, Strindberg returned to health after six months and continued anew to produce literary work for the next 15 years without interruption, although his religious conviction remained.

Summary

The concept of vulnerability promotes an interest in attempting to find causal factors for every psychotic breakdown. A first episode has usually been triggered by some kind of frustrating distress. With some slowly evolving conditions it may not be possible to identify clearly the triggering factor. If the psychosis returns, the triggering stressful event is often less evident than it was the first time round – one sees a lowered threshold for vulnerability to psychosis. Trigger factors may include non-specific stressors of a physiological kind which lower the threshold for tolerating the deeper, more specific frustrations which often lie beneath. To understand their nature in greater detail it is necessary to get to know the person well: watching for maturation crises, separations, acute conflicts or violations. It seems that relapses may reinforce themselves as defensive strategies. This is borne out by the increased risk of subsequent psychosis after each relapse.

Chapter 9

Protective factors

How is it that more people do not become psychotic? Our brains are sensitive instruments and the process of building up an inner representational world includes many misperceptions and distortions, which may collide when confronting reality. We allow ourselves to be influenced by drugs, alcohol or rituals that disturb our awareness and identity. Yet after some hours we are back to our old selves with an intact ego apparatus. Our perceptions and interpretations of reality again allow us to find a place from which to function and communicate with the surrounding world.

There are certainly strong genetically determined mechanisms that support our reality testing: their survival value is indisputable. One may hypothesise that, like aeroplane computers, there exist hierarchies of security systems which take over if one mechanism gives way. A constant reconnecting and assertion of control takes place automatically, not least via the ego's protective mechanisms. We can correct our dreams and desires or manipulate and deny our realities in sophisticated ways. What is important is that we should create a continuity of meaning within the stream of stimuli that we encounter.

Knowledge of both the brain's 'data processing' functioning at a cellular level and the nature of biological factors that protect against psychosis are still rudimentary. Before long we may be in a better position to know what constitutes protective and not just vulnerability factors in our genetic inheritance: for example, how can we better protect against prenatal and perinatal damage in the development of the brain? How can we stimulate the development of the brain through an early trusting parental relationship?

The psychosocial protective factors against psychosis are non-specific. They not only include protection against psychosis but also against overall loss of orientation and control. The same factors that protect our psyche also appear to function to strengthen physical health. The bridges between the psychic and the somatic lie in the endocrinological and subcortical neural systems. We know that sorrow, loss, stress, hopelessness, etc. have somatic correlates and can potentiate somatic illness. Accordingly, the protective factors that I will take up here have a general value: they include somatic just as much as psychic health.

Psychosocial protective factors

I now consider three groups of psychosocial protective factors that are well established by international research:

- a functioning network
- meaningful employment or creative activities
- experiences of coherence and meaning.

A functioning network

The social network is defined as the close circles of both an informal (private) and formal (public) nature within which the individual moves, which can offer:

- emotional support, appreciation and love
- information and help towards personal orientation in the surrounding world and for coping with problems
- recognition, friendship, shared interests and values
- material support.

A good social network acts as a psychological protective factor in that people who have grown up in such an atmosphere should have stronger ego functions and thereby greater defensive capacities.[1] Social relationships within adult networks can also act as buffers in crisis situations and frustrations. A functioning network can also encourage a person in need to find professional help at an early stage. Naturally, our knowledge is greater around the effects of the breakdown of protective factors than of the opposite.

Individuals with limited resources

The quality of the social environment is especially important for people who have a poor capacity to care for themselves. These people include those who have suffered from illnesses and disabilities; the unemployed and the homeless; and those who are involved in or affected by crime and substance misuse. Teenage parents and single parents, especially in certain areas, can also be exposed to stress as can immigrants and refugees. As more and more stress factors exist, mental illness becomes increasingly likely.

Ill health promoted by social disintegration

Social disintegration occurs when both formal structures in the community (public services) and informal structures (family, friends, neighbours) are insufficient. This interacts with the mental health of the community and both may spiral downward as a result (Leighton 1963). Areas easily hit by social disintegration can suffer from depopulation, becoming the new low-status housing estates. The affected areas can mushroom on the peripheries of large towns. Segregation for negative reasons is high: there is an over-representation of unemployment, immigrants, the mentally ill, misusers of alcohol and drugs along with other people with few resources. Studies from Nacka outside Stockholm (Cullberg *et al.* 1981) and from Oslo (Dalgaard 1980) clearly describe what are known as the 'new low-income areas'. They feature rapid high-rise developments with poor social services that show much evidence of social disintegration. Subjectively experienced poor mental health is found among 30 per cent of the adult inhabitants. There is a high level of dependence on social services for provision of care. The children of parents in these compromised social situations may be greatly affected. The parents, often single and uneducated, struggle to cope with their parental roles. Nurseries are crowded and many children have specific educational or care needs. The schools have difficulties with discipline and there is a rapid turnover of teachers, resulting in poor academic performance. Youth crime, violence and drug abuse are common. Suicide and relapse into psychosis occur more frequently (see Figure 9.1).

The people who live in these areas are trapped in a Catch-22 situation where their low capacity to build up a functioning supportive network is worsened by the high turnover rate of the population. Those who have the energy and financial resources to move form part of a 'creaming off' of the more able population and such areas disintegrate even further (see Figure 9.2). Even so, after 10 or 15 years occasionally positive initiatives take effect, the area then stabilises and takes on a higher status.

Many people with long-term mental illness are rehoused in these kinds of estates. Since there is a lack of support networks and the social services are understaffed, often those who are discharged from hospital receive too little or unorganised support. Much greater resources are needed in the form of an appropriate place to live, social contact and a meaningful occupation if they are to recover (see further Chapter 26).

The circumstances in the older low-income areas are often quite different to the new low-income ones. Here we find well-established, informal networks in a community with three generations present in addition to social services. The same is true for the older high-income areas. People living on these estates have an ability to mobilise support and to help each other in times of crisis. The toleration of mental illness is admittedly limited and as a result it may be concealed. With regard to the new high-income areas it is

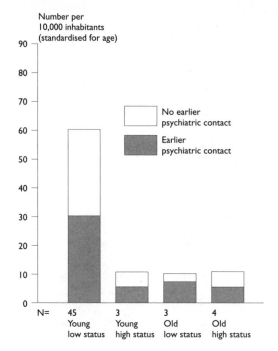

Figure 9.1 Number of suicide attempts in suburban areas per 10,000 inhabitants by accommodation type (Cullberg *et al.* 1981).

noticeable that there is a low tolerance for mental illness. Younger families with good finances and opportunities to find the services they need live in these neighbourhoods. Since there is less rented accommodation people with mental illness are less likely to be placed in these areas. In addition attempts to set up homes for the mentally ill often result in opposition from the local community.

Meaningful employment or creative activities

For most people, work has positive meaning beyond that of bringing in an income: for example, the mental stimulation inherent in problem solving can strengthen self-esteem. When work is fulfilling a function it provides the feeling of being needed. Work also has important social functions by providing opportunities to develop new relationships and encounter new environments. Work gives a foundation and structure to life. Amongst other things, working gives value to an individual's free time.

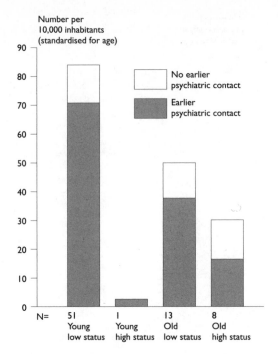

Figure 9.2 Number of patients with psychosis in a suburban area per 10,000 inhabitants by accommodation type (Cullberg *et al.* 1981).

Lack of work or occupation

This can have many consequences: lack of rewards for one's accomplishments, lack of challenges or goals to aim for, not having work mates, an alternative place to go or to have demands made on one's day. These things could, for most people, eventually result in a breakdown. This experience of being excluded can create a depressive reaction where passivity is prominent.

Today, poor mental health is an important reason for early retirement on the grounds of ill health. Three-quarters of those who are diagnosed as schizophrenic are given early retirement within five years (Svedberg *et al.* 2001). Their quality of life is usually poor, as much because of isolation as from the lack of appropriate activities. These factors in turn worsen mental health. This is not only a cause of suffering for the person concerned, but also a waste of potential economic resources. It is not usually possible to expect those who are mentally ill to compete on the open market for employment. For these reasons, meaningful work should be created which is appropriate to their needs and capacities. Although in many countries communities are obliged by law to find an occupation for these individuals, it is still a widely neglected issue.

Experiences of coherence and meaning

The concept of a *sense of coherence* (SOC) has been defined by the Israeli sociologist Aaron Antonovsky (1987) as a result of studies that he made on survivors of German concentration camps. He discovered that those people who had survived a psychically extreme and disturbing experience with an eventual lower degree of psychiatric ill health than others had an inner sense of coherence which was able to supply them with motivation and hope, even in confined and threatening circumstances. Using a scale, Antonovsky attempted to rate the degree of a person's sense of coherence and then cor-related the result with different health factors. The validity of this idea has been criticised but clinically it stands out as important, not least for someone working with psychoses. The incipient psychosis is often accompanied by a deep feeling of alienation and incomprehension of outer and inner events. The pre-psychotic person chooses regressive, magical solutions (in the form of delusions) in the face of a loss of coherence, and as a result becomes all the more excluded from the community. Those things that help to create and strengthen a realistic sense of coherence and meaning are therefore essential in the recovery of psychosis.

We know little about the relationship between the existential, philosophical vision of the world and psychosis; only that some become ill after a long period of fruitless musings. The consequences of *rapid social mobility*, both national and international, need to be considered. Disturbances in cultural patterns and values and in historical, religious and linguistic traditions may result in increased alienation, even in the children of migrants. These younger people appear more vulnerable to psychosis as a result of these shifting and sometimes competing traditions.

Therefore, a cultural development that must be monitored with care is the rapid secularisation of the western community. Traditional communities may have a high level of self-conviction derived from their historical roots, which greatly contributed to its inhabitants' defined sense of self. However, these communities have much to lose from secularisation. Those bridges between the inner and the outer world, which were described in Chapter 1, are in danger of being affected by this loss of cultural roots.

Summary

Three different psychosocial protective factors have been described: the social network, meaningful work and activity, and an inner sense of coherence and meaning. Each is a means of protection against psychosis and mental ill health and the three factors may work synergistically together.

It is essential to understand that these factors contribute to the increased risk of mental illness under certain conditions. Recognition of these factors is also essential if psychosocial conditions are to be provided that maximise the potential for recovering health and social rehabilitation.

Chapter 10

Psychotic disorders I

First-episode psychosis – three clinical types

Neither the ICD-10 nor the DSM-IV provide guidance for treatment or prognosis in first-episode psychosis. I have found it practical to consider that one is faced with one of three possible disease courses. Roughly speaking, they each encompass a third of those with a first-episode psychosis. I shall briefly describe the clinical pictures. Naturally the future course is never possible to predict with certainty. This three-type grouping is not intended to be a new diagnostic tool but an aid in the clinical discussions about treatment and prognosis.

After that I shall introduce the various psychotic disorders as they are categorised in the DSM-IV system. The term schizophrenia is controversial and in Chapter 11 I provide an historical description of its development so that those who are interested will be able to follow the theoretical discussion.

Psychosis Type A: single-episode psychosis

This usually develops quite rapidly from a 'normal' mental state over one or two weeks. The psychosis can be relatively inconspicuous, with paranoid symptoms and perhaps some auditory hallucinations. It can be more extreme with grossly disturbed behaviour, schizophrenia-like symptoms with more bizarre manifestations, such as prominent hallucinations and ideas of reference. Clear trigger factors of a psychosocial nature are often found. With good psychosocial treatment the psychosis passes within a few weeks or months. Antipsychotic medication in modest doses will often be of assistance but is not always necessary if the psychosocial treatment and environment are satisfactory. A relapse, if it occurs, is an isolated event.

Psychosis Type B: recurrent psychosis

Here one often finds that prior to the appearance of the psychosis the person has suffered from a borderline or schizotypal personality disorder. The triggering events can be minor relative to the severity of the psychosis and are sometimes, especially in the later outbreaks, difficult to identify. Substance misuse often contributes, where even a short period of use can be enough to trigger a relapse. Schizophreniform symptoms are not uncommon and can include intense hallucinations and/or bizarre delusions. A genetic vulnerability and a disturbed childhood are common – often several relatives have suffered from mental illness. Those with cyclical affective psychosis or schizo-affective illness are treated accordingly. In these cases relapses may be very sudden.

As is the case with Type A, the psychosis usually passes without perceptible changes in the personality. However, there is a greater risk of relapse and the new psychotic episode should be regarded as a reminder of a recurring vulnerability. Most require antipsychotic medication at intervals, or long-term medication as a preventative measure. Persons with recurrent psychoses with affective features often benefit from mood stabilisers such as lithium. Supportive, educative, as well as in certain cases insight-oriented or cognitive psychotherapy, which may involve the family, should be available.

Psychosis Type C: with long-term functional disability

Sometimes the chronic nature of the illness only becomes evident after several years of recurrent illness. These persons often undergo fundamental changes in their personality. These can be minor or major changes; for example, the person appears veiled by a very thin 'film' of detachment. Sometimes, although not always, this change can accentuate a trait or traits that have been present for years prior to the development of psychosis.

Recovery is all too often incomplete, but it can be enhanced by supporting the often deficient network of relationships. Antipsychotic medication usually has a beneficial but not curative effect. Balancing therapeutic effects of medication against side effects requires a good working relationship with the patient. If given in excessive doses the mental state can deteriorate as a result of increasing passivity, restlessness or non-adherence. It is essential to inform the patient and their carers about the nature of the illness and the possible treatments that may minimise disability. Psychotherapy with Type C psychoses is predominantly of a cognitive nature designed to help the patient counteract his delusions and/or hallucinations. (See Table 10.1.)

Diagnosing the psychotic syndromes

I wish to emphasise that there are no clear boundaries between the different types of psychosis that I have described. Overlaps between these types are more common than typical syndromes. The following aspects will probably be crucial in the future, giving us more useful guides into treatment and prognosis:

Table 10.1 Prognostic indicators in acute psychosis

Better prognosis	Worse prognosis
Clear triggering factors	No clear triggering factors
No prodromal symptoms, or short duration of untreated psychosis	Long prodromal period
DUP (duration untreated psychosis) < 1 month	DUP (duration untreated psychosis) > 12 months
Depressive or hypomanic features	No affective traits
Few negative symptoms	Negative symptoms apparent
Earlier good social development	Earlier adjustment problems
No substance or alcohol misuse	Substance misuse
Good insight about the psychosis subsequently	Denial of the psychosis

- the presence of pre-existing maladaptive personality traits or personality disorder
- the level of organisation of the personality (ego strength)
- degree and type of cognitive deficiencies
- brain injury or aberrations
- abnormal neurotransmitter receptor function
- amenability to different types of treatment.

We still have no overall or comprehensive theoretical system that allows for absolute diagnostic precision. However, we must describe what we see in as clear and reliable way as possible. The differences between DSM-IV and ICD-10 are relatively small. DSM-IV's criteria will be followed in this exposition (the ICD-10 criteria can be found in the Appendix).

Brief psychosis

Key features

In a population of 100,000 inhabitants perhaps three or four cases of acute, short-term psychosis per year are cared for in the psychiatric services. The total incidence is probably significantly higher as many may never reach the mental health services. This is in part due to the self-limiting nature of brief psychosis. In addition many people have a high threshold when it comes to seeking psychiatric help. Some make do at home, or survive in other ways without any psychiatric intervention. Some may commit suicide without the psychosis being detected. However, the symptoms can be florid and often necessitate psychiatric attention. Usually the psychosis does not return, but one or two relapses can occur over the course of a couple of years with the same good prognosis.

Even if such a psychosis usually occurs in people under 35 years of age, short-term psychosis can occur in old age. Failing cognitive function, reduced hearing, other physical ailments or medical treatment are also common factors that lower the threshold for psychosis.

Symptoms

Two types of symptoms are often linked together: disorganisational and paranoid. *Disorganisation* is perhaps the most common, manifesting a state of *perplexity-filled anxiety*. In this state one feels bewildered but also desperate to find out what is going on and why. Questions that are not satisfied by answers are asked over and over again. The patient is often poorly orientated in time, place or person. This disorientation differs from the acute confusional state, which points to an organic cause such as endocrine problems, other somatic illness, poisoning, or the onset of dementia (see Chapter 13). With such states one finds a more random kind of wrong or made-up answer to questions concerned with orientation.

Sometimes a patient can become very disturbed, smearing their surroundings with excreta or menstrual blood. If the person is stopped they can become very aggressive. In addition undressing and wandering naked can cause distress to both staff and fellow patients. The psychosis that occurs after childbirth – puerperal psychosis – may present like this. There are powerful literary depictions of brief psychoses. Perhaps the most well-known examples are in Goethe's *Faust* when Gretchen is deserted by Faust and in Shakespeare's *Hamlet* when Ophelia becomes disturbed when she is deserted by Hamlet.

Brief psychosis can be distinguished from acute confusion by the level of consciousness. In acute confusion the level of consciousness tends to fluctuate from hour to hour, with the patient drowsy at one time and then hyperaroused at another. Memory for recent events is usually also disturbed. In brief psychoses auditory hallucinations can occur but do not always dominate the picture. Often the voice belongs to someone who is well known to the patient or famous. It is noticeable how the patient sometimes stops and seems to be listening to the voice or voices.

Brief periods of catatonia, sometimes with attendant fever, can complicate the situation, especially if the patient is very anxious. Catatonia refers to a range of unusual motor system disturbances seen in psychosis including stupor, excitability and posturing. There is evidence to suggest that catatonia diminishes the subjective experience of anxiety. The motor disturbances can prevent a patient from eating and drinking, and from receiving basic personal care. If this is prolonged for more than a few days the patient's life may be endangered from dehydration.

On not knowing the child after its birth

Ulla, a 25-year-old assistant nurse, had given birth to her first child after a complicated pregnancy. During the final months she had protein in the urine and high blood pressure. The delivery was drawn out and painful. When Ulla was given her child to hold after the birth she was surprisingly indifferent towards it. Her apathy increased. Although clear psychotic symptoms were not present, Ulla told the consultant psychiatrist that she was not sure that the child was hers. When it was time for her to go home her anxiety intensified. She insisted that someone else's child had been thrust upon her. In spite of this she breastfed the baby. Her husband thought that the problem would sort itself out at home with the help of Ulla's mother. However, when they got home the situation worsened. Ulla began to wash the child roughly and there was a fear that she might harm it. She was admitted to a psychiatric ward and the baby was cared for on a neonatal ward.

Ulla deteriorated into an acute psychotic episode. She tried to break out of the ward and had to be detained compulsorily. Her husband brought the baby to her and initially she managed to breastfeed. However, the breastfeeding had to be abandoned because of concerns for the child's safety. Attempts to reach Ulla using psychotherapy failed. The situation in the ward was complicated by the fact that it was summer and the hospital was mainly staffed by temporary workers. Ulla refused to wash herself and several times when she was not being watched she wandered out onto the ward naked. She also had obstetric complications, with infected vaginal fissures from the delivery, which were difficult to treat. She attacked staff on several occasions. Ulla was treated by force with neuroleptic injections, without much success, in an attempt to reduce her level of arousal and treat her psychosis. Electroconvulsive treatment (ECT) was resorted to. She responded after two treatments and a few weeks later was able to leave the hospital completely recovered.

During a return visit, Ulla said that she was sorry she had to abandon her breastfeeding and complained bitterly about the unprofessional treatment that she had experienced in the psychiatric department. Her relationship with her child did not appear to have suffered any deep long-term damage. Her husband became depressed and needed psychotherapeutic help in order to regain his trust in his wife.

COMMENTS

The psychosis was triggered by a combination of psychological trauma created by the difficult delivery and the somatic disturbances that occur after childbirth. It may be that the situation would have improved sooner with a more consistent group of skilled staff. In refractory brief psychoses, especially when the patient or others are at risk, ECT can offer advantages over more conservative treatments when used with care. Ulla's next pregnancy went well and the birth took place, at her request, by caesarean section.

In brief psychoses a range of paranoid symptoms may be seen. These may include beliefs that one is being pursued by alien forces, that one's food is poisoned or that one's home has been burgled and objects rearranged or tampered with. Transient illusions, auditory and sometimes visual hallucinations confirm these experiences.

Brief paranoid psychosis after group therapy

Maria, an immigrant, was 30 years old. She was married and had an 8-year-old daughter. Her husband had been arrested for drug-related offences and was undergoing residential treatment for substance misuse. During a week of family treatment, where members were asked to work in groups 'with their personalities' and their nearest relations in an intense way, Maria developed difficulties in sleeping. On returning home she began to believe that a friend was poisoning her and that she had drugged her coffee. Maria also became frightened that her husband wanted to kill her. She thought her telephone answering machine was bugged and on one occasion she heard a threatening voice. She also believed that someone had made copies of the keys to her apartment. An emergency psychiatric assessment was carried out. They observed that she appeared guarded with incoherent speech, paranoid ideas and a flattened affect. She was admitted for observation.

After some weeks the paranoid symptoms resolved without antipsychotic medication. It transpired that the previous month whilst standing on a train platform she had taken several steps forward as the train pulled in. At the last moment she had realised the danger thinking, 'What am I doing?' and had stopped herself.

Maria's childhood had been traumatic. She grew up in a southern European country and had been sent to Sweden when her mother died when she was 6 years old. While waiting to emigrate, she had been sexually abused by her uncle with whom she was staying. She had grown up with many different foster parents. This had made her 'hard' she said, but the group discussion opened up her feelings in an uncontrollable way. Her underlying fear was that her daughter would be taken away from her. This child was now the same that age Maria had been when she was sent to Sweden.

After her psychosis Maria felt a strong need to talk over what had happened to her. She went into psychotherapy for several years and was also treated with antidepressant medication, because of the severity of her depression. She was able to get her social conditions more organised and separated from her husband who, it transpired, had lived with other women for most of their marriage.

COMMENTS

Maria had a clear psychological vulnerability after her traumatic childhood. Her breakdown was not unexpected, partly because of the serious suicidal impulses which she experienced. Her ability to deal constructively with her feelings of abandonment and rejection, along with her fear of the future was low from the start. The identification with her daughter and the fear that she should be taken away from her were reinforced by the fact that her daughter was now the same age as Maria when she had been sent away from her home country. This way of dealing with her childhood traumas – by emotional isolation and maintaining a 'stiff upper lip' – is common with those who develop a psychosis after their emotional barriers have suddenly been disrupted. On the one hand it would be easy to criticise the family therapy for lack of care. However, it is not always possible to know how vulnerable to psychosis a person who appears in control might be. The typical symptoms are non-bizarre paranoid delusions and possibly some hallucinatory experiences. The triggering stress may itself be worsened through the revival of old traumatic memories.

Brief psychosis can also feature schizophrenia-like characteristics where the delusions are bizarre, perhaps with delusions about outside forces influencing the brain. The hallucinations may also be more intense, with many voices interacting. In order to be classed as schizophrenia the illness must have been endured for at least one month according to DSM-IV.

Triggering factors

It is common to find a clear *psychological stress* preceding the brief psychotic illness like a loss, violation or other extreme events (for example, see the case of Angela in Chapter 2). It may be that one has to explore a person's background and circumstances in order to understand why a particular event has acquired such powerful significance that it could act as a trigger for psychosis. Occasionally, *isolation* or *somatic illness* can contribute to the onset of psychosis. Cortico-steroid medication in high doses can sometimes trigger psychoses, especially of an affective nature.

The menstrual cycle may be implicated in women, especially premenstrual tension, which can lower the threshold for psychosis. In the same way, women in the post-natal period are particularly vulnerable for hormonal as well as psychological reasons. In both cases, perplexity and disorganisation are typical and suggest to an organic (hormonal/receptor) component. In acute brief psychoses it is important to look for *organic factors*, such as brain disease, systemic illness or intoxication of any kind. The fact that an organic factor has reduced the threshold for psychosis should not deter one from seeking out the psychological aspects which have added to the trigger. Knowledge about these can be used preventitavely in future crisis situations as it adds to a better understanding of the overall situation. However, there are always some brief psychoses where the cause may be difficult to discern.

Progress and prognosis

According to DSM-IV criteria, a brief psychosis should not last more than a month. A well-adapted premorbid personality and clear precipitating stressors increase the chance of a rapid and complete recovery. It is important to ensure an environment that facilitates healing and the task of working through.

However, as we have stated earlier, a short-term psychosis can herald a deeper long-term illness, either affective or schizophrenic. In the former case one often finds marked emotional fluctuations in the early history, together with depressive or manic states. In addition a close relative is often found to suffer an affective illness.

Affective psychosis

Recent history reveals just how much the classification systems for psychosis do change. Many who in earlier decades, especially in the USA, were diagnosed with schizophrenia, would today be diagnosed with an affective psychosis. Before DSM-III, which was introduced at the beginning of the 1980s, the concept of schizophrenia in the USA was closer to the general concept of psychosis. For that reason, the prognosis connected with

'American schizophrenia' was understood to be unrealistically positive for those who worked with the stricter European diagnostic conventions. This may also account for many of the good results reported with psychotherapy for this kind of 'schizophrenia'.

In classification systems, the affective psychoses are today not categorised as psychotic illnesses. In spite of this, I have included them in this book because most acute psychoses do have an affective element. That is to say, they have depressive or manic elements. In-between forms are common. An artificial border is therefore set up between those psychoses which have a low content of affective symptoms and those with a high content. A period of marked depressive or hypomanic symptoms can herald both brief psychoses, schizophreniform and schizophrenic psychoses. In an affective psychosis the underlying disorder is depression or a bipolar illness, where the person, during a period of their illness, develops a clear psychosis. In affective psychoses the preceding deterioration in mood may act as a trigger for the psychosis. This would support the idea that there is not necessarily a categorical distinction between affective and non-affective psychoses. These psychoses usually resolve without any residual deficit, and so the prognosis is usually better in comparison with a schizophrenic psychosis. Another dynamic interpretation for a better recovery is the fact that the inner representations of the surrounding world and the self (see Chapter 4) have reached a higher developmental level in the affective psychoses.

A bipolar illness which starts with a short-term psychosis

Yvonne, a musician, was a 35-year-old single woman. She had warm and good friendships. In recent years her life had been entirely taken up with a relationship with a married man. When he separated from his wife Yvonne thought that they were going to move in together but he had suddenly declared that he did not want to continue their relationship. Some days later she went to her best friend's wedding in the country. During the ceremony she began to behave strangely, talking symbolically and in rhyming verse. She tried to play charades with children that she did not know. For several nights she hardly slept. One night she awoke in a state of anxiety and, convinced that her life was in danger, she fled into a wood wearing only her nightdress. After a police search, she was found and taken to a psychiatric unit. Her speech was disorganised and she appeared very anxious. After a period of treatment with antipsychotic medicine her mental state settled and it was possible for her to return to her home town. However, she did not improve further; rather, she sunk into a deep depression with persistent suicidal ruminations and again had to be taken to a psychiatric unit. After treatment, Yvonne was able to return to work but six months later she was ill again, this time with prominent manic symptoms. She did not sleep, dressed bizarrely and conceived unintelligible plans. To prevent her from ruining her career and because of the suicide risk if she were to switch to a depressive phase, she was immediately detained and admitted to hospital. She was successfully treated with lithium and entered into cognitive psychotherapy.

COMMENTS

This acute brief psychosis turned out to be the first presentation of a bipolar (manic-depressive) illness. Yvonne was not able to resume her career as a musician for a long time. Her self-confidence was low and she felt self-conscious in the face of the surrounding world. She experienced her psychosis as if an emotional lid had been blown away with a great force letting her repressed feelings emerge, chaotically. Two years of intensive cognitive psychotherapy had a significant and meaningful influence on her ability to accept and work on her vulnerability and to increase her insight. The choice of therapy was dictated by Yvonne's marked dedication to seeking out a systematic way of helping herself. Several years later she was able to safely discontinue lithium therapy.

Occurrence

The *frequency* of affective psychosis is uncertain, not least because of the difficulty in defining it diagnostically. Yet it is no more unusual than the other forms of psychoses mentioned above. It mainly affects people over 30 years old.

Symptoms

In addition to affective components of depression or bipolar (manic-depressive) illness, the patient also experiences a simultaneous *psychosis*, which is shorter lived than the affective illness. Delusions, as well as hallucinations, can occur for a substantial period of time, but they do not replace the affective symptomatology. (Cases where schizophrenic and affective symptoms occur but do not always occur simultaneously for a longer period than two weeks are known as schizo-affective psychosis.) Psychotic experiences can be 'congruent' or not congruent with the affective state of mind. *'Mood congruent' delusions* may feature thoughts of worthlessness, earlier misdemeanours, death, destruction and guilt.

In *'mood incongruent' delusions* there may be beliefs that the mass media singles one out, spreading false information about mistakes or shameful sexual deeds. Occasional auditory hallucinations of accusatory voices can be experienced. Also, more bizarre delusions occur, such as the belief that thoughts are implanted in or withdrawn from the brain. Although such delusions are considered to be typical for schizophrenia, the disorder may be classified as affective if these psychotic features are short-lived and in the longer term the other features correspond to the criteria for an affective illness.

The *risk of suicide* can be high during acute psychotic episodes. Even in the later phase of the depression when the psychosis is resolving, the risk is high as motivation and energy levels increase enough for one to act on one's suicidal ideas. (For an example, see the case of Helen, Chapter 22.)

Triggering and background factors

A deep depression or manic state can trigger a psychotic reaction. Often it is discovered that there is a first-degree relative who has had an affective illness. Sometimes too early difficult separations are uncovered, also deaths or childhood abuse. These early experiences have usually been hidden away or their influence has been denied until they have been brought to life by a real or symbolic traumatic event in the present.

The foreign scholarship

Charles, a 25-year-old, newly qualified engineer had been awarded a scholarship to study at a foreign university. He had several close friends that he could contact but he was shy and anxious, especially with women, in spite of an active sexual interest. Charles was bullied during his high-school years. He had grown up in a Nonconformist religious tradition with many strict moral codes. However, he had moved away from religion. Charles felt tired and stressed even before leaving Sweden as he had had several reports to complete. When he arrived at the university he was quite isolated on the campus. However, he would go out for a drink in the evenings (there was no evidence of alcohol abuse). His sense of dejection increased. On one occasion he stumbled and fractured his ankle which had to be put into plaster. His tutor was a religious fundamentalist and both he and Charles quickly became close. Charles suffered from increasing insomnia and lay awake at night ruminating over questions regarding his existence.

Early one morning, about three weeks after his arrival, he heard someone – 'Was it Satan?' – calling him through the window. Nobody was there, but he felt compelled to go out. He went and stood beside a field just outside his residence and was suddenly filled with an ecstatic feeling. He saw a light shining from the sky in the shape of a cross. When he returned indoors he hit his head against a tap on purpose and with such a force that he cut open the skin on his forehead and had to be taken to hospital for stitching. From here Charles was taken to a psychiatric clinic as he appeared perplexed. He was put on high doses of antipsychotic medication and was flown home after a week or so. When he arrived in his home country he was disturbed and dejected but there was little evidence of psychosis. Therefore, Charles's medication dose was reduced. However, as he still suffered from unpleasant side effects the medication was stopped. This allowed Charles to reflect on what had happened to him. He realised how the combination of overwork, isolation and intense conversations about religion awoke conflicts within him about his religious beliefs. Memories of the days in the psychiatric clinic plagued him for a long time. He continued with psychotherapeutic treatment for another six months and even his parents joined in on several sessions. His depression eased up during this period and he was able to return to his ordinary work. At follow-up three years later he felt well and was able to look back on his period of psychosis with insight and understanding.

The delusional disorder

Occurrence

Even delusional disorder constitutes a heterogeneous group of disorders. The patient is more commonly a woman over 35 years old, but the disturbance can occur in younger people and in men. Of those affected few seek psychiatric help: each year two or three new patients with psychosis per 100,000 inhabitants receive this diagnosis. As a result of their symptoms, people usually first come into contact with primary care, social services or other community institutions such as the police or the Church. When the symptoms overstep a socially acceptable level, urgent psychiatric referral often follows. Delusional disorders are particularly resistant to treatment and may run a protracted course.

Symptoms

Often the delusions revolve around one isolated psychotic idea or a group of interconnected delusions. According to DSM-IV, delusions need to be present for at least one month (three months according to ICD-10). The presence of delusions distinguishes this condition from *paranoid personality disorder*, which only occasionally develops into psychosis. One can see a smooth transition to paranoid schizophrenia in a number of cases. Sometimes it can take three to five years before it becomes clear that a schizophrenic illness is developing. Delusions then become more bizarre, more intense auditory hallucinations occur and/or personality and behaviour become more disorganised.

Usually, delusions persist for many years – sometimes for the rest of the sufferer's life – even if the intensity fluctuates. Sometimes a minor injustice can trigger a crisis and hence the illness. Delusional ideas can be persecutory (a gang which is plotting against you, academic enemies who secretly spread rumours, authorities which conspire against you, etc.). A series of letters and petitions may be produced in order to take care of these miscreants or to see to it that they are prosecuted. In extreme cases serious allegations such as child sexual abuse may be made against relatives or neighbours.

Pathological or morbid jealousy may become delusional, with the patient becoming obsessed with the notion that their partner is unfaithful. They may harangue him or her with supposed evidence to prove it: every night the husband discovers semen stains on his wife's nightdress. Or as soon as her husband leaves the house, his wife is convinced that he is enjoying secret trysts with the female neighbours. It may be hard to differentiate these cases of delusional disorder from paranoid personality disorder. An association with alcohol misuse has been observed with morbid jealously.

Often you hear about how ill-intentioned people wish to 'upset' or 'trick' the patient in some way or another. The reason for this may be more or less clearly defined by the sufferer. The persecutor or enemy can be someone well known who has never even met the patient in question. The patient may harass the object of their delusions to such a degree that compulsory care is required. A popular elderly singer was persecuted by telephone and in letters by a woman with a delusional disorder. Although they had never met, she insisted that he should marry her – she believed he was proposing to her through his songs. The woman was so jealous of his family that she even went to the lengths of setting fire to his summer house, which burnt down. After that she wrote about the many injustices she had experienced in a book which she had published at her own expense.

The contents of the delusion are often very personal in nature: for example, believing that one smells, or that people are insinuating that one is homosexual, or that one has a bodily malformation. These delusions may be hard to distinguish from hypochondriasis or paranoid personality disorder. They are resistant to treatment but important to detect if unnecessary medical treatment or corrective surgery is being sought. *Irritability or depressive states of mind* are associated – presumably as a consequence of the subjective suffering. The *risk of suicide* is then greatly heightened, particularly at times when the psychosis diminishes.

The poisoned photographer

Szandor, a 38-year-old immigrant who was a photographer, asked for emergency help at a psychiatric clinic. He was unemployed but received state benefits in order to continue with his work. He had began to worry that he was being poisoned, partly by the fumes from the chemicals he used in developing his photographs, but also from the metal from tins of food and from cooking utensils. He also feared that important substances were being lost in his urine, and so he had begun to drink his own urine every morning.

Szandor was well organised, competent and appeared to be able to make good emotional contact. He reported that six months prior a four-year relationship with a woman had ended. They did not have any children, but he missed her. He thought that his mistrustfulness and jealousy had largely contributed to her ending the relationship.

Szandor was hospitalised for some days as he was anxious that someone had got into his flat. Who this might be, or why, he was not able to say. He was put on a moderate dose of antipsychotic medication. On his follow-up visits he was even less willing to talk about his problems. He still believed that someone wanted to 'spite' him, to interfere with his flat and change his lightbulbs. However, he did not want to commit to any future treatment. On several occasions his doctor tried to get in touch with Szandor by telephone to see how he was but without success.

Eventually the local police discovered that Szandor had taken his life by cutting his veins and throwing himself out of his seventh floor apartment. They also found unopened bottles of medication. This occurred exactly one year after he had originally sought help.

COMMENTS

Without knowing for sure whether there would have been a different outcome, there are certain factors which can be considered: no active attempts were made to find out if there was a support network which might have been available to this patient. His quiet ways and need for privacy were never discussed. No visit was made to his home where one might have explored his beliefs about the mysterious visits from outside. Little respect was paid to his delusions about being harmed and poisoned. Instead of trying to explore more closely the basis for these beliefs, something which could easily been initiated with a home visit, a diagnosis of delusional disorder was quickly made and he was simply put on medication.

Of course, Szandor did not take the medication. This polite patient hid his deep mistrust of the psychiatrist and may have felt violated and accused even though he had been treated in a friendly way. He probably regretted his initial openness. The diagnosis of delusional disorder was not in itself a difficult one to make, but perhaps it was too early to be certain. The symptom of drinking his own urine makes one wonder if this might have been an incipient schizophrenic illness.

It is important to distinguish transient from persistent auditory hallucinations, as the latter suggest a schizophrenic illness. Bizarre delusions such as one's thoughts being inserted, broadcast or removed have similar implications.[1] It may be difficult to determine whether an individual's preoccupations are truly delusional. Many delusional ideas are plausible and cannot be dismissed without corroboration from family or friends. It is also important to treat a patient's delusions with respect, whilst not actively colluding with them. It can be especially difficult when the patient recounts how other people have avoided him and or how he or she has been the victim of sexual maltreatment. Psychiatry owes the patient the respect of avoiding a quick diagnosis. This is less of a dilemma when the psychotic nature of symptoms is self-evident (e.g. delusions of thought insertion). But even here it is important that the patient is not contradicted or made to feel his beliefs are dismissed, questioned too quickly or in a way which is felt to be intrusive.

Spying neighbours

Vera had had a fairly successful career as a journalist. She was 40 years old when she failed to place a report from the former Soviet Union. It had been difficult to confirm the information that she had gathered for her article on child prostitution. Hurt and disappointed by this, Vera withdrew to her flat, which she left less and less frequently. Instead she began to compose letters to authorities and reported neighbours whom she considered had behaved badly towards her and who probably were spying on her.

The police had abandoned the investigation into her reports as they were unable to corroborate them. At night, Vera began ringing relations that she had lost touch with and accusing them of sexually abusing children. Eventually they reported her to the police. By this point she depended entirely on financial support from her parents and on the food that they placed outside her door. She would not even open the door to them.

This eventually led to a home visit from her local GP. Vera appeared to be quite collected and lucid. She did not seem to be experiencing hallucinations. However, when she did not improve the concern about her increased and she was eventually taken into hospital by force. She underwent compulsory treatment with an antipsychotic medication. The dose had been low but after some weeks Vera had become warmer, more amenable and, fortunately, insightful. She left in a positive state of mind. After some months Vera stopped taking her medication. The symptoms gradually returned over the following six months and Vera was admitted to hospital again – this time with her consent. After much argument she was able to be persuaded to take the medication again. Some months later she was able to return part time to her old job on the newspaper. The improvement with antipsychotic medication prompts one to ask whether the nature of her disturbance might not have been the early stage of a schizophrenic illness along with the relapse when off medication, but the ability to return to a high-functioning job would go against this.

Progress and prognosis

The course of delusional disorder is variable. In some instances it resolves within six months and in others it persists for many years and even for the rest of one's life, albeit with fluctuations in intensity. In the first year it is difficult to know whether it is an early phase of schizophrenia. Sometimes this presents with increasingly bizarre, disturbed behaviour and a reduction in the capacity to function, perhaps over five to ten years. In these cases it is important to treat with appropriate doses of antipsychotic medication. However, the challenge is to establish sufficient rapport with the patient whose insight into their problems is often at best marginal.

Psychosis not otherwise specified

In around 10 to 20 per cent of first-episode psychosis patients there is insufficient information to make a diagnosis with a high degree of certainty. The symptoms may be too non-specific. Also it is often felt to be too early to make a definitive diagnosis, especially of chronic illnesses like schizophrenia. Instead, a non-specific diagnosis is often used which, in due course, can be replaced by a definite diagnosis according to the course of the illness. There may be auditory hallucinations without any clear evidence of delusions, or a situation where one suspects that an organic factor might be involved. This diagnostic category is also used if one is unclear as to whether the affective component should be seen as determinant in a psychosis. Generally, around half of those with a non-specified psychosis are given a diagnosis of schizophrenia after one year and most of the others recover.

Dissociative (hysterical) 'psychoses'

Often it is hard to differentiate between true psychosis, where the ego is no longer able to integrate reality, and a *dissociative* or, in classical psychodynamic terms, *hysterical psychosis*. Such a patient manifests apparent signs of 'madness'. Their speech may appear disorganised and incoherent or simply illogical. They may make mysterious movements which appear to have some symbolic meaning, and can appear to be experiencing both visual and auditory hallucinations. There is however a communicative and dramatic element to this presentation that unconsciously avoids a situation which triggers internal conflict. What would be considered as true psychoses are not usually related to a clear primary gain from the illness. Just as conversion hysteria mimics different physical illnesses such as paralysis, muteness or blindness, etc., in hysterical psychosis the patient appears to present with a psychosis. They will have a more integrated personality, often with neurotic traits. It should also be pointed out that there is a continuum between 'hysterical' psychosis-like conditions and pure psychoses. DSM-IV does not describe dissociative psychosis though it is related to multiple personality disorder (MPD).

Aetiological factors

Often a number of early traumatic experiences with, for example, sexual abuse or significant early losses are found in those with dissociative psychoses. Being a victim of or witness to repeated violence is also common, as is early abandonment or neglect. The traumatic content of these experiences does not integrate with the 'normal' functioning self because language is still not developed or because the experiences are too painful and for that reason they are repressed. They are split off (dissociated) from the personality to a 'foreign' part of it, but can emerge during psychosis-like personality changes when under stress in adult life. Certain people enter into dissociative 'psychoses' very easily and mistreatment can cause the condition to become chronic. Early traumas can also weaken the development of the ego and can, for that reason, contribute to the development of a psychosis if there is a vulnerability to it.

Many claims of speedy psychotherapeutic successes in the treatment of psychosis concern dissociative conditions, which often react well to intensive psychotherapy when provided by an experienced therapist. For this reason it is important that this diagnosis is made early on. Treatment is first and foremost psychotherapy orientated both towards the individual and if possible the family. Antipsychotic medication is usually not indicated.

Delusions and disorganised behaviour – but not a psychosis

Nina, a married woman in her thirties, was taken into a psychiatric unit as an emergency. She was in her seventh month of pregnancy, had a 4-year-old daughter and a son of 16 months. Her problems had started soon after she had discovered that she was pregnant. She began to believe that unknown persons tried to inject her with HIV-infected syringes whenever she went out. The anxiety that accompanied this idea, which she knew to be unrealistic, became so powerful that she was unable to go out or take her children out. Her husband, who was a computer consultant, was forced to take leave from work for ever longer periods of time. A private psychiatrist believed that she was psychotic and put Nina on a low dose of antipsychotic medication. The dose was increased by degrees without having any effect and, due to her obsessive ideas, she was also given SSRI medication. When her condition worsened the couple was referred to a unit for first-episode psychosis patients.

At our first meeting Nina was not well integrated: she was withdrawn and very anxious. She said that she wore her raincoat so that she would know if someone secretly tried to perforate it with a needle. After a while she asked if she could search through my pockets as I might be carrying syringes. Nina also displayed small fresh sores on her skin. Her husband described how she would cut off small slices of skin which she thought had been pierced in order to study them under a magnifying glass. During the conversation she suddenly jumped up and searched behind the chairs because she was convinced that someone had come in and hidden himself or herself somewhere in order to inject her later on.

In spite of the chaotic situation I was not so certain that she suffered from a psychosis and suspected that Nina was able to control herself more than she allowed me to see. She was invited to make frequent visits together with her husband. To begin with, and also in view of her pregnancy, she was taken off the medication – a daily dose of 6 mg of haloperidol together with antidepressant medication. This markedly improved communication and already by the third visit Nina felt that her mind was clearer. By degrees she was able to describe her chaotic and insecure childhood as well as her powerful and guilt-filled protests about her pregnancy. She had worked freelance in an occupation that she very much enjoyed but had not been able to get back to it in the last four years. For emotional reasons Nina could not contemplate an abortion: 'I love children.' All the same, she repeatedly dreamed that the foetus had died. She also dreamed that her youngest child, who was now one and a half years old, grew so fast that he no longer recognised her.

She still breastfed her son so that he should benefit from the best form of nourishment (in spite of which she had become pregnant). Nina began to admit that she felt consumed by her pregnancies – she had no life of her own. Her husband, who had felt very guilty for being responsible for her pregnancy, corroborated Nina's views. At the same time he maintained a firm psychological control. Nina felt from the beginning that she could not express any complaints because it was not fair on the unborn child and on her husband who had given up so much for her sake. Nonetheless, she began to hurl strong accusations against him. Later she was able to take greater responsibility for her part in their situation. She accepted the interpretation that she felt herself to be hit by a mortal illness as a punishment for her incriminating thoughts with deep feeling and increasing relief. Nina was able to remain alone with her children for increasingly longer periods during the daytime. Her obsessional thoughts disappeared and her husband returned to his work, which had suffered badly. After two months she was fully restored. She gave birth to her child without difficulty some months later. Supportive therapy continued during the following year intermittently.

COMMENTS

This case shows the importance of a correct early diagnosis. The key difference between a pure psychosis and a dissociative and essentially neurotic reaction is that the obsessive thoughts or 'delusions' express a symbolic reinterpretation of the patient's inner repressed conflicts. The affective contact was also more available than one finds in a psychosis in spite of the use of medication. In a psychosis the ability to accept reality would be more disturbed and the ability to work through the conflicts would be greatly diminished.

Chapter 11

Psychotic disorders II

Schizophrenia – the sickness of the self

> We see the schizophrenic as one of us who has abandoned the struggle which we all share; about a self, about a personal existence which no longer adapts itself to reality's inner contradictions.
>
> Manfred Bleuler 1984

Historical development of the concept of schizophrenia

Dementia praecox versus affective disorders ('Kraepelinian School')

At the end of the 1800s, the German psychiatrist Emil Kraepelin (1855–1921) described a group of illnesses which he called *dementia praecox* (Kraepelin 1971/1919). The term had been used for many decades and Kraepelin's contribution was that he distinguished the prognostically more benign affective illnesses, such as 'manic-depressive psychosis', from those with catatonia, hebephrenic and paranoid psychoses. He claimed that this group regularly progressed towards an early dementia, that is to say, a chronic lowering of mental capacity. This view has been considerably modified today.

Schizophrenia constitutes a heterogeneous subgroup of the psychoses which often has a worse prognosis. The disturbance of the sense of self is much deeper than with the other psychoses which in turn affects the capacity to relate and adapt to the future. The definition and diagnostic boundaries vary between different schools of thought and scientific points of view. Thus, there are no clear boundaries such as those we might otherwise expect from the medical world. I will give an overview of the characterisation of the concept of schizophrenia which, in principle, corresponds to the European psychiatric tradition. Later in the chapter I describe the schizophrenic disorders more systematically.

Fundamental symptoms ('Bleuler School')

The term schizophrenia was first used in 1911 by the Swiss psychiatrist Eugen Bleuler (1857–1939), the father of the author of the citation above, Manfred Bleuler. He was a contemporary of Freud's and at times they collaborated. Bleuler (1950/1911) described the schizophrenias as a group of illnesses with certain typical symptoms which he called fundamental symptoms. Bleuler's diagnostic criteria for schizophrenia, known as his 'four As', make up the 'fundamental symptoms':

1   *Associative disturbances*: these are disorders of the patient's ability to think logically. The observer will notice an altered logic, a private symbol or word, a tendency to think concretely, vagueness, a disturbed integration and splitting of logical concepts. (Note that these formal thought disorders should not be confused with disturbances to the *contents* of thoughts such as delusions and hallucinations.)
2   *Affective disturbances*: these include an affect that is inappropriate to the content of one's thoughts (e.g. laughing whilst discussing the death of a loved one), increasing indifference, loss of interest, apathy and lack of desire.
3   *Ambivalence*: the wavering between different impulses, something which can result in the impairment of the capacity to make choices.
4   *Autism*: a withdrawn state and disturbances in being able to interact with one's physical and emotional environment. It consists of a lack of concordance between the individual and the surrounding world. One key feature is the 'lack of intersubjectivity' necessary for understanding other people's minds which is necessary for social interactions.

In addition, there are other well-known psychotic symptoms, but these are not diagnostic of schizophrenia since they may also be seen in other conditions. They are hallucinations, delusions, language and speech alterations, and changes in behaviour and other symptoms.

Basic symptoms ('Phenomenological School')

Whilst fundamental symptoms are only observed, the phenomenological concept of 'basic symptoms' refers to subjective psychological experiences which can be described by the patient (or whose behavioural counterparts can be observed). This approach was formulated by the phenomenological psychiatric school lead by Gerd Huber in Bonn. Phenomenology stresses the value of what is experienced, or directly observed, without interpreting or making use of any theoretical model to understand the phenomena.

Normally patients with schizophrenia report several of the following non-psychotic disturbances of experience:

1 *Disturbances of the self* include alterations in the experience of having a cohesive identity, being alive and being autonomous. De-realisation (feeling detached from reality, for example, having the feeling of being on a stage set) as with depersonalisation (feeling detached from oneself, that one does not exist, or is not physically integrated) is common, especially in the early phases of psychosis, but are not true psychotic symptoms. The boundaries of the ego are permeable or flagging and the dividing line between oneself and what is not oneself are unclear. This too can be seen in the marked anxiety and exalted experience of an uncontrolled involvement with the surrounding world.

2 *Disturbance of attention and perceptual processing* presents as difficulty in concentrating and in carrying through plans. The capacity to filter out non-essential stimuli is impaired. Perception of sound and light can be heightened or reduced. Attention is reduced and the capacity to shift attention to different stimuli is affected. Some people are unable to perceive their environment as an integrated whole; rather, their perception is fragmented and so less coherent.

3 *Disturbance of cognition.* Disturbances in concentration are common. Many complain that alien thoughts suddenly appear for no reason and disturb their concentration. Some find themselves stuck in meaningless ruminations over what they have just thought or said. Others complain of feeling crowded in by thoughts. Thought blocks are often reported, where the patient feels his stream of thoughts is suddenly interrupted or disappears for a second or more. Patients can also experience saying something they had not thought of saying.

4 *Disturbances of actions and movements.* Patients may make movements against their will – grimacing or moving their arms or fingers in a specific way. Movements, previously automatic, now come under scrutiny. For example, whilst walking, the patient is aware of thinking out the action first – having to put the left foot forward, and then the right, etc.

5 *Conaesthesias* are brief (seconds long) bodily experiences of weakness, pain, and heat or numbness. Such feelings may become the subject of a delusional misinterpretation.

6 *Non-specific disturbances in the sense of self.* A marked sense of loss of energy is common. To the non-specific experiences we can add feelings of depression and anxiety.

Psychotic symptoms consist of a loss of proper understanding of reality. When the basic symptoms become psychotic in nature they contribute to deep-seated personality change because they are no longer experienced as alien to the ego but as ego-syntonic. What happens is that the person goes from experiencing the disturbing discontinuity within himself to understanding it as an influence coming from the outside world. The anxiety-ridden experience of an imminent disintegration of the self now tries to 'repair' and explain itself by means of the construction of delusions.

First- and second-rank symptoms

Kurt Schneider, who also belonged to the school of phenomenology, distinguished between 'first- and second-rank symptoms' in an attempt to separate symptoms deserving more serious prognostic attention (Schneider 1967). They are not unlike Bleuler's differentiation between fundamental and accessory symptoms.

First-rank symptoms include the person whose psychic experience of integrity becomes disturbed in a bizarre way. He or she hears her thoughts spoken out loud, hears voices in the form of running commentaries, experiences thoughts as inserted, withdrawn or broadcast, and delusions (known as passivity phenomena) that others are influencing their movements, feelings, instincts and desires. These symptoms reflect the schizophrenic's loss of experiential integrity with hallucinations and delusions representing an increased permeability between the ego and the surrounding world. In the same way, sometimes 'compulsive thoughts' can be felt as an invasion. For example, ideas or visions with sadistic or promiscuous content are 'inserted into' his or her normal thinking.

According to Schneider *second-rank symptoms* are of lesser diagnostic importance. They concern delusions such as being watched by a helicopter or aeroplane, hearing messages directed to oneself through the radio or television, that someone at work moves the furniture around or arranges meetings in order to express criticisms. Second-rank symptoms include perplexity, depressive or manic moods, etc.

Schneider asserted that first-rank symptoms were especially important for a diagnostic distinction between schizophrenic and non-schizophrenic psychotic phenomena and affective disorders. They are also central when it comes to the criteria for schizophrenia according to ICD-10. However, more recent research by Shepherd *et al.* (1989) has shown that these symptoms do not have such a high prognostic value as Schneider imagined. They do not differentiate a group that has a poor prognosis. Nevertheless, first-rank symptoms characterise a more deep-seated psychosis, even if the patient may recover completely.

The implications of DSM-IV and ICD-10

As we can see in the Appendix, the diagnostic systems not only regard schizophrenia as a long-term psychotic illness but also as a *group of illnesses* which is characterised by disorders of thought and association, bizarre experiences of being influenced, and/or greater or lesser disturbances of psychosocial functioning. Most importantly, DSM-IV, which is more derived from Kraepelin, suggests a poor prognosis and the development of a functional deficit together with certain well-defined symptoms (akin to the Kraepelinian concept of dementia praecox). To connect the concept of schizophrenia so emphatically with a bad prognosis goes against a set of long-term studies which find that, at presentation, schizophrenic patients, in 50 per cent of cases or more, have a good or relatively good prognosis.

ICD-10, which is closer to Eugen Bleuler's and Schneider's definitions, offers a set of somewhat wider and less exact criteria. Overall the similarities between the systems are greater than their differences. No matter the diagnostic criteria one uses, the prognosis of the illness in any individual case is hard to predict in the first few years.

Positive and negative symptoms

The division of schizophrenic symptoms into positive and negative ones has been used a great deal during recent decades. Over a hundred years ago, the English neurologist John Hughlings-Jackson (1958/1894) observed *negative* 'deficiency symptoms' in mental illness such as introversion, decline in language and loss of will, as well as *positive* 'productive' symptoms such as delusions, hallucinations and bizarre behaviour. Aside from his theory of how the brain functioned when damaged, Jackson maintained that the negative symptoms are a manifestation of a loss of brain tissue occurring in the process of the illness. Positive symptoms result from secondary adaptations in brain function – higher organisational centres which had previously inhibited more primitive functioning no longer exert the same degree of control.

This view came to the forefront in the 1970s (Strauss *et al.* 1974) when it formed the basis for a model (Crow 1980) where schizophrenia with overwhelmingly positive symptoms (*schizophrenia type 1*) is seen as referring to a genetically caused pathological excess of dopamine receptors in the brain, while schizophrenia with overwhelmingly negative symptoms (*schizophrenia type 2*) is seen as a form of subtle, early onset brain damage. This theoretical dichotomy has not, however, been confirmed: most patients with schizophrenia have features of both types to varying degrees. The negative symptoms outweigh the positive in the later stages of the illness. All the same, it is worth distinguishing between positive and negative symptoms, not least because the negative symptoms are similar to the side effects of neuroleptic medication and must be distinguished from them. Negative symptoms may also be the result of the long-term isolation and lack of stimulation which are so common in the case of patients with schizophrenia. In other words, there is a risk that side effects of treatment or social consequences of symptoms might be interpreted as signs of the illness. Even depression can be misdiagnosed as negative symptoms.

Schizophrenia spectrum disorders and schizotypal personality disorder

The concept of schizophrenia spectrum disorder is linked to an increased genetic vulnerability among the patient's biological family members. In these relatives, an increased frequency of *schizotypal* personality disorder has been observed: that is to say, individuals who have a tendency to magical thinking or 'strange' perceptions, 'verging on delusional' thinking and eccentric, although not psychotic patterns of behaviour. Schizophrenic basic symptoms (as described by Huber and the phenomenological school) include an accentuation of schizotypal thinking. Schizotypy is seen as a risk factor for developing schizophrenia later in life. Some researchers claim that *paranoid* and *borderline personality disorders* occur more often in these families (see Chapter 6). Thus the concept of schizophrenia becomes, from the spectrum viewpoint, a little wider. However, this is in accordance with the view about ground and basic symptoms which I advocate in this book.[1]

Schizophrenia as an illness or a functional disability

The concept of psychosis is less prognostically (and emotionally) charged and should, in my view, be used during early and acute phases. The concept of schizophrenia becomes more useful in the longer term psychic dysfunction that certain patients go on to develop. Even if the characteristics of an *illness* are easy to ascertain in an acute psychosis – whether it is of a schizophrenic kind or not – it is no less correct according to WHO (1994) criteria to denote its further progression as a functional *disability* (of a cognitive or emotional nature). This functional disability can result in a handicap when the world imposes its conditions and makes its demands. The community's capacity or incapacity to compensate for a person's functional disability determines the nature and degree of the specific handicaps. Those with a long-term schizophrenic disorder have to adapt to a partly altered state of mind, to the residual hallucinations, delusions, attention deficit, problems of making contact or/and behaviour disorders. At present, 20 to 30 per cent of people with chronic schizophrenia need some kind of daily assistance in order to cope.

The notion of handicap is an improvement on the concept of illness because it allows the individual to be regarded as a person who has reached his or her full potential in spite of the disability. It also places a legal obligation on the community to provide financial and social support.

Schizophrenic syndromes

Epidemiology

Every year, around five to ten individuals in 100,000 inhabitants develop an illness which will ultimately be diagnosed as a schizophrenia spectrum disorder. This means that 50 per cent of all those who become psychotic for the first time will fall within the group of schizophrenias, that is to say, also schizophreniform and schizo-affective disorders and the rare simplex form. It has been suggested by several research studies that the incidence (number of new cases per year in a given population) of first-episode illness in schizophrenia has decreased during the last decades (Der *et al.* 1990; Munk-Jørgensen and Mortensen 1992). There are also many signs, until now scientifically unverified, that with increased accessibility to and effectiveness of psychiatric care in the early phase, the frequency of the more serious conditions lessens. Some studies indicate that the natural history of the illness has been changing over the last century. A good example of this is the catatonic form of schizophrenia which presents with psychomotor (movement disturbance) rather than psychotic symptoms. Today catatonia is seen less often in western countries than in the third world. However non-industrial societies are thought to be more tolerant and accommodating of such illnesses which have a less florid presentation. Thus schizophrenia with mild symptoms may be underdiagnosed because its lack of acute severity does not necessitate hospital care and thus the case will not be recognised. Since the prognosis for more florid cases of acute schizophrenia is better than for the patients with milder symptoms there may be a false impression of better prognosis in these countries than in the industrial west (see Figure 11.1).

More men than women become ill. The proportion is around 60:40. On the whole, men fall ill at least one year earlier than women at an average age of 24 years as opposed to 25 years in women. In some ways, this distinction between the sexes tends to even out because more women are diagnosed with schizophrenia after the age of 50 (although it is fairly unusual to see schizophrenia present for the first time at this age). With regard to the prevalence (that is, the amount of people suffering within a given community at any one time), large towns have the highest and rural areas the lowest (see Figure 11.2).

Between 0.5 and 1 per cent of all people suffer from a schizophrenia spectrum disorder of which around half develop a chronic illness. This means that in Great Britain with its population of 60 million inhabitants between 150,000 and 300,000 have a disabling schizophrenic disorder. In a population of 100,000 inhabitants one can expect that there will be between 250 to 500 people diagnosed with schizophrenia who need some form of support from the community.

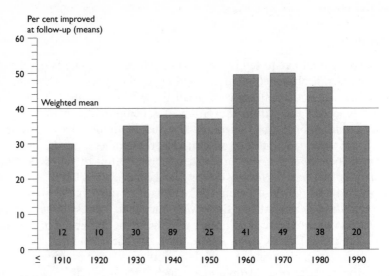

Figure 11.1 Rate of improvement over three (four) decades for individuals retrospectively diagnosed with schizophrenia at ten-year follow-up. The improvement seen during the later decades is probably a result of the introduction of narrower diagnostic criteria in DSM-III in the 1980s (after Hegarty *et al.* 1994).

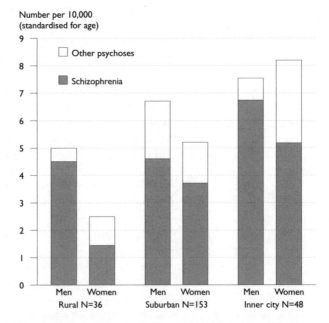

Figure 11.2 The prevalence of chronically psychotic individuals stratified by age over a year in different types of area (Widerlöv *et al.* 1989).

The development of the illness is more chronic when it comes to men, who therefore also have a higher prevalence than women. It is unclear as to whether differences between the sexes result simply from hormonal factors (there is a theory that oestrogen protects against the development of schizophrenia). Other proposed factors include differing perinatal risks for both genders, and the contribution of social expectations and gender roles.

Data relating to schizophrenic illnesses

- Around 300,000 people in Great Britain (4–6 per 1000 inhabitants) suffer from a functional disability related to schizophrenia.
- Of these, at least 75,000–150,000 are markedly handicapped and in need of social support. The cost to the community for the treatment and social care is around £7 billion per year.
- Every year 6000–9000 people develop psychosis for the first time.
- Of these, around 50 per cent will develop a long-term disability.
- The average age of onset of illness is 24 years for men and 25 years for women.

Symptoms

Earlier I gave an account of the clinical and phenomenological expressions of schizophrenia. With DSM-IV's operational diagnosis of schizophrenia it is necessary to differentiate between three groups of symptoms that occur in different combinations:

- Positive symptoms (delusions and hallucinations)
- Negative symptoms (paucity of speech, blunting of emotional responses, introversion)
- Disorganisation symptoms (disorganised or chaotic behaviour and social habits, unintelligible speech which may reflect thought disorder).

Positive symptoms

As mentioned in Chapter 3, the delusions should be *bizarre*, that is impossible within one's own culture or belief system. There are a number of bizarre themes which are frequently seen. For example, the belief that one can control a TV reporter's speech or movements, that people or satellites are controlling one's mind, inserting or withdrawing thoughts, perhaps using 'rays'. Another example is that tiny transmitters have been inserted into one's body, perhaps by a dentist. All of these delusions can be seen as attempts to explain the experiences of being controlled as described above, and/or the presence of auditory hallucinations which echo one's thoughts or comment on one's actions.

Certain kinds of delusions create acute anxiety: for example, being ordered by God to prevent the world's destruction by carrying out certain acts, or feeling that one is a pawn in a game between good and evil forces. Another example would be the belief that to prevent a catastrophe it is necessary to have the correct thoughts a particular number of times or about certain letter combinations. Such compulsive psychotic phenomena are very exhausting and painful for the patient.

Hallucinations are often experienced as a commentary with someone criticising or (less commonly) praising everything that one is thinking, doing or is planning to do.[2] Voices can also comment on one's various actions. This is very exhausting and disturbing to one's concentration. Command hallucinations can sometimes drive a person to self-destructive behaviour or to harming someone else. Some people experience a host of different voices, which may be coming either from people they know or from strangers. These voices can persist for years on end and more or less dominate thinking processes. It is not unusual to find ten or twenty such identifiable inner personalities. Often the hallucinated voices can be more dramatic and filled with symbolic messages during the acute phase while they become nagging and more needy as the illness develops.

Auditory hallucinations are the most common (discussed further in Chapter 3) while sensory and visual hallucinations also occur. In the latter cases the hallucinations are less defined even though they are intrusive. Visual hallucinations may suggest an organic cause or a dissociative 'hysterical' background. Olfactory hallucinations (smells of gas, rotting, etc.) are not unusual in the acute stage.

The quality of the voices experienced varies from being as distinct as if they came from a radio station or from a living person to sounding like a mumble in the background. If the patient listens carefully to this mumbling the voices soon appear more clearly. In acute psychosis the voices are more apparent, while during the calmer phases they lie 'somewhere in the back of the head'. They can disappear altogether.

Negative symptoms

Negative (defect) symptoms include apathy, indifference, difficulties initiating tasks or speech, negligible emotional contact, social withdrawal and introversion. They indicate a worse prognosis than the positive symptoms, especially if they are present when positive symptoms disappear or if they persist long term. They belong to the fundamental symptoms. However, similar symptoms, as mentioned earlier, can occur when neuroleptic medication doses are too high, if the patient is depressed, as a response to positive symptoms and as a result of understimulation in an institution. These causes should be differentiated from true negative symptoms.

Disorganisation symptoms

Disorganised behaviour can express itself in bizarre, fixed postures known as catatonia. It can also be encountered in vague, incoherent, disjointed speech that can be hard to understand. 'Paramimics' such as little grimaces or tics that accompany speech, appear. Sometimes behaviour can be more frightening: 'obscene' or threatening. For example, a young man who has become ill for the first time gets into his mother's bed and gropes for her breast. He may suddenly launch into a physical attack on either of his parents. He may complain that his life has been ruined by them, that they are responsible for all his past disappointments and unpleasant experiences. This is common and painful, since few parents would feel wholly free from blame especially with regard to their child's mental illness.

Another example would be sexual disinhibition: a young girl might visit her neighbour, undress and invite intercourse. It is not unusual in the acute phase for masturbation to take place, openly in front of others. Such behaviour takes place in such an aberrant and absent-minded fashion that it seldom results in sexual violation. It is more likely to lead to other people seeking out psychiatric help. On the other hand, in the early period of acute psychosis sometimes more risky sexual acting out occurs. A woman who does not appear to be disturbed can have a multitude of sexual encounters with men before she presents with overt signs of acute illness, perhaps of a catatonic nature. It is possible that these experiences would have increased the distress thereby worsening the illness.

Subgroups

Since the days of Kraepelin, four subgroups have been differentiated. In spite of much research, it has not been possible either to discover whether each subgroup has a different aetiology (set of causes) or whether they require different treatment. In clinical practice, in-between states are more common. The same individual can have different kinds of symptoms over different periods of time. However, the prognosis might differ between the subgroups. I will list them here in order to relate to the classical literature on the subject.

The most common form is *paranoid schizophrenia* which is dominated by bizarre and often persecutory delusions and hallucinations. The prognosis of this form is often said to be better since a higher level of functioning in other areas is maintained.

Hebephrenic (disorganised) schizophrenia is diagnosed where deep, unmanageable emotional changes and behavioural disturbance dominate. An 'unnatural' giggling, grimacing or manneristic behaviour with deep self-absorption often appears dominant. Hebephrenia is often reported to come on in late adolescence or early adulthood, and as having a poor prognosis. The latter may be due to this early onset before the personality has fully developed.

Catatonic schizophrenia appears less frequently today than it did 50 years ago and is characterised by psycho-motor disturbances such as a fixed posture or tendency to move in a stereotypical way or respond to commands in an overcompliant, resistant or opposing fashion. Such behaviour can last for less than a week or for weeks or months. A young man held his hands so tightly clenched over a period of several weeks that he developed a fungal infection in them. There are descriptions of catatonic conditions that lasted for many years but which have later resolved.

Undifferentiated schizophrenia cannot be placed in any of the three previous groups because it features elements from all of them.

ICD-10 includes the rare group (one that is not widely accepted) of *simple schizophrenia*. Here there are no positive symptoms, delusions or hallucinations, but instead a creeping but deep-seated deterioration of the personality occurs. One sees progressive negative symptoms with loss of interest and aims along with increasing self-absorption and social withdrawal. These must be present for at least one year before making the diagnosis.

Residual schizophrenia is a common presentation seen later in the illness. It is another name for the *functional disability* that some patients develop. It is characterised mainly by negative symptoms, which develop after one or more acute episodes. The symptoms, according to DSM-IV, will have endured for at least a year. Behaviour and appearance is eccentric, dress and hygiene are often neglected. Speech may be jumbled, containing words and sentences that are hard to understand or reduced in content and spontaneity. This condition may be made worse by a lack of engagement with rehabilitation. Auditory hallucinations are often also present – sometimes in a distressing and disturbing way, but sometimes the patient is not particularly concerned about them.

Delusions may persist, but reduce in their overt intensity. Many patients learn to cope with their ideas (as with their voices) in such a way that they do not outwardly affect relationships too much. The residual form of schizophrenia can, in some cases, be so well integrated with the healthy personality that one has to get to know that person very well before discovering that he or she is experiencing auditory hallucinations or having bizarre delusions.

In a project with rehabilitated people who have had a schizophrenic illness, I interviewed an engineer who maintained a good and non-psychotic contact in every way. But when the interview was about to come to an end it transpired that he was waiting for an X-ray investigation of his head which he had requested. Since the inception of his acute psychotic illness five years previously, he was convinced that a little piece of metal had been secretly inserted into his brain and was still there. He believed he could be used as a receptor for radio signals by means of this piece of metal. However, he said that no such signals had been sent over the last two years.

Functional disability in unrehabilitated patients with schizophrenia

- Fear of contact.
- Tendency to live in a world of one's own.
- 'Morose' behaviour.
- Occasional unintelligible speech.
- Unusual conceptions of the world.
- Deficient ability to make plans.
- Strange clothing.
- Untidiness.
- Worsening with stress or lack of stimulation.

However, it should not be assumed that these experiences are always painful; sometimes their contents give a reassuring meaning to life. The voices, for example, can be well intentioned and supportive and can (in rare cases) give rise to pleasurable sexual experiences. All the same, behaviour may be sullen and with a tendency towards angry outbursts. These might be triggered by unintentional and well-meaning intrusions by those who do not know the patient well. However, it is essential to look after and support these people as they can have difficulties feeding themselves, along with maintaining their personal care and accommodation. Without some intervention several times a week, the house can pile up with dust, rubbish, ill-smelling, rotting food and left-overs. These problems can be worsened by institutionalisation, if patients have not been encouraged to care for themselves as much as possible.

The painter Inge Schiöler

Inge Schiöler (1908–1971) is one of Sweden's most well-known painters. He had already had several exhibitions when he developed a schizophrenic illness in 1933 and was taken to hospital. During the years that followed, for most of the time he lay in bed in a catatonic state until 1942 when he spontaneously took up drawing and painting on lavatory paper. To begin with he used coal and simple colours but eventually he managed to obtain better materials. During the 1950s he was treated with the new neuroleptic medicines. This helped him to leave the hospital more often. At the beginning of the 1960s he was allowed to leave, on a trial basis, to resume life in his own house on the island of Koster. He became engaged and his partner moved in with him in 1967. His creative activity continued uninterrupted and brought him much recognition.

A resident of Koster has described his memories of Inge Schiöler: Inge was both demanding and shy towards the people he met. If one got too near his flowers he would yell, if one walked too close to the carefully ordered stones in his garden he became furious, but when he was allowed to show his newly planted reindeer moss, the wild roses or the apple tree, his smile appeared again. Then he was happy.

Inge inhabited a realm outside his pictures. It was a world of animals and plants. Here he was king and here nobody would control him. When the subject of conversation died – and it often did – one could talk about animals. Why doesn't the woodpecker fell any trees? Of course they do. The other day, just after you had gone out a woodpecker appeared and felled a fir tree just outside the window. Yes, it was just a little after you had left. The shopkeeper's horse is called Hyacinth. We said: 'Strange name for a horse.' 'Strange? Not at all. When I visited the market in Strömstad I saw thirty-four horses. Every one of them was called Hyacinth.' When the conversation turned to flying fish in the sea he claimed that a shoal of such fish had flown right into his sail. 'There were so many that I was forced to bail out the boat otherwise it would have sunk.' Just as one is not allowed to question children about the games they play, so we were not allowed to question his stories. It would have pulled the carpet from under his sovereignty over this realm he had built for himself. Here he lived a thrilling life. Although no one had seen a snake on Koster, it happened that when he was picking roses a nearby branch turned out to be a 'thorn snake'. (Cappelen-Smith et al. 1994)

Stages in the development of a schizophrenic psychosis

Sometimes it is hard to judge the exact onset of a schizophrenic illness. Several studies point to the fact that many people with schizophrenia had functioned poorly for years before they were first treated (Loebel et al. 1992; McGlashan and Johannessen 1996). It is not unheard of for people to have been quietly psychotic for ten years and still managed to cope in the community. The development of schizophrenia can be divided into two types. In the first group the inception is clearly defined, with a prodromal loss of functioning. The second group's whole lives have been filled with an increasing social withdrawal and lack of capacity to hold their own amongst friends and colleagues at school and work. Shyness and a lack of a physically active life as well as lack of ambition are often reported. There is often a history of stigmatisation and exclusion, resulting in a downward spiral of their limited social skills and circumstances. Over time, there is a worsening of odd behaviour, hygiene and self-neglect.

In a British research programme a cohort consisting of all children born on a certain day in 1946 was studied (Jones *et al.* 1994). The 30 children who were eventually diagnosed with schizophrenia were compared with the rest and, overall, were found to have delayed development from early childhood. These delays included learning to walk, speech problems, inadequate school performance and tending to play alone from around the ages of four to six. If the figures are studied more closely, around half have undergone delayed development as described, whereas the development of the rest up to the onset of illness is no different from the control group. Thus the study suggests that the picture of schizophrenia in certain cases must be understood as a developmental disturbance of the brain that can result in a lifelong functional disability. A Finnish study has confirmed this finding (Isohanni *et al.* 1999). Here, 11 per cent of the pre-schizophrenic boys had very high school reports against 3 per cent of the comparison group with which the comparison was made. This illustrates the high degree of heterogeneity in those diagnosed with schizophrenia and that the vulnerability can be bound up with a high level of giftedness.

Before the onset of the actual psychosis often one finds *prodromal symptoms* for months or sometimes years. These are symptoms of a non-psychotic nature that can be seen in retrospect to have heralded the illness. They include increasing worry and decreasing ability to work or to concentrate on school lessons. They can be seen as the beginnings of the basic symptoms as described earlier in the chapter. The person concerned can withdraw from their circle of friends. Some have peculiar experiences such as feeling that life is strangely different. People describe perceptual disturbances, heightened experiences of colour, light and sound. The tendency to react more intensely than others in response to different kinds of stimuli is also described (Chapman 1966). Some have likened the prodromal stage to an irreconcilable guilty feeling that one has committed a terrible crime that no one else knows about (Conrad 1958). There is also a deep feeling of isolation and of being different from others. The prodromal phase contains a diffuse feeling of approaching breakdown in the ability to understand and to deal with reality. These descriptions, in my experience, convey the sense of emotional overload that many of these patients express (see Chapter 5 for further descriptions of the phases of acute psychosis).

The *onset of psychosis* itself can either be gradual or more acute and very dramatic. With the *acute process*, the development of psychosis is dominated by an affect-filled sense of anxiety or paranoia and persecution, which can escalate into panic and threats of impending catastrophe (such as death or 'world war') or inner disintegration. Secondary depressive symptoms are commonly seen. This depression is best described as one which is filled more with a sense of meaninglessness and existential chaos than of a personal sense of worthlessness and self-contempt, which is more typical of primary depressive illness. Unexpected and frightening outbursts of fury can be triggered and friends and relatives watch powerless as the condition progresses towards catastrophe. For a family member to seek help from outside is experienced by the sufferer as a betrayal. Even so, this 'betrayal' must happen sooner or later, as more bridges connecting the sufferer to the community collapse. Sometimes the condition explodes in an act of violence but, in retrospect, the development of the psychosis can easily be recognised. Usually however the schizophrenic condition develops by degrees.

As we have said, the *full schizophrenic illness* may develop in many different ways. During a five-year period, Shepherd and his colleagues studied a large group of first-time sufferers and outlined four typical forms of development. However, it should be added that the diagnostic criteria were wide and quite similar to an overall definition of first-episode psychosis (Shepherd *et al.* 1989).

In over half the cases one or more psychoses were found without there being any long-term disability. Amongst the others, none returned to a normal life after their first psychotic episode. In many cases the disability increased after each subsequent psychotic relapse. These findings correspond quite well with results from other studies where chronic psychoses have been studied. Manfred Bleuler (1974) maintains that after five years the risk of relapse decreases. The illness seems to level out and become less dramatic. Both Bleuler (1972) and Ciompi (1980) found that around half of all patients with schizophrenia recover their health, while the rest develop a greater or a lesser handicap (Figure 11.3).

The American nurse and later professor of psychiatry C. Harding and her colleagues (1987) have made a well-known 30-year follow-up of over one hundred patients with chronic schizophrenia, discharged from a psychiatric hospital in Vermont, USA, when a number of wards were closed at the end of the 1950s. After their discharge, these patients, who were later rediagnosed as suffering from schizophrenia according to DSM-III criteria, had all been given a carefully thought out rehabilitation programme with residential, occupational and psychiatric aftercare. It transpired that 68 per cent of the previously chronic patients (from the beginning the study focused on patients with longstanding 'illness'), now lived what the author termed a 'full life' where they no longer had symptoms or were not significantly bothered by symptoms. They maintained good communication with other people and had meaningful occupations. Fifty per cent were still prescribed antipsychotic medication but only half of them actually took it. Many still had what can be called delusions or heard voices, but without being troubled

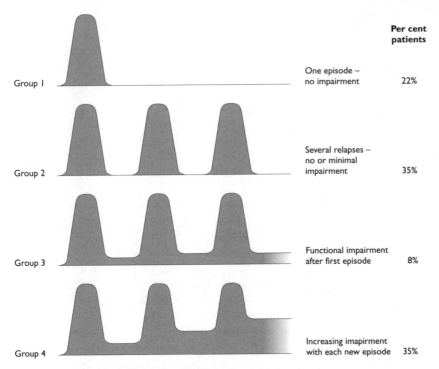

**Per cent
patients**

Group 1   One episode –
              no impairment   22%

Group 2   Several relapses –
              no or minimal
              impairment   35%

Group 3   Functional impairment
              after first episode   8%

Group 4   Increasing imapirment
              with each new episode 35%

Figure 11.3 Typical progress during the first five years after first presentation of schizophrenia (Shepherd *et al.* 1989).

by them. The study gives a significantly more hopeful picture of the prognosis of chronic schizophrenia than other studies, especially as it argues for
the importance of creating a thoroughgoing and long-term rehabilitation
programme in order to ensure good results (Figure 11.4). We still do not
know how many we might be able to help at an earlier stage with judicious
use of the many interventions available. But this study suggests that even late
interventions are valuable.

Schizophreniform disorder

Nowadays this diagnosis only appears in DSM-IV. It refers to an attempt to
define a subgroup of patients with schizophrenic symptoms who had a good
prognosis. According to DSM-IV, the diagnosis schizophreniform psychosis
is made when the schizophrenic symptoms have been apparent for at least a
month and the symptoms, including the prodromal stage, have diminished
over a period of six months. However, its relationship to a schizophrenia
diagnosis is unclear. Is schizophreniform disorder a form of schizophrenia
that responds well to early interventions resulting in curtailment of the

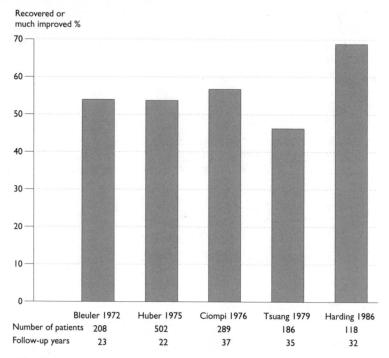

Recovered or
much improved %

	Bleuler 1972	Huber 1975	Ciompi 1976	Tsuang 1979	Harding 1986
Number of patients	208	502	289	186	118
Follow-up years	23	22	37	35	32

Figure 11.4 Five more or less contemporary long-term follow-ups of patients diagnosed with schizophrenia (Bleuler 1972; Huber *et al.* 1980; Ciompi 1980; Tsuang *et al.* 1979; Harding *et al.* 1987).

chronic disabling disease process? Or is the schizophreniform psychosis a different form of psychosis that carries a good prognosis irrespective of treatment? Both these interpretations seem possible.

Schizo-affective disorder – cycloid psychosis

The central feature of this disorder is the presence of symptoms of schizophrenia along with manic or depressive symptoms at the same time. There are specific diagnostic criteria. The schizophrenic symptoms should have been present for at least two weeks without prominent affective symptoms. However, the latter should be actively present during a significant part of the total period of the illness.

The diagnosis is often hard to make with any degree of reliability (i.e. in such a way that others would come to the same conclusion). There are many reasons. Are the affective symptoms significant enough? Are the psychotic symptoms in keeping with the criteria for schizophrenia? Is it more an affective psychosis, which can commonly feature bizarre psychotic symptoms in young adults? Or is it a schizophrenic psychosis which has presented initially with hypomanic excitation? This is not unusual and does not necessarily mean that the affective component will be an essential feature of the subsequent illness. These are questions to do with classification which can easily distract from the more important questions in terms of treatment: how great is the affective illness and how enduring will the schizophrenic symptoms become?

As with other psychotic conditions one should not make a definitive diagnosis before one or two years have passed. By then it is often possible to see if there is a chronic psychotic illness with functional disability or if it is a bipolar illness where the psychotic features are only significant during acute exacerbations, if at all. This distinction has important treatment implications for pharmacological treatments (long-term antipsychotics versus mood stabilisers) and assessment for psychotherapy.

German literature often refers to a *cycloid psychosis* in this connection. This diagnosis stresses the affective traits with the recurrent aspect of psychotic illness, the good recovery that occurs between psychoses, and the common incidence of affective illness in the family. A special feature is the often strong affective swing between euphoria or ecstatic feelings and the experience of horror ('Glück/Angst-Psychose').

The important fact is that schizo-affective psychoses often have a better prognosis than schizophrenia, in the sense that the residual disability is less in spite of the acute psychotic symptoms. However, the prognosis is not as good as that for bipolar disorder as some residual symptoms may be seen. A manic component in acute exacerbations may involve significant levels of arousal and aggression. For this reason, these acutely psychotic patients are among the most provocative to treat and often create mayhem on the ward: fellow patients can feel frightened and harassed. The schizo-affective disorder, in contrast with schizophrenia, often results in a favourable outcome with lithium treatment or similar drugs when combined with antipsychotics (see Chapter 24). For the description of a relevant case see Beth in Chapter 2.

Conclusion

Schizophrenia must be seen as a non-categorical concept, that is to say, diagnostic definitions according to DSM-IV and ICD-10 do not mirror the actual indistinct transition between normal and pathological seen in clinical practice. Similarly these definitions do not reflect the transitional forms between the different psychoses. The latter are in fact more common than the categorically described forms in DSM-IV and ICD-10.

It has been shown that the degree of bizarre thinking in psychoses (Schneider's first-rank symptoms) is not closely connected to the prognosis. There are also psychoses of a non-schizophrenic kind that can become chronic (for example, delusional disorder). The potential for change in relation to the clinical picture is also great during the first years, so there is good reason to use a *descriptive concept of psychosis* during this period instead of the prognostically all too negatively imbued concept of schizophrenia.

In 1984, Manfred Bleuler put together his vision of schizophrenia and maintained that perhaps there was no such thing as a single, specific cause. 'Schizophrenia represents a final adaptation after a long-term struggle to hold together different inconsistent aspects of the mind.' This internal perspective emphasises *the person* with schizophrenia, who might otherwise easily become lost within the diagnostic niceties. But it does not mean that the importance of biological vulnerability should be neglected.

The schizophrenia syndrome disorders consist in practice of an ill-defined group characterised by bizarre delusions, hallucinations, mild cognitive impairment and disorder of thought and behaviour. The syndromes usually develop over a considerable period, giving rise to a long-term functional disability – otherwise the disorder is known as schizophreniform. The idea that outcome is necessarily negative is, however, contradicted by a number of long-term follow-up studies showing that around half the cases have a good or fairly good prognosis. Evidence suggests that the prognosis can be influenced by early supportive as well as later rehabilitative work.

In practice, the diagnosis of schizophrenia often includes a mixture of three types of symptoms: positive symptoms (bizarre psychotic ideas), disorganisation symptoms (disorganised speech and behaviour) and negative symptoms (reduced motivation and long-term personality change). The presence of some of these factors in the first years of illness may lead to a premature diagnosis of schizophrenia. This is especially important in those whose negative symptoms are either marginal or actually secondary to medication, social isolation or understimulation. In such cases the label of schizophrenia can diminish both the extent of the treatment offered as well as the optimism of the patient, their family and the treating team. This pessimism can then become a self-fulfilling prophecy, inhibiting constructive therapeutic work and positive self-development.

Chapter 12

Autism spectrum disorders and childhood psychoses

It is important to give an overview of these conditions in order to illustrate the indistinct boundary between psychosis and non-psychosis. Adult patients with autistic spectrum disorder are still misdiagnosed as suffering from schizophrenia and consequently given inappropriate treatment. In 1943 the American Leo Kanner described a condition which he termed childhood autistic disorder. The children he described usually had a marked intellectual disability together with various disturbances of communication and interaction with other people: an autistic isolation. In 1944 the Austrian Hans Asperger described a similar syndrome except that the child was of normal intelligence or exceptionally gifted. It is still not clear whether these two syndromes represent variations of the same basic disorder or if they differ from one another. Today we work with a spectrum of autistic disorders. Our understanding of autism is far from complete: it is not clear if and how childhood autism corresponds to the autistic-like disorders which are found in schizophrenia. So it is important not to draw definitive conclusions with regard to childhood autism syndrome and adult schizophrenia. However, it does seem, at least with Asperger's syndrome, that there are cases of intellectually highly developed children who develop schizophrenia. Childhood autism has only been tentatively linked to childhood schizophrenia.

Up until the 1980s it was thought that these syndromes were to a large extent the fault of the mother for not having provided an emotionally satisfying relationship with her baby. The child would react by withdrawing into him or herself, and as a result their development would be severely disturbed. Consequently, the treatment would consist of the mother entering into psychotherapy. However, this theory has now been discounted. On the other hand, powerful tensions can occur in family relationships which may worsen the symptoms.

The suggestion that mothers 'cause' autism led to much suffering in families who were already suffering from the pain of having a child who is unable to make contact or who may be very difficult to care for. Treatment has now changed, offering support and educational advice for parents, siblings and teachers. There is still a need for individual therapy or family therapy in many of these cases, but often using behavioural or systemic approaches with the goal of reducing difficult behaviours.

Key features of the autistic syndrome

The autistic syndrome usually presents in affected children before the ages of two or three years old and can be detected by the following:

1 *Difficulty in normal social communication and interaction.* Certain children are especially easy to care for from the beginning and need very little extra attention. Others can be extremely difficult to please and cry day and night. They avoid eye contact and do not respond by stretching out their arms to their parents to be picked up and held. They do not reciprocate smiles or cuddling and do not play with other children.

2 *Disturbances in the development of speech.* These children have a diminished understanding of language and their speech has a marked concreteness. Half of children with autism never learn to speak. Around 80 per cent of this group are learning disabled. Certain autistic children have circumscribed skills such as being able to learn long pieces by heart, sing songs, etc. in a mechanical way.

3 *Behavioural disturbances.* The autistic child has a strong dislike of change and is often acutely obsessed by rituals that they feel obliged to perform. Hand waving and other stereotypical and repetitive physical movements are common. These may take the place of imaginative play which is often absent or impaired. For example, an autistic child may arrange toys in rows rather than play with them. Strong affective reactions occur if regular routines or the environment are disturbed; for example, if a vase is moved from its usual place or if a mealtime is changed. Many children become obsessed by a specific object such as a tuft of hair or a flashing toy car and will constantly carry such objects with him or her, sometimes until adulthood. It is important to remember that this is a heterogeneous group of individuals and that many have a lively and sensitive appearance in spite of their low functional ability.

Epidemiology and aetiology

Infantile autism is relatively common – about one child per 1000 develops this disorder. For this diagnosis symptoms from all three categories described above must be present and onset must be before the age of three. If the diagnosis is widened to autistic spectrum disorders, which only include two of the three criteria outlined above, the group becomes five to seven times larger.

Around a third of all children with autism develop epilepsy during their lives. Their autistic symptoms often diminish during later childhood but they are still unlikely to live independently. Many different causes of non-specific brain damage have been found in many of these patients. Certain chromosomal abnormalities have also been identified in some sufferers. As with schizophrenia in adults, it is assumed that it is not a question of a simple cause or set of causes.

Asperger's syndrome

Asperger's syndrome is differentiated from autism by the absence of learning disability (an IQ greater than 70). People suffering from this disorder have also been described as suffering from high-functioning autism. The syndrome cannot be diagnosed before the age of two or three years. Key features include indifference to contact, eccentric behaviour and speech, and a lack of emotional responsiveness. The symptoms can be summarised as follows:

1 *Disturbances in relationships with others and indifference to interaction* with a lack of understanding of what others think and feel. On the whole, their capacity to fantasise is poor. These children cannot play with other children and appear aloof or eccentric.
2 *The development of speech is normal* or very good in specific areas, but their *understanding of language* and symbolic comprehension is *concrete*. If a person with this handicap is asked if he can help move a chair he will answer 'yes', but doesn't understand that he is meant to move the chair. He only hears the concrete question and not the implicit requirement. Speech can be *monotonous or scanning* with unusual use of grammar. Some learn to speak several languages fluently.
3 *They develop restricted, repetitive and stereotyped patterns of interests.* They can learn bus timetables, mythology or military history to the exclusion of other interests. They may have a remarkable memory, particularly for their specific interests.
4 Some of these children also have marked *motor clumsiness.*

Epidemiology

Asperger's syndrome is not sharply distinguished from what might be termed normal but can, in its less disabling forms, be seen as a variation in personality.[1] It is important not to be too ready to diagnose Asperger's syndrome. The idiosyncrasies of children can all too easily be labelled as an expression of pathology, which might lead to rejection instead of supplying the support necessary for adaptive development.

The syndrome occurs in three to ten per 1000 children. It is three or four more times as common in boys. The prognosis is usually good in that most are able to look after themselves in adulthood and some can do well in professions where there is no specific demand for a deep involvement with others. A few will manage to form and sustain a partnership and have children. All the same, during puberty some individuals with Asperger's can deteriorate psychically and it is not unusual to find a psychosis developing. For instance, it can happen as a result of the young person having been misunderstood or frustrated over a long period of time. These people should not be given neuroleptic medication. As adults, they can sometimes be wrongly diagnosed as borderline psychotic, paranoid schizoid or the like. Presumably many with Asperger's syndrome are hidden behind what is known as 'simple schizophrenia', causing them to be treated painfully and fruitlessly with neuroleptic medication.

Postulated causal factors include genetic damage or chromosomal damage as well as insults to the foetus during the mother's pregnancy. However, the findings in the area are as non-specific as those in schizophrenia.

Schizophrenia in children and other psychoses

Schizophrenia is very unusual before the age of ten years, however cases have been described in five-year-old children. In one study by Baron *et al.* (1983) it was found that 14 per cent of all patients with schizophrenia develop symptoms before the age of 14 years and 55 per cent after they are 20 years old. As with adults, it is often difficult to identify the exact time at which the schizophrenic psychosis first develops. Retrospective reports from family may misidentify normal phenomena as pathological or vice versa, making these estimates unreliable.

The main symptoms are the same as for adult schizophrenia: hallucinations, delusions and behavioural disturbances. The prognosis is similar to the one we have found in adult psychiatry with a quarter recovering, half improving and a quarter unimproved. However, those who become ill before 10 years old suffer a worse prognosis (Eggers 1978, 1989). There are also organic causes of psychosis which are relatively specific to childhood and adolescence. These include viral infections such as infectious mononucleosis and encephalitis. They tend to cause a more benign, affect-laden psychosis.

Today, during adolescence, *toxic psychoses* are increasingly common. They are triggered by central nervous system stimulants such as cannabis, ecstasy, etc. An acute onset with visual hallucinations together with paranoid delusions suggests a drug-induced psychosis. It is important not to forget that there is a growing body of evidence that cannabis misuse increases the risk of subsequently developing schizophrenia (Allebeck *et al.* 1993).

The onset of first-episode psychosis in young people aged 15 to 18 presents the same diagnostic and prognostic dilemmas which are seen in other age groups, and have been described elsewhere in this book. This includes the problems with clarification of psychobiological vulnerability, and triggering factors, along with the classification of the symptomatology, diagnosis and subsequent choice of methods of treatment.

Chapter 13

Delirium, confusion and organic psychosis

This chapter gives an overview of the conditions that can be confused with what is traditionally called *functional psychosis*, the forms of psychosis which have been defined in earlier chapters. The essential difference is that the symptoms result from an identifiable organic disturbance or from damage to the central nervous system (CNS). The concept of delirium is used to cover these conditions both in DSM-IV and ICD-10. In Scandinavia it is closely associated with delirium tremens and 'confusion' is often used as a synonym.

Characteristic symptoms of delirium according to DSM-IV and ICD-10

1 *Fluctuating level of consciousness* with a diminished capacity to concentrate and to maintain attention.
2 *Cognitive impairment with disturbances of memory and orientation.* Disorientation not only affects the sense of time but often also affects the sense of space and person as well. Patients are not sure of the date, where they are or whom they are talking to. In contrast, awareness of self-identity is not usually disturbed.
3 *Disturbance of perception* with illusions or hallucinations. These may vary from fleeting ill-formed illusions to distinct visual hallucination (auditory and tactile hallucinations can also occur). Visual hallucinations are strongly suggestive of an organic cause of psychotic symptoms.
4 The condition develops rapidly and tends to *fluctuate in intensity* during the day. Often the night proves to be the most disturbed time.
5 The condition is caused by *CNS disturbance* due to a medical illness, brain damage, poisoning, alcohol or drug intoxication or withdrawal.

The degree of alertness may be heightened, reduced or unchanged. This will also often fluctuate. The visual hallucinations are vivid, and in this sense they differ from hallucinations that usually occur in the functional psychoses. In schizophrenia visual hallucinations are sometimes reported but they are usually less distinct and less intricate: for example, a light, the effect of a ray of light, a shape, and so on. This contrasts with complex, realistic and intense visual hallucinations that the delirious person can experience. They may feature anything from dancing girls to huge spiders that try to creep into the bed or snakes which lunge at you out of a television screen.

The combination of tactile and visual hallucinations can bring with it anxious fidgeting which may be a response to the need to pick off the insects felt to be creeping over the skin. In acute delirium the person is deeply involved with and terrified by his experiences. Hallucinations are often of a 'protean' type in that they can continually change. Objects, textures or spaces multiply, change size and colour, disappear and reappear – the kinds of experiences which many of us have lived through during a high fever.

Auditory hallucinations are fairly impersonal. In this way they differ from the commentating voices heard by the person with schizophrenia which want to control and influence. Pieces of music playing or a voice singing a melody are common. After the acute phase the experiences may persist even though the patient is no longer delirious. This is seen in alcoholic hallucinosis where auditory hallucinations persist in the absence of the other signs of confusion seen in delirium tremens.

Transient hallucinations and delusions can create potentially dangerous situations on medical wards. They can result in the patient trying to abscond or even throw himself out of the window in order to be free of his persecutors, whether they are people or animals. Other clinical findings can include a moderate *increase in temperature, sweating* and restlessness. Sometimes a light or moderate *tremor* can be detected. Emotionally the person may also fluctuate between feeling dispirited, irritable, fearful, and sometimes euphoric.

Perplexity is characteristic of confusional states. It features musing, uncertainty and a lack of recognition of his or her environment. He or she can stand around, contemplating a passer-by with questioning, empty eyes, perhaps pleading for some answer as to what is really happening or asking why something is being done in a particular way. He or she may reveal fears of impending mistreatment, execution or a great catastrophe.

Causes of confusional states

Confusion can be characterised as a non-specific reaction to an underlying deterioration in the functioning of the brain. The corollary of this is that many different causes have the same final common endpoint – the confusional state. Medical causes include the following:

1   *Pathological changes associated with ageing.* In old age *arteriosclerosis* is common and results in a reduction in blood supply to the brain. This

can be exacerbated by a fall in blood pressure at night. Heart failure can, for the same reason, produce confusion.

2   After an *epileptic seizure*, confusional states can occur (post-ictal confusion). Rarely the person can behave mechanically (automatism) and assault others. More commonly classical confusion is seen together with agitation. Temporal lobe epilepsy can cause hallucinations in any sensory modality.

3   *Intracranial infections* such as encephalitis (infection of the brain tissue), meningitis (infection of the brain's covering, the meninges) and abscesses can all cause confusion. Head injury can result in a broad range of intracranial pathologies, including gross brain tissue injury (with or without skull fracture), intracranial haemorrhages, and generalised microscopic damage (known as diffuse axonal injury). Infections elsewhere in the body may be severe enough to impair cerebral function, especially in the elderly. Common examples include pneumonia and urinary tract infections.

4   In *metabolic disorders* there are significant changes in the blood concentrations of biochemically active compounds and/or their toxic waste products. Examples of such biochemically active compounds would include glucose, calcium and sodium. Examples of toxic waste products include urea and ammonia. Metabolic disturbances may result from organ failure (e.g. high urea and potassium in kidney failure, high ammonia in liver failure) or from endocrine disease. Endocrine diseases produce disturbances in hormone levels which may in turn disturb metabolic or psychological factors. For example, a diabetic may become very dehydrated as a result of prolonged high blood glucose, or in an overactive thyroid extreme anxiety and agitation may occur.

5   *Intoxication or abstinence.* Alcohol and other substances that cause dependence such as benzodiazepines can produce delirium either as a result of direct intoxication or from sudden withdrawal. This may be complicated by malnutrition, dehydration, head injury and a specific vitamin deficiency (thiamine) which causes a specific form of brain injury (Wernicke-Korsakoff's syndrome).

6   *Hallucinogenic* substances such as LSD, cannabis, magic mushrooms, etc. have to be considered when young people present with delirium. Medication such as corticosteriods can produce confusional symptoms as well as affective psychoses, as can some medications, which reduce blood pressure. The same is true of medication for the treatment of Parkinson's disease as well as overdoses of anticholinergic medicines, used in the treatment of side effects of antipsychotic medication (see, for example, the case of Elizabeth in Chapter 2).

Common confusional states in hospitals

Post-operative confusion

This occurs in 20 to 30 per cent of people after major operations, especially heart and lung surgery. It may present with visual hallucinations alone, or persecutory delusions and secondary anxiety and arousal. Management involves reassurance, reality orientation, consistent nursing in a well-lit side room, and avoiding under- and overstimulation. A member of staff holding the patient's hand or talking to him about family members may offer an immediate relief. Low doses of benzodiazepines and/or antipsychotics may be needed if agitation cannot be contained, but runs the risk of worsening the confusion. The degree and length of the confusion is often connected to the use of narcotic analgesia and to the level of fear experienced by the patient prior to the operation, but may also be related to some of the causes described above and so warrants careful investigation.

'Queen Silvia is experimenting with patients'

Simon, a 60-year-old prominent Jewish civil servant, underwent major cardiac surgery. The evening before the operation he got into a small disagreement with the ward nurse, a woman who spoke with a German accent. Simon had the impression that she would be reluctant to give him enough medication to treat any post-operative pain. In the days after the operation, which had been carried out successfully, Simon developed — in his physiologically compromised condition — the belief that he was part of a cruel experiment. Outside his window he saw a poplar tree and so believed he had been made a prisoner on a Swedish country estate. He believed that he and the other surgical patients were to be exhibited at a conference, under the direction of Queen Silvia, as examples of how it was possible to operate without anaesthesia. When the staff came to care for him in his ward he complained bitterly that they had subjected him to an unethical experiment. The staff simply shook their heads and left. Simon decided that he must flee; from his bed he began to look for a means of escape through the window of his room.

His fellow patients began to ask him why he was inspecting the room in this way. As Simon explained, he became embarrassed as he realised that it was probably due to a delusion. Everyone laughed at the story. One of the other patients who had just undergone an operation suddenly looked serious. He pointed at the opening to the ventilation over the door and said that it was still a fact that strange things were happening in their room – all the people who had emerged from the hole and searched through his papers should not have been there.

COMMENTS

The confusion, which occurred while awake, was construed like a nightmare by this Jewish patient. The day's vestiges were incorporated into the delusions: the German nurse was symbolically construed as Sweden's German-born Queen Silvia. Post-operative confusion is not an unusual or remarkable condition as we can see from the fellow patient who did not understand that he too was experiencing 'hallucinations'. Neither did the staff understand what was happening, which is more worrying. If Simon had been left alone there was a risk that he might have detached himself from his drips and monitors and tried to abscond through the window.

Night-time confusion in older patients is often encountered in hospital. There are many theories as to its causes, including arteriosclerosis combined with low blood pressure resulting in a reduced cerebral blood supply. The illness(es) for which they have been admitted, cognitive impairment and the unfamiliar environment may also contribute. (for an example see the case of Elizabeth in Chapter 2).

The boundary between confusion and psychosis

The concepts of confusion and psychosis should not be mixed up. If the function of the brain is disturbed, *acute confusion* will be a direct and usually fairly non-specific consequence. Typical symptoms produced by disturbance in the brain are visual hallucinations, disorientation and alterations in level consciousness. With *psychoses* we have less reason to believe that the brain might primarily have been under acute physiological or toxic pressure. Here the personality is under psychological stress. The continuity of the self has been threatened by an anxiety-filled loss of control resulting in reparative attempts to create coherence with delusional explanations that ultimately lack rationality. The presence of a biological or psychological vulnerability lowers the threshold further, and psychosis develops more readily.

Sometimes we can see confusional components in psychoses and vice versa. In *acute schizophrenic psychoses* confusion can occur temporarily. It is usually seen as a prognostically good sign. *Short-term psychoses* may also have some features of acute confusion such as perplexity and loss of orientation. Sometimes symptoms of confusion could be a sign that a functional psychosis might be a misdiagnosis and that it is necessary to search carefully for an organic cause. It may be an endocrine disorder or a toxic reaction, perhaps due to medication. Occasionally it can be the first sign of a brain tumour or a brain metastasis. This diagnostic uncertainty underlines the importance of a thorough medical investigation when assessing a patient with first-episode psychosis.

However, it may result from a combination of psychological and organic stressors, for example, in long-term alcoholism, perhaps following a divorce or during a holiday alone in a warm country complicated by dehydration and diarrhoea. In these situations a combination of paranoid and confusional symptoms is common. Figure 13.1 demonstrates a multifactorial way of thinking even with organically determined states, where the physical factor is an essential cause, but where confusion can be worsened or strengthened by the person's emotional state and the lack of containment in the social environment.

It would be an oversimplification to say that confusion corresponds to a disturbance in the hardware of a computer – its mechanism – while psychosis is a disorder in the software which is insufficiently or wrongly programmed. Ultimately the brain and the psyche are inseparable. We have no knowledge of a consciousness that functions separately from a biological substratum. The brain and the psyche cannot be translated into each other in spite of the dreams of those who research into the workings of the brain. There is an epistemological abyss between mind and brain which we are, as yet, unable to bridge. In spite of this, modern psychiatry strives towards a monistic view of the human mind.

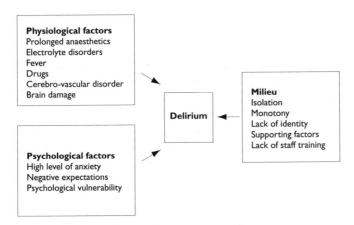

Figure 13.1 Model of interacting causes in organically based deliria.

Chapter 14

The two critical periods in psychosis and the potential for recovery

When, as staff on the wards, we meet someone who has developed a psychosis for the first time, one should be cautious about making an absolute diagnosis (McGorry 1994). The overall picture of symptoms change, the affective aspects diminish or become more marked, and delusions can suddenly resolve as the patient finds his way out of his psychotic world. Alternatively the psychosis can worsen with increasing difficulties in making contact. At one time catatonic symptoms may be prominent while at another paranoid symptoms may dominate.

Even if the acute symptoms prove important for making decisions about immediate treatment and what level of care is indicated, experience still points to the fact that acute psychoses resolve, sooner or later, except in rare cases. The traditional way of treating psychosis has, for better or for worse, been entirely directed towards treating and containing the psychotic state. However, our more recent knowledge suggests that the acute psychosis is flanked by two critical periods, each in their own way demands serious consideration:

1   The period preceding psychiatric treatment must be made as short as possible in order to diminish the psychological and social damage caused by the psychosis, that is to say, *the time from the inception of prodromal symptoms.*

2   In order to lessen the risk of relapse, *the period after the superficial healing of the psychotic symptoms has occurred* is just as important. Here, the traumatised vision of the self as well as the damage to the social network must be repaired. An understanding of what has occurred must be integrated within the personality including insight into possible new prodromal symptoms, to ensure that steps are taken to prevent a relapse. These are hard tasks, but they are essential for prognostic reasons. In this part an overview will be given of the two periods (see Figure 14.1). They will be discussed in greater detail in Part II.

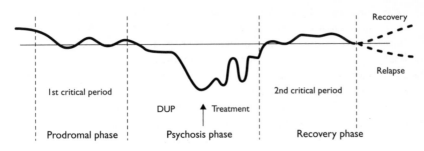

Figure 14.1 A psychosis model – the critical periods of a psychosis.

The first critical period: prodromal symptoms and untreated psychosis

In most cases the person experiences a clear breakdown in his or her self-experience and this occurs within a range of a few weeks to some years before the onset of psychosis. Prodromal symptoms express themselves first and foremost in an increase of mental distress and a diminished ability to relate to others and to live up to the requirements of school and work.

In the case of a more slowly developing psychosis an almost imperceptible transition can take place where the normally perhaps shy and slightly eccentric person presents with a prodromal condition which by degrees turns into a manifest psychosis. As explained in Chapter 11, for some people who are diagnosed with schizophrenia (DSM-IV) it is possible to find – if careful attention is paid to their developmental and personal history – that the person has been impaired since early childhood by difficulties in making friends and in dealing with the normal expectations of school.

It is important that too much time must not be allowed to pass between the first psychotic symptoms and the time when the patient is offered adequate psychiatric help (*duration of untreated psychosis DUP*). A psychosis that continues month after month, even if it is mild and does not demand immediate psychiatric intervention, will result in increased isolation and will reinforce delusions, which can make a complete recovery more difficult.

More recent theories on the neurobiology of psychosis suggest that untreated psychosis may have a toxic neurodegenerative effect on the brain, resulting in a more chronic illness (Verdoux and Cougnard 2003). Scientific corroboration for this has not been available. This hypothesis originates from the common clinical observation that an increased DUP is associated with a worse prognosis (Loebel *et al.* 1992). A reasonable alternative explanation for this is that those who are treated at a late stage have lost contact with more of their psychosocial network and become isolated.

There is much to suggest that these patients represent a subgroup with less acute positive symptoms, more negative symptoms and more neuro-psychological disorders. It also appears that their response to antipsychotic medication is poor. It may be for a combination of these reasons that they have a worse prognosis than those who develop a more acute type of illness do and who are treated more quickly.

In a concrete biological view a 'toxic psychosis' presupposes that a toxic or other damaging biological process would be created by the psychotic symptoms.[1] We do not know of any such 'psychosis-toxins'. Such ideas have been launched through lecture campaigns by the pharmaceutical industry's experts, who maintain that immediate neuroleptic treatment is the essential form of treatment in psychosis. On the other hand, presumably with pro-dromal symptoms, early intervention is of significance in order to put a stop to illness which might occur later on, especially in the case of those forms of schizophrenia which are manifest early on in perceptual disorders, lowering of function, etc. (see Chapter 21).

The second critical period: the recovery process – rebuilding hope

Of those with a first-episode psychosis 75 per cent recover within a few months or years. All the same, most people remain anxious for years about those experiences that have not been worked through, during or after the period of the illness. In the same way family and colleagues might find it difficult to talk about the painful events which have happened and an 'unseen wall' often builds up around the person. In some cases it can mean that the supportive network dwindles and the risk of relapse increases.

Many – around 70 per cent of those who have suffered a first-episode psychosis – will relapse if they do not have appropriate interventions. When residual symptoms are present, relapse is very likely during the first or second years and so antipsychotic medication is indicated. Various psycho-therapeutic interventions have significant effects during the period after psychosis. Psycho-education such as teaching the patient to note early signs of relapse are useful, as well as helping the family to gain greater insight into and understanding of what has happened. Psychotherapy of a dynamic and cognitive nature can give an increased sense of self-awareness and an ability to work on key experiences, as well as working through depressive problems or residual hallucinations and delusions. The goals are however usually more limited than when used for 'neurotic disorders'. Usually the kind of psychotherapy offered contains, to varying degrees, different components of these forms of assistance according to the patient's needs and capacities. See Part II for further details.

What needs to be healed?

The work that lies ahead for someone suffering with psychosis can seem insurmountable:

- The trauma encountered within the self should heal. As we shall see (p. 186), often what is known as a *post-traumatic stress disorder* occurs after an acute psychosis. Working through here concerns the reparation of a destroyed vision of the world. The myth concerning the view of the self as invulnerable, which was previously clung to, no longer protects. The psychosis itself has been such a traumatic factor. Another is the potential damage to the personal integrity, which may have been incurred during hospitalisation such as the fear evoked by being forced into intimate dealing with others who are mentally ill.
- The impaired *relationships with family* and *colleagues* must be restored. Increased loneliness is often present.
- One may need help or treatment for any *residual symptoms* such as hallucinations and delusions, anxiety and depression.
- Careful review of *prescribed neuroleptic medication* is necessary: the doses may be too high or medication may continue for too long. Others can be mistakenly left *untreated* when medication might have proved necessary to restore functional capacity.

Requirements of treatment

The first requirement necessary for competent treatment is the awareness that knowledge of the person's psychological world is no less important with psychotic conditions than it is with other disorders. Here, as with other conditions, we find behind the symptoms defensive and adaptive mechanisms, unconscious conflicts, a need for improved self-esteem and help to find the motivation for change (i.e. personality traits). Insight into these aspects influences the outcome. Dynamic functioning is tied up with vulnerability and eventual cognitive functional disabilities. The implication is that (along with Eugen Bleuler and others) we must view psychotic symptoms as dynamic attempts to adapt to the underlying vulnerability factors.

An important psychological experience that we have realised from working in this field is that alongside psychotic functioning one often finds a non-psychotic part of the personality that one must try to co-operate with directly or indirectly. This non-psychotic part may have to be inferred: for example, in a patient with intense, complex persecutory delusions who, in spite of their denial of mental illness, presents themselves to mental health services, often for non-psychiatric reasons requesting help.

Another requirement for successful treatment is that one should realise the *importance of encouraging optimism*. Comparative psychotherapy research shows that the capacity to maintain a realistic hope is the most powerful single therapeutic factor behind a successful therapist–patient relationship (Luborsky *et al.* 1975). There is also a positive relationship between the encouragement of hope and the ability to maintain a biological immunity to infection and other somatic healing processes (Solomon 1987). Even if we do not know how immunity plays its protective role in the recovery of acute psychoses, it gives us insight into the psycho-physiological significance of hope as a vitalising factor. We must think too of the unacceptable fact that many handicapped people with schizophrenia live their lives impoverished by the lack of hope and motivation. For that reason research into these factors is significant for improving rehabilitation.

The psychiatrist John S. Strauss (1989) has provided a longitudinal interview series with patients after the onset of acute psychosis. He differentiates three typical patterns (Figure 14.2) encountered in 'coping' procedures that appear after an acute period of psychosis:

- the low turning point
- 'woodshedding'
- a fluctuating course.

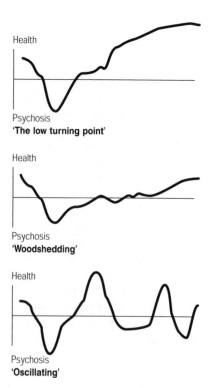

Figure 14.2 Three types of progress – freely adapted from Strauss (1989: 22–28).

The low turning point

This state contains a classic response to a crisis. It is often applicable where a breakdown into an acute psychosis has occurred as a result of a clearly defined cause. Sometimes it is quite easy to see how, before the psychosis, the person had maladaptive personality traits which were functioning less and less efficiently with the increasing demands of their situation. Eventually with an acute stressor a psychotic *disintegration* occurs. This is followed by a *reorganisation* where, in some cases, a more flexible organisation of the personality is built up during the subsequent process of working through. Within psychiatry we see this happen more often than is acknowledged. It is our job as carers to maintain within ourselves a life-affirming attitude of meaning and coherence, so that we – even without words – can inspire a 'vicarious hope' in those who need it. In our treatment of the patient, we attempt to help both the patient and his closest family to internalise such an attitude.

Sometimes we can see how closely interwoven the breakdown is with the adaptive process of rehabilitation. It is even possible to ask, in certain cases, whether the psychosis might have represented a potential impetus for the development of their personality in the future. Someone who is stuck in deadlocked, enmeshed and dependent relationships may need to encounter a crisis in order for the personality to alter or grow. Similarly those around them may need a crisis to enable them to recognise and change their habitual roles.

Such an attitude is very important when it comes to finding a meaningful perspective from which to offer hope in the face of a psychotic illness. Of course, this does not mean taking a romantic attitude towards the psychosis as something desirable in itself. Psychosis is a painful and deeply hazardous state of disorganisation. However, in certain cases it can bring with it a remarkably positive development, which could hardly have happened without the psychotic reaction. But, usually it also requires long-term psychotherapeutic work following on the recovery from the psychotic crisis (for example, see the case of Beth in Chapter 2). Without this there is a risk of distorted forms of healing.

Woodshedding

'Woodshedding' is a term used by American jazz musicians who, when they wanted to practise together, used to gather in a hut in the woods where they could play uninterrupted, until they felt they had achieved their aim. The expression is close to the concept of 'moratorium'. It denotes something like a waiting or rest period necessary for developing something new, where life makes as few demands or expectations as possible – but without loss of hope.

As soon as the patient has improved he or she can sink into a low state of functioning for a long time, perhaps for years. This plateau phase often occurs after the patient has left the hospital. The patient himself, together with his carers and family, wonders if he is ever going to get well again. Sometimes improvement can take place in small steps, interrupted by occasional relapses. However, if looked at more closely, it can be seen how the patient at times begins more frequently to talk to others, or take up new activities, how self-esteem begins to grow, lingering symptoms become less bothersome and the person's identity no longer consists of being primarily a mentally ill person. Return to work or study begins to take on a new importance. There are two key risks in this period: on the one hand, the patient never dares to leave the unproductive plateau phase but remains within it and on the other he or she is rushed out of it much too quickly, resulting in a relapse.

Measured in psychiatric terms it can look as though negative symptoms such as apathy and indifference are dominant, and there is a risk that the condition is judged to be chronic all too quickly. Behind what one might see as a sign of a serious functional disability is hidden the ongoing, albeit fragile, healing process.

One must be aware that introversion may be the expression of low self-esteem rather than simply negative symptoms. Another and more positive way of looking at this state can be by seeing the person as intuitively decreasing his contact with the environment in order to protect himself against disaster, excessive demands and too much stimulation. It is obviously hard to define what exactly might constitute a reasonable and adaptive degree of introversion as protection against the risk of increased or new psychotic symptoms. In any case one should be aware that recovery following a psychosis can take many years.

The woodshedding phase can take place under the protection of supportive family members and friends or in a psychotherapeutic residential home. Ideally every patient will be given time and the expectations of treatment will relate to the person's ability and situation. It can also take place alone, but the risk that the person might get caught up in a vicious circle of understimulation and isolation will be greater. With today's brief treatment periods and lack of sufficient psychotherapeutic resources, it is not easy to find places where such a recovery can take place. Ensuring a positive interest in an active support system for woodshedding is of great importance. Perhaps the greatest enemy still found in psychiatry is a pessimistic attitude towards psychoses. Such an attitude does not just obstruct investment in therapeutic environments but damages the patient's will to improve as well.

Medication or rehabilitation

Joanna had gone through a turbulent adolescence. She had tried out several different training courses none of which proved fulfilling. When she was about 20 years old she began to isolate herself more and more. Delusions about being poisoned developed and she believed that she was being followed and dared not go out. For long periods she withdrew into herself. Clearly defined hallucinations did not occur. She was admitted to a psychiatric clinic and treated with higher and higher doses of antipsychotic medication without any noticeable effect, even in depot form. Joanna did not want to take the medication, but the doctor did not dare comply with her wish. As the situation became more entrenched and a chronic illness began to take hold, her parents contacted a psychotherapeutically orientated treatment clinic to which Joanna was admitted. She wanted to get better by seeking insight into herself. As it turned out, her admission lasted for three years while her state of mind fluctuated, and the medication was slowly reduced to a low dose. Joanna was helped to make friends with the other patients and she was allowed to start training for a few hours a day as an office worker. Eventually she moved to her own home.

A fluctuating course

A rapidly fluctuating illness can be even more difficult to contain, both for the patient and for the carer. In these cases it is all the more important to see how the biological and dynamic factors are woven together and may influence each other in a progressive worsening. Some people alternate between complete health and acute psychosis. These fluctuations can sometimes happen quickly and frequently while at other times they can occur after long intervals. Sometimes the process is best understood from a biological point of view – especially with bipolar disorder where treatment with lithium or other mood stabilisers can often effectively control these fluctuations.

Sometimes the biological factor may easily be triggered by psychosocial conditions. A deep-seated lack of self-confidence together with a personality disorder reinforces behaviour that might be seen by others as senselessly oppositional, and the resulting crisis triggers an acute depressive reaction which in its turn may develop into psychosis. In other people a 'neurotic' inability to tolerate success can create a heightened anxiety towards a very positive state of affairs. This may trigger or contribute to an episode of bipolar illness.

Sometimes you meet people who, just after they have 'hit the bottom', can 'allow themselves' to accept the help which is offered. This can be seen as a form of self-inflicted punishment. It can be seen in gifted people who have strong guilt feelings perhaps related to drug misuse or antisocial activities.

On 'hitting rock bottom'

A 25-year-old woman came to the acute psychiatric outpatient's reception with an acute psychosis, which had been worsened by occasional substance abuse. Many times over the past seven years she had presented in a similar state, sometimes after having made suicide attempts. She was a gifted person with a borderline personality disorder and a tendency towards psychosis. On numerous occasions she had been offered psychotherapeutic help by a psychologist at the hospital but each time she refused it. However, on this occasion she agreed to come for regular talks. This became the start of a very stormy five-year psychotherapy, during which she managed to regain her health and reached a degree of social functioning. When she was asked in a follow-up examination why she had not accepted help earlier, she replied, 'It was not the right time. I had to feel that I had reached the bottom line. From there I would only have one way to go.' It transpired during her psychotherapy that when she had been a child she had suffered incestuous abuse. These memories were suppressed resulting in an unbearable diffuse feeling of guilt and shame. Only when she broke down completely was she able to allow herself to accept help.

The defence mechanism of *denial* can also interfere if a biological fluctuating mechanism is dominant. Many find it difficult to recognise that they have suffered a psychosis in the past. Instead they turn away from reality or maintain that they have been the subject of other people's abuse. As a result it is hard for them to seek psychiatric help when signs of relapse develop. In such a fluctuating situation there is a demand, not just for medical assistance, but also for support along with educational and psychotherapeutic interventions in order to overcome the denial. The person must get to know his or her biological and psychological vulnerability in order to help the development of better ways of dealing with the illness.

Many who talk about a 'turning point' in their illness return to this state when they decide actively to counter their illness rather than let themselves passively continue in a pathological spiral. The question as to what it is that constitutes the conditions for such a turning point is a central one in psychiatry. It can certainly not be simply 'determined' from outside. In a positive sense, to tire of dependence on inner destructive forces and to decide to depend on one's own potential is a process which sometimes bears a resemblance to Christian parables of conversion. Often the event is conveyed through a personal relationship with a carer, a partner or someone who believes in the person's potential and who does so at the right time. Not enough research has been done on these questions.

We still do not know to what degree it is possible to counter the functional disabilities that occur later on in schizophrenia as a result of optimal early support and well thought out rehabilitation. The results of most treatment that we see today lie well below an acceptable level – and this is not just because we are awaiting better medication. Above all, we have reason to be optimistic when we see good results in individual cases that have received an early intervention together with sensitively prescribed medication and the provision of a therapeutic environment over a long-term period with the appropriate resources for rehabilitation.

Chapter 15

Cognitive disorders and the psychotic thought process

Dear Servants
I cannot get any peace here in this institution because of Nurse A's gentle care. Her mild eyes persecute me day and night. Can you not take me to a rough place? I would prefer to go the following way: twenty stabs in the stomach (big and small), clinical treatment from Dr. Brünicke (suicide anticlinical), active service, being drilled through the back hole and up out through the front passage with a sword, then crucifixion to a tree, finally, a duel in Skagen [a small town in Denmark] followed by deep cuts made by a doctor's hand or a clinician, having my right leg sawn off high up as well as being thrown to the lions and being boiled alive. I am a little unsure about this way but naturally I am always at your service.

Signature
Quoted from Rosenbaum and Sonne 1986

This letter, written some fifty years ago by a patient with schizophrenia, is an example of how a formally correct letter can express a strange distortion in the relationship between the sender and the recipient. One assumes that warm feelings for a nurse had been awakened in the author. These feelings are painful for him for unknown reasons and he wants to be moved to a stricter place and to be given the most terrible punishment – perhaps to prevent his further seduction. He starts with a soft tone where he seeks help, but by the end of the letter he is discussing the different aspects of his execution in the tone of a formal and relaxed businessman. The letter also shows how bizarre distortions of thinking may be revealing of the existential position of the writer.

What is a thought disorder?

Both Emil Kraepelin and Eugen Bleuler maintained that the basic disorder in a patient with schizophrenia is an organically determined disorganisation in thought processes (see Chapter 11). Kraepelin maintained that what was primarily at stake was disturbance in memory. The concept, dementia praecox (a term meaning early dementia), is an expression of this, but in later publications of his textbook he emphasised instead the decisive deficit of attention and will.

Bleuler suggested that the primary factor in the illness was an organic disorder, which affected the sufferer's thinking in such a way that loosened or split associations occurred. The mental apparatus worked through or later interprets this primary disorder by forming psychotic symptoms (delusions and hallucinations) or protects itself with an autistic withdrawal from the world. Both Bleuler and Kraepelin wrote that a lowering of a cognitive level (that is, the capacity to think and organise perception) occurred in nearly all cases, although Kraepelin tended to place emphasis on a rapid progression of dementia. This view, put forward in the first decades of the 1900s, greatly contributed to the pessimistic attitude towards schizophrenia. It is a view that has been taken over especially by the neo-Kraepelin-inspired DSM-IV diagnosis, which includes a long-term functional handicap in the criteria for diagnosing schizophrenia.

State and trait phenomena

When a person is acutely psychotic their interest is not directed towards the outside world. Instead, they are more or less preoccupied with delusions and hallucinations. The psychosis is a temporary condition, a *state phenomenon*. Any observer can see that a psychotic person, with their disturbed awareness of what constitutes reality for others, will express a number of deviations in thinking and responding to a conversation in a neuropsychological test situation. A more difficult problem concerns the degree that *trait phenomenon*, that is, the long-term functional disability which occurs prior to the breakdown into psychosis and persists *after* recovery, is an expression of the cognitive disorder. These cognitive disorders affect day-to-day interactions and so further increase the stress which can trigger psychosis.

Research into schizophrenic symptoms can lead to contradictory conclusions unless care is taken to avoid undue generalisation. There are psychotic conditions that become a lifetime disability and others which appear to have a good prognosis, and yet both fulfil the criteria for schizophrenia. The problem lies with how to distinguish between them from the outset.

Another problem is the influence that antipsychotic *medication* has on cognitive abilities, especially neuroleptics, and those medications which treat extra pyramidal side effects. Patients can be on high doses in a given situation and in another be given no medication at all. Most reports, as well as clinical experience, suggest that classical neuroleptics particularly influence attention, concentration and processing speed. The medication's effect on cognition in schizophrenia can be positive in low doses but essentially negative at high doses. The so-called new neuroleptics have a slightly different profile (see the section on pharmacology, Chapter 24, for further details). In the literature on schizophrenia spectrum disorders concerning *cognitive capacity* (the ability to think), impaired function has been described in the following areas:

* memory
* concentration
* processing speed
* precision of thinking
* attending to simultaneous tasks.

At the same time, specific disorders are found in *the structure of thought and in its contents*:

* logical errors in thinking, syntax and expressive language use
* impaired abstract thinking and reflective (meta-) thinking, i.e. thinking about one's own or other people's way of thinking
* fixed and rigid patterns of thinking resulting in 'unreasonable attitudes'.

I will now touch on the current 'neuro-cognitive' research, centring on the two first points, in order to distinguish discrepant contents of thinking.

Neuro-cognition and schizophrenia

An objective, biologically determined discrepancy specific to schizophrenia has long been sought, but so far without success. However, certain psycho-physiological findings have repeatedly been recorded in schizophrenic research. Unfortunately whilst these markers are relatively sensitive for detecting schizophrenia, they are non-specific (i.e. they are present in non-schizophrenic individuals frequently enough to prevent them used as discriminating signs). Examples include:

* *Pre-pulse inhibition (PPI)*. We know that everybody jumps and blinks when they are suddenly surprised by a loud noise. However, this reaction is diminished if, just before the loud noise, a soft less surprising noise is heard. This inhibiting of the reaction of surprise is less marked in schizo-phrenic people. One explanation for this is that their sensory threshold is constantly lowered and so they have difficulty in adapting to new events. (Pre-psychotic people often describe strong sensory impressions.)
* *'Eye-tracking'* is another finding. People with schizophrenia have diffi-culty in smoothly tracking a moving object with their eyes in the way that a healthy person does; instead their eyes move in a jerky manner. Furthermore, it has been found that 40 per cent of relatives of first-time sufferers of schizophrenia have the same problem. In other words, there is a genetic factor which is as yet undefined. Naturally, this kind of finding must be researched further.

There are numerous methods for testing cognitive functioning. When the results from these studies – known as intelligence tests – are gathered together, a general diminishment of intelligence quota (IQ) can be found in groups of patients with schizophrenia. Even though intelligence is a somewhat controversial concept because of the contribution of cultural and educational factors, precise and replicable neuropsychological tests have been designed. The best known is the Wechsler Adult Intelligence Test (WAIS), which assesses different aspects of cognitive function. There is good evidence to suggest that diminished cognitive functioning makes social life more difficult. Those diagnosed as schizophrenic often present the following cognitive deficits (Green 1988):

1 *The ability to process sensory data arising from the external world is diminished* at an early stage in the perceptual process. This results in difficulties in maintaining a stable inner representation of a percept as these are easily altered by other percepts or illusions.

2 *The ability to maintain concentration is diminished.* This has been calculated by observing a person's reactions to certain signals over varying periods of time. For example, he or she must react to a specific number that is briefly displayed but not react to others.

3 *Disturbances of memory* both in terms of long-term memory and in terms of what is called working memory. The latter can be studied in many ways, for example, by attempting to match a symbol, memorised a few seconds previously, with its likeness in a mixed group with other symbols.

4 *Executive functions* refer to both planning and problem solving as well as the ability to alter approaches to thinking and to alternate between assignments. This is a complex area with many different aspects. One of these aspects is the ability to 'set shift', that is to move from one set of rules to another. One method of researching this complex function is with the Wisconsin Card Sorting Test (WCST; see Figure 15.1). Here, the subject has to match different cards. The matching is done according to one of either shape, colour or number, but the subject must work out which rule is currently being applied by the tester (for example, matching

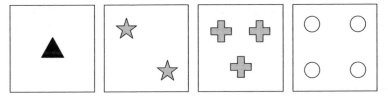

Figure 15.1 Wisconsin Card Sorting Test (WCST). Examples of cards that are sorted by colours, form and number of symbols.

by colour) and be able to follow alterations in the rules. Damage to the frontal lobe results in difficulty with this test. Another method of studying executive functioning is through different maze tests where the degree of difficulty is varied.

Are cognitive disorders primary or secondary?

Many researchers have emphasised the fact that schizophrenic functional disabilities include impaired function in perception, sustained attention, concentration and memory. However, the one-sided claim offered by followers of Kraepelin needs to be questioned since this is directly linked with neuronal damage, corresponding to the atrophied cerebral cortex found in Alzheimer patients. We cannot point to any straightforward neuro-anatomical changes that correspond to dementia.

During superficial contact with schizophrenic patients, such as that which occurs in a laboratory, it is easy to get the idea that their mental activity – slowness, poor concentration and impaired 'working memory' – might result from a specific dementing process. After many decades of working with people who have been diagnosed with schizophrenia, I find it difficult to concur with this attitude. The findings from laboratories studying neuro-cognitive disorders have been obtained in an artificial environment that does not take account of these patients' subjective experiences. Patients who are often more concerned with their inner illusions and hallucinations unsurprisingly show a diminished motivation or capacity to take in and work together with the test leaders' instructions. They may look as if they are interested, whereas in actual fact they might only be using a small part of their concentration. The rest is directed elsewhere as a result of these inner disturbances. The fact that they are regularly assessed as having poor attention and memory is hardly surprising. Under more relaxed circumstances, I find that they show a markedly good memory which they do not use as other people do. With their limited interest in the surrounding world, they are not interested in specific events or the requirements of daily life while other things that appeal to them have a much greater significance.

With the growing intense interest in neuro-cognitive disturbances and the renewed interest in Kraepelinian views, there is the risk that schizophrenia will again be seen as a neuronal dementia. But this neglects the fact that most patients with schizophrenia improve over time if their external situation allows for it. Moreover, there is a significant group of people with a diagnosis of schizophrenia who have normal or above normal intellectual functioning.

By questioning the 'dementia' component of theories in schizophrenia one does not have to dismiss the importance of biological factors. Why is the surrounding world partly shut out in schizophrenia? And why does it remain so for a lifetime with some while with others it can pass? It appears that one of the central problems lies within the ego's loss of the capacity to integrate outer with inner stimuli, where the inner world begins to dominate over the outer resulting in a distortion in the interpretation of reality. Adaptation to the demands of the outside world will suffer. As a result, there is an interference with the ability to communicate, to make relationships, and with speech and adaptation. The low degree of specificity of neuro-cognitive findings challenges the idea that there are determining organic factors which may deepen our understanding of these severe disorders.

Schizophrenic thought disorders

The 'concrete attitude'

Since the publication of an article by Kurt Goldstein in 1943, it has been possible to trace the development of many of the ideas he broached, concerning neuropsychological aspects of schizophrenia. Goldstein maintained that schizophrenic symptoms can be best understood as *an expression of a concrete attitude*. The surrounding world's stimuli become abnormally determinate. Also words used by someone with schizophrenia are often associated with a part of a concrete object or a situation; there is no general representation for the object. It is easier to understand the meaning in what a person with schizophrenia is saying if we understand it in a concrete way; that is to say, what the person is associating the word to. The word for a certain colour – for example, green – is expressed by healthy people in terms of the category to which the individual colour belongs. According to Goldstein, for the schizophrenic, when the word green is used, it will refer to an aspect of an identifiable individual object, as in 'the grass in Kentucky', 'the grass in Virginia', 'the bark of a tree'.

The difference between schizophrenic and traumatic brain damage

Goldstein claims that we should not just see schizophrenia as an organic illness. The cognitive disturbances can be produced by both psychological and organic factors. Goldstein points out that an important difference between patients with traumatic brain damage and those with schizophrenia is that the world, in the case of brain damage, is emptier, smaller and simplified. In schizophrenia the alteration is at the level of the person's other inner representations and fantasies. The disturbances, which one sees in certain tests, do not depend primarily on general difficulties in following the instructions but on the fact that the person's inner representations disturb his or her behaviour. So the inner world in schizophrenia is richer and more animated by his or her personal ideas than in the case of brain damage. Often, the strangeness becomes less pronounced when we understand how poor our speech is in finding expression for the unusual experiences had by schizophrenics, which cross the borders of common understanding. The 'healthy channels' for articulate speech are neither sufficient nor comprehensive enough for the verbalisation of these experiences. The individual with schizophrenia is forced to build up a language which can seem absurd for a healthy person, but which is wholly adequate for his or her own experiences, making communication with other people more difficult.

Illusions consist of perceptual misinterpretations of a given situation and may give rise to delusions as a consequence. They can be described by a psychologist of perception as a situation where passing events are given a misconstrued and central significance through a loss in the 'filtering function'. A shout from the street becomes especially significant rather than remaining part of some background noise, which would normally be filtered out. The significance of certain concrete objects or stimuli appear in the foreground in an abnormal way, while the person does not seem to react to other more usual stimuli, which now become part of the background (Figure 15.2).

Without denying the relevance of these facts about altered perceptual mechanisms, it is important to hold on to the fact that an inner logic also contributes, especially to delusions and hallucinations. It is logical to understand an individual's increased awareness and lowered threshold for stimuli in certain situations, but if approached from a psychodynamic point of view, one must also ask why particular interpretations are placed on these perceptual disturbances. A common example is the schizophrenic patient's paranoid experience of constantly feeling pursued. It is not simply a nonspecific lowering of thresholds. We must also ask why it is that the threatening experience occupies the mind to such a degree.

Today, thanks to the stress-vulnerability theory, we do not need to see the

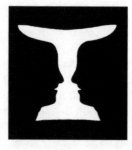

Figure 15.2 Rubin's vase. This classical picture is an example of how one person can absolutely insist that a figure represents a certain image while someone else is just as certain that it represents another. It depends on what one chooses as figure and what one chooses as background. The perceptions that ground what we call our reality always undergo a fast, unconscious interpretative process. This interpretation evolves out of our entire past experiential world.

causes behind schizophrenia as mutually exclusive, rather we can see the illness as a result of a combination of stressors which trigger a vulnerability to react with abnormal and often concrete thinking.

To 'desymbolise the metaphors'

One of the major names in psychoanalytic schizophrenia research is that of Harold Searles (1965), who originally worked at the Chestnut Lodge Hospital in the USA. Searles stresses the schizophrenic's 'flight' from abstract to concrete thinking with a loss of distinction between the concrete and the metaphorical.[1] The schizophrenic does not think either in genuine concrete terms, free from animistic superstructures, or in terms which are comprehensively metaphorical. This implies that the schizophrenic does not clearly differentiate between the three classes of objects in the surrounding world: (a) dead things; (b) living but not human objects; (c) human beings.

On an occasion when his patient was distressed and had temporarily relapsed into a psychotic state, Searles writes that he said to this patient: 'You can't have your cake and eat it too!' The patient replied that he wouldn't want to eat a cake in this hospital. The psychoanalytic notion of *desymbolising* refers to a situation where a metaphorical meaning, which was once able to function as a symbol, is no longer put to use symbolically: that is to say, to represent anything else. Instead, it is now experienced and treated as literal and the metaphor becomes concrete. This is what is happening in a psychosis. It is the work of psychotherapeutic treatment to support the *resymbolisation* of language and reality.

According to a psychodynamic view, the concrete literal thought process is designed to act as a protection against affect that cannot be dealt with. The condition constitutes the final result of the schizophrenic thought process, where the ego regresses from the painful affect and there is a lack of capacity to differentiate between the concrete and the metaphorical. Consequently psychosis involves setting up a barrier against the experience of feelings of sadness, longing, or hatred.

A man with a schizophrenic functional disability who lived alone used to ring up his family at night and shout at them for persecuting him. It transpired that, on awakening, he felt himself to be lonely and would then hallucinate the voices of his family before ringing them. His need for contact was far too threatening to admit to and this conflict produced aggressive feelings in him. His family were able to learn little by little what these nightly procedures were really about. Thus, instead of protracted mutual accusations, in the telephone conversations the

> relatives were able to bring warmth and friendliness to relieve the misery of being alone.

Even the most concrete behaviour is metaphorically tinged and can become symbolically loaded by psychotic thought processes resulting in delusional misinterpretations. People who give you looks can be experienced as persecuting and intrusive as daggers, so it is necessary to hide behind dark glasses or to gain control over these 'looks' by some method such as drawing eyes on the walls.

> A 40-year-old woman had the illusion that her dentist had operated on her and placed a microphone into her tooth and that by this means he could control her thoughts. Behind this lay the vague but powerful feeling of not being able to understand the voices she heard inside and the feeling of being controlled.

The following example is taken from a video interview with a patient carried out by the psychoanalyst Murray Jackson and presented in his book *Unimaginable Storms* (1994). This shows how, with psychodynamic methods of interviewing, one can reach a deeper understanding into the different meanings that symptoms have. In the following conversation, Jackson meets a 28-year-old man who had been diagnosed with a schizophrenic illness that had lasted over ten years. He was admitted to hospital after having set fire to himself as a result of unrequited love. We enter the conversation at a point where the patient is describing his recurrent anxieties and his fear that God is about to abandon the world.

Pat: I was anxious about being institutionalized or becoming a werewolf or possessed, you know.

MJ: What would possess you?

Pat: What I was afraid of was becoming septic. Like gangrene, where once you have a healthy leg and then rot sets in and you just become cancerous and take . . . just suck the juice out of life without giving anything back again. It wasn't just a possession, it was just about me becoming evil because I had such an unhealthy response to life that instead of giving out I was taking in and distorting it. I wasn't really doing it, but that's how I felt. I was becoming a bad influence, becoming destructive.

MJ: You felt you were becoming septic. That would be like gangrene or cancer?

Pat: Yes. I would become cynical. Septic. Sceptic. You know septic-sceptic.

Sceptic is looking askance at experience. Sceptical, doubting it, not thinking it is very good – that's it, sceptic and septic, they're related.

MJ: They are not the same.

Pat: Not the same, but related. I think sceptic is . . . what's that word . . . phonetically like septic. Or it has the same origins.

MJ: What would be the state in which something started happening inside you? You talked of it as a body getting gangrene or . . .

Pat [interrupts]: It's an emotion. My emotions are doing it.

MJ: How might it be if your emotions became gangrenous in that way?

Pat: I'd have to be institutionalized. I'd have become very unhealthy and have to stop myself from becoming totally rotten.

MJ: And the rottenness would be an emotional rottenness? (Jackson 1994: 50–51)

We suspect that a private use of words is revealed when the interviewer gets the patient to stop and explain himself. The metaphor concerning infection and contagion is seen by the patient as a concrete expression for his mental state. During the conversation a resymbolisation begins to take place.

Jackson also cites a female patient who underwent periods of extreme dieting when she would suddenly decide to become a vegetarian. Her explanation was: 'When you love someone, you have to stop eating meat, otherwise the earth will devour you!' The same work discusses a series of conversations with a young priest who became acutely ill with a catatonic schizophrenia after his father was murdered. The patient could sit for long periods of time in a penitent pose or lie motionless as if he had been cruci-fied. His own explanation was that he wanted to be one with God. Perhaps the catatonic symptoms were secondary to a delusional guilt about res-ponsibility for the father's death? Jackson comments that a non-psychotic religious person who carries out rituals related to regret and punishment can also take up stereotypical poses. In this case, however, the person in question is aware that it is a ritual and can leave the situation when the ritual is over. In spontaneous stereotypical poses in catatonic schizophrenia there is no such freedom of mind.

Lack of 'theory of mind'

Christopher Frith (1995), a British researcher in the field of modern neuro-psychology, writing half a century after Kurt Goldstein, maintains that there are three principal abnormalities in schizophrenia which together explain the central symptoms:

1   *The difficulty in generating conscious activity*. This lack of capacity – 'negative symptoms' – can also trigger goal-less activities such as perseverations (monotonous repetitions) or mindless reactions to

outer stimuli, as seen in the behaviour of those with frontal lobe damage.

2   *Lack of self-monitoring.* This leads to experiences of being controlled by others, of believing that thoughts are coming from outside or are inserted into the mind or withdrawn from it. Frith suggests that this can be related to temporal lobe damage.

3   *Impaired ability to gauge other people's emotions and intentions* which creates paranoid misinterpretations. Frith explains that it is unclear where in the brain this disturbance might be located.

Frith sees these symptoms, put together, as a defective *meta-representation*. A meta-representation is an inner representation of inner representations, meaning that there are difficulties in the person's capacity to reflect over his or her own or other people's thinking. Lack of meta-representation, also described as lack of 'theory of mind', is a concept taken from research into autism (see Chapter 12). According to Frith, three situations are character-istic for the autistic person: autistic aloneness, discrepant communication and lack of pretend play. The autistic child is not able to understand other people's way of thinking as different from their own. The person who does not have a 'theory of mind' is not able to create the sort of pretence neces-sary for playing or understand when other people are playing because the ability to symbolise is impaired. With an autistic person, people are not differentiated from other exterior objects and this leads to isolation.

Frith's theory is that schizophrenia is like autism in its incapacity to use a 'theory of mind', which he says is an ability the schizophrenic has had up until his breakdown. Whereas earlier he had been able to imagine other people's ways of thinking for himself, now the ability to form such judge-ments has broken down. Instead, the delusions and other psychotic symp-toms come to express the resulting misinterpretations. Primary autism does not have psychotic symptoms because the autistic person has never been able to understand that other people have intentions and a represen-tational world. However, they might acquire such understanding with difficulty.

Frith also observes how very sensitive processes, which normally remain unconscious, influence the schizophrenic person's behaviour. This explains divergent aspects of language use as well as the difficulty in distinguishing between irrelevant and relevant stimuli. In contrast to many others, Frith does not claim that the 'stimulus barrier' is too low. Instead, he sees the phenomenon as being due to a lack of the control normally asserted by processes higher in consciousness ('supervisory attentional system'), the lat-ter not functioning so efficiently in a person with schizophrenia. In this way 'lower processes' gain a greater dominance than higher processes. (These formulations are closely allied to psychoanalytic structural models even if Frith is not using their specific terminology.) This is demonstrated by the breakthrough of primitive impulses, just as it is with a general lack of control over thinking.

The lack of a capacity for abstract thinking described by Goldstein expresses the same observation as Frith does where he describes the schizophrenic's lack of meta-thinking. Goldstein nevertheless leaves the door open for the possibility that the schizophrenic's thinking can also express an unconscious strategy for solving an existential threat. In my opinion, this is a fruitful perspective and is clinically supported in many cases of both schizophrenic and non-schizophrenic psychoses.

In this latter conception, the fact that the acute psychotic patient lacks the capacity for meta-thinking is built into the definition and is connected to psychosis viewed as a 'Copernican revolution' in the psyche, where he or she becomes the centre of their own world (see Chapter 5). By contrast, in my experience, people with a long-lasting schizophrenic disorder often express a marked ability for meta-representation insofar as they have an intuitive feeling for what is happening in other people. However, they often cover this up with an indifferent or 'disorganised' attitude, or perhaps do not reveal it outwardly other than in metaphorical circumlocutions or in a subtle but ready irony.

So I think that the comparison between autism and schizophrenia is all too mechanical. Many schizophrenics have an exceptional empathic capacity. They have recourse to humour and subtle irony in a way that is hardly seen in autistic people. Nonetheless, I think that Frith's formulations come close to the central questions in the search for an understanding of the essence of schizophrenia.

A semiotic theory

An interesting yet relatively underutilised area for research lies in the use of semiotic research (the theory of the meaning of signs) within the psychiatric field. The semiotic concept *deixis* means 'to point to'. It is connected with how elements of speech and other forms of expression (writing, non-verbal gestures, etc.) orientate communication in the mental area around an 'I-here-now'. The speaking subject becomes the origo in a co-ordinated system. Deixis is the part of the person's expressed statement, which refers to the speaking subject. This is placed in a world of other subjects as a collective phenomenon. The deixis function develops and is trained right from birth to be clearly verbalised by the age of three. It expresses the child's growing competence for intersubjectivity, the ability to place oneself in how others think, and to adapt oneself to it. Earlier we have seen how intersubjective competence is distorted in the early stages of psychosis as well as in chronic schizophrenia. The lack of 'theory of mind' that Frith speaks about refers to aspects of the same phenomenon.

The Danish psychiatrist and psychoanalyst Bent Rosenbaum (2000) has studied the function of deixis in schizophrenia. He believes that the patient with schizophrenia does not understand him or herself in a stable sense as originator or organiser of his or her own speech. He or she does not establish the relevant deixistic circumstances in their speech or written texts, but uses syntax and word meanings in a private way with references that remain unexplained. As a consequence, their statements do not sound coherent and become unintelligible for the person who is hearing them. The person with schizophrenia also has difficulties with thinking in hypothetical terms so that he or she is able to readjust his or her earlier delusions about whether events, which he or she assumed had happened, really did occur. Moreover, he or she does not reckon with the way other people evaluate a statement. Consequently symbolisation assumes uncertain points of reference.

Examining the disorder within a science of language, in a deixistic capacity, offers a new way of studying the schizophrenic's loss of reality. This research is still in its infancy, but one can see how it might help develop our knowledge of both how the schizophrenia spectrum disorders should be understood, and how they might be treated with psychological methods.

Thinking with fractals

How much of what we call schizophrenic thinking and behaviour is the result of isolation and could be modified by countering the tendency to shut out the surrounding world? Until recently, a person who had developed a psychosis was, after only a short time, treated as a hopeless case: someone to be medicated, guarded and cared for. The opportunity for staff to have a real and personal relationship with their patients was remote. With this attitude, the psychotic world remained shut away from communication and insight, and the psychotic patient continued undisturbed, following his or her own internal logic. As the person's psychotic processes become more entrenched, their condition becomes chronic and divergent, accentuating the need for ongoing care from those who are healthy. Unchallenged thought systems of a metaphorical nature began to fill the inner world. Emptiness in the outer life renders the inner life all the more rigid and compulsive.

Personal statements, in speech, writing, picturing, etc., become broken up and are expressed in stereotypical repetitions. For example, the pattern in a picture can repeat itself in different scales. Classical psychiatry has often interpreted this tendency as wholly primary and a typical sign of the illness. Instead, I think there is good reason also to view this as a symptom of understimulation and incorrect treatment. The notion *fractal*, which I have borrowed from mathematics and chaos theory, following inspiration from the Swiss Professor of Psychiatry Luc Ciompi (1997), expresses this idea fairly well. A fractal is a process with constant, broken up quantities which have a characteristic structure as a result of repeating themselves. Fractals have a potential for growth and for filling out empty spaces with no other goal. This stereotypical filling out of an area of paper with a pen is sometimes called schizophrenic art if it is appealing and carried out with talent. It can also refer to the unintelligible controlled or uncontrolled and repetitive talk best described as a word salad. You see these manifestations most commonly with isolation, lack of treatment and an impersonal attitude towards the schizophrenic's flight from meaningful relationships (Figures 15.3, 15.4, 15.5).

The psychoanalyst Wilfred Bion (1967) has shown how schizophrenic thinking consists of a constant inner attack on linking between the inner and outer object or in speech. Schizophrenic people are unable to allow themselves to create symbols or gather words constructively in order to form a meaning that relates to the surrounding world. If the schizophrenic is left to his or her own ways, he or she will continue to break up meaningful thoughts and create a world of his or her own without outer meaning and without pain. In order to avoid this, every schizophrenic person must be helped to gather around them people with whom they can develop relationships. To begin with, in certain cases, this can prove to be difficult and trigger outbursts of fury or strengthen the symptoms. This problem lay behind earlier hospital treatment where strict proscriptions were issued to prevent subordinate staff from developing friendly or close relationships with patients. As a consequence, the patients' recovery of capacities in relating was restricted. Nowadays, we know that a foundation of treatment is the creation and maintenance of meaningful relationships, and a need to respond to autistic thinking that could otherwise develop in a 'fractal' way. But certain schizophrenics do get caught up in this kind of thinking in such a manner that finding a way out of it can seem impossible. All the same, even in these cases the person can usually be reached and influenced to a greater or lesser extent if one has patience and tolerance. This is where a well-functioning social worker can become significant in helping the ill person to be seen as a person in his own right; just as, for example, the laying of the groundwork in rehabilitation by helping a person manage their own home can mean so much. Psychotherapy in its classic psychoanalytic meaning has seldom proved useful in these cases. Instead, methods must be used that protect and encourage the person's capacity to work with others step by step.

Summary

Certain people have lower thresholds than others in their vulnerability to react with psychosis in response to different kinds of stress. In those who develop a schizophrenic functional disability a variety of neuropsychological impairments is found, affecting memory, attention and executive (problem solving). These all add to the difficulties in solving certain kinds of problems and help explain why primitive attempts to solve them, as represented by psychotic thought processes and symptoms, are seen.

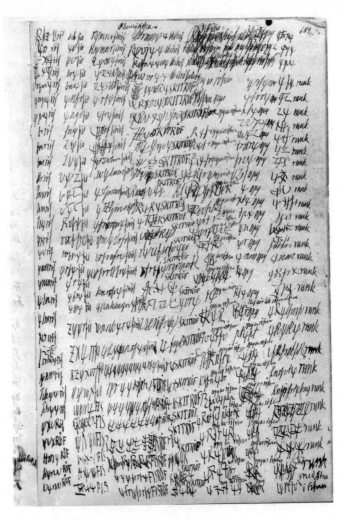

Figure 15.3 The Swedish painter, Carl Fredrik Hill (1849–1911), who developed a lifelong schizophrenic illness in 1878, produced a quantity of pictures during his illness. His writings, called 'Verse Manuscript' which are many hundreds of pages long and in folio format, vary between rhymed poetry, ornamentally entwined words, and rhythmically repeated signs or words. The form of these musings reflects his fluctuating mental state and suggests that the manuscript was produced over a long period of time. The contents are often obscene, and can be understood as a loss of inhibition in this shy but sexually charged person.

From a psychoanalytical viewpoint, the difficulties that the schizophrenic person encounters in differentiating between symbols and their concrete contents have been described. The disturbance in the ability to maintain a 'theory of mind', expressed by a lack of intersubjectivity, has been pointed

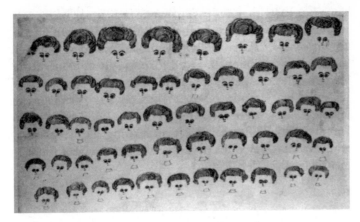

Figure 15.4 This picture drawn by a psychiatric patient one hundred years ago, shows a rhythmic, stereotypically repeated face similar to the sort of jottings shown on the page of Hill's 'Verse Manuscript'. (The original picture measures 46.7 × 71.2 cm.) These kinds of pictures exist in great quantities from the days when mentally ill patients were isolated without having anything to occupy them. With the active treatment offered today they have disappeared. (Photograph: Hans Thorwid, National Museum, Stockholm.)

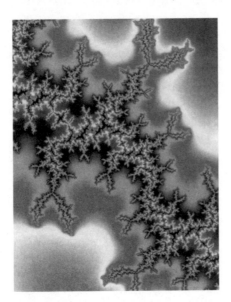

Figure 15.5 'Fractal' similar to an ice crystal which contains a rhythmic 'eternally' repeated, meaningless pattern. (Photograph: Masterfile Corporation/Pressens Bild.)

out by many researchers. To a greater or lesser extent, this function should be open to the influence of different psychological and social conditions.

The schizophrenic person's thought disorder is strengthened by social and physical isolation and moulded into a compulsive and stereotypical pattern. In these cases, they are more likely to be the result of a lack of or an incorrect treatment rather than an expression of the illness.

Chapter 16

The construction of the identity of a 'chronic schizophrenic'

Factors that hinder recovery

First, I will offer a short recapitulation of what happens within the person who is affected by psychosis. The three main players in the process of healing are:

- the individual himself
- the family–staff network component of treatment
- medication.

The ways in which these work together or counter each other will be decisive as to whether mental health is recovered, or to what degree a functional disability is reinforced into a chronic psychiatric handicap.

I have highlighted how the coherence of our mental reality – our picture of the world – is open to attack through fantasies, wishful thinking, threatening experiences and physiological disorders. As a result, reality – that is to say, the meaningful interaction between the inner world and outer events – is permanently threatened with destruction. At the same time, through the work of the ego, there is an interaction between the outer stimuli and our inner representations of the world about us (memories) which result in a constant continuation of and reconstruction of our world view.

In acute psychoses, the ego's capacity to create meaning and to integrate the surrounding world with the inner world has broken down or become fixated at an ineffectual level. The healing process now has to restore the ego, which can resume this ability and has to provide an understanding as to what happened during the psychosis. I will examine some factors that hinder the ego's capacity to carry out this work, with the result that the ego becomes entrenched at a wholly or partly psychotic level.

Post-traumatic stress disorder and post-psychotic depression

The presence of post-traumatic stress disorder (PTSD) is one important factor that forms a hindrance to the development of a healthy ego's ability to resume control. It occurs in over half of those who have been treated for acute psychosis. It remained present in one-third after one year (McGorry *et al.* 1991). PTSD has specific features, in addition to any persistent psychotic symptoms. These include anxiety, depressive symptoms, painful reliving of the onset of the illness in the form of flashbacks, nightmares along with a fear of being recommitted to hospital. The underlying trauma in PTSD following psychosis stems from the experience of what it means to be psychotic as much as from the frightening and sometimes integrity destroying experiences around the admission to hospital. Presumably, the PTSD is often subsumed within what is usually called the *post-psychotic depression*, but which has its own diagnostic code.

Prescribing pitfalls

Another important factor in the work that needs to be carried out in order to regain health is that the medication dosage should be appropriate. If too high, it can result in subjective side effects such as apathy, fatigue and impaired concentration. Sometimes such a situation has been preceded by a struggle between the doctor and nurse and the patient regarding the strength of the medication and the patient has given up struggling after a series of forced treatments. The patient has then been treated with high doses, usually 'for safety's sake', and sometimes as a depot preparation, in spite of his or her complaints. The patient might also have been given *too little treatment* and for that reason will have remained psychotic for longer than necessary.

The process of stigmatisation

Another potential complication is connected with the *process of stigmatisation and rejection* that can follow from the community seeing the person having a diagnosis of 'ill'. The response of the community to the individual's detachment from reality often leads to that person being automatically placed under a specific kind of protection or treatment and becoming cut off from normal company, as well as from the expectations and rights enjoyed by the normal world. The medical and legal establishments have readily taken over responsibility for those who are defined as different or not fully able to take responsibility. These steps are taken both for the sake of the 'ill' person and for the sake of the community. The problem is that if this view of being an outcast from society is not countered as quickly as possible, it automatically exacerbates the person's already poor self-esteem and makes the work of regaining control over the real world even more difficult for

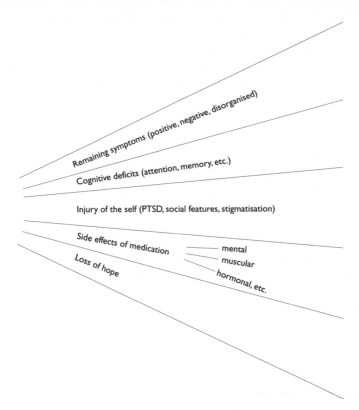

Figure 16.1 Different dimensions of acquiring a chronic identity, which vary strongly from person to person.

him. This process, built up by the person's view of events and the attitude of the community, can be experienced in the following way:

> Others crept about me looking fearful and full of hatred. They talked about me assuming that I didn't understand. They conspired. When I was taken forcibly to the hospital the police and my parents aided each other. My rights are gone – the notice, which has been put up on the wall in the ward about how to complain, is just bullshit. They want to poison me with some substance, which is going to alter my mind. Naturally, I say, 'No.' Who wouldn't? Then they hold me down and inject it into me. My mind does become seriously altered. I can no longer think, can't get myself together, become rigid and strange and feel much worse than I did before I came in. Others say I have improved. This is how they want me to be.
>
> I can't fight it any longer. I give up and adjust myself to their world. I suppose I am ill.

You do not need much experience to see that this is about two views of the world fighting each other, where one wins and forces the other into subjection. Instead of the need to rush the patient into treatment and attempt to force upon him another's view of normality, one can create a situation which allows for respect and take an interest in the patient's view of the world. In this way, it is often possible to find that a constructive working together can ensue.

During recent years, the sense of stigma arising from mental illness has been confronted more and more often in order to emphasise the high risk that the person who has suffered a psychosis might later see themselves as ill, inferior and permanently excluded. This negative picture of the self is strengthened by the attitudes and prejudices of the environment, just as the negative picture of the self in its turn strengthens the attitudes and prejudices of the environment. Eventual functional disabilities and perhaps neuroleptic side effects accentuate this and become all the more fateful. The workplace loses interest in reclaiming him or her. Friendships dwindle, social life no longer quite includes the former family member or friend as they did before. This can result in a downward spiral, which needs to be countered with information, support, psychotherapy and work with the family and social network. Cognitive behaviour therapy (p. 285) especially has been used in order to counteract the lowered self-esteem that follows the experience of stigmatisation.

Institutional treatment

Until the 1980s, institutionalisation in a ward had been seen as the obvious answer for a patient with a long-term psychosis. However, with the social psychiatric movement during the 1950s de-institutionalisation started, since it was beginning to be accepted that institutional treatment had damaging effects (Wing 1960). In these settings the tendency towards psychotic thinking as well as negative symptoms were encouraged and the healthy aspects of the personality retreat into a passive, chronic identity. This is created by the psychosocial attitudes and possibly by impaired neuro-cognitive functioning, these two factors reinforcing each other. The identity of being a chronically ill person is examined below.

A strategy against mental pain?

First, we must remind ourselves of some psychological factors that increase the risk of a psychotic reaction:

1   A tendency in the personality to the kind of thinking where symbols are understood as concrete events and where the line between the inner and outer world is often blurred.

2   In certain cases, this tendency can combine with latent cognitive disorders in the brain's capacity to handle information which become
marked by heightened affect and stress. This is especially so with regard
to the capacity for strategic thinking and the use of certain memory
functions. Sometimes, this lack can be enough to cause the person to
develop serious and increasing social and functional disabilities.

3   At the same time, the difficulties in working through the central existential conflicts within close relationships, separation and aggressivity, are
increased. It is a problem for everyone, at different levels, but even more
dominating in the psychotically vulnerable. It concerns the ambivalence
between the intensive need for closeness, intimacy and symbiosis and
the deep fear of the consequences, such as having to give up autonomy
and responsibility for the self (which, in concrete thinking can be translated into being annihilated). If this usually unconscious and 'insoluble'
conflict is actualised in the vulnerable person, the sense of the self's
continuity threatens to break up (a situation which can become
cemented during psychotic disturbances). It can take place in relation to
the family, a therapist or in relationships, and is not just played out on
the level of fantasy.

The autistic defence

Those who easily find themselves in this dilemma, characterised by panic
and mental pain, can react by getting entrenched in a world which is partly
psychotic as a defence against finding themselves in this state again. In the
same way, the distressing environment encountered over long periods in
psychiatric wards where there is too little stimulation for the healthy part of
the personality has the same effect.

The resulting interruption in the process of healing makes the ill person
feel that he or she is fixed in a state where it is impossible to function in
relation to other people. After some years, other people's efforts to
approach, to communicate and question the psychotic way of thinking and
the identity of the person as 'ill' usually meet with strong opposition. The
resumption of relationships with others is not free from risk either. There is
the fear of the return of a state filled with potential for further overwhelming
pain and failure. The impulse towards self-abnegation and hatred can be
hidden behind a chronic identity of apparent turning away. If someone tries
to break through this barrier with a deeper, eventually sexual, loving relationship or with some other abrupt bid for closeness, there is a risk that
uncontrolled feelings will break out with an increase in psychotic symptoms.
Many an attempt at psychotherapy has been stopped because the patient's
anxiety, self-destructiveness and psychotic symptoms have worsened. Such
psychotherapies are often begun with great hopes, but lack know-how
and experience. The therapist has not understood that the chronic psychosis

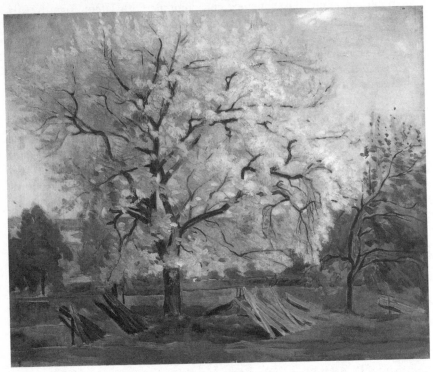

Figure 16.2 Carl Fredrik Hill (1849–1911) is considered to be one of Sweden's best land-
scape painters. Having worked in Paris from 1873, he succumbed to an illness in
1878 which was later described as schizophrenia. From 1883 he was cared for
at home by his mother, a sister and their housekeeper. During these years he
produced a large quantity of very expressive drawings: apocalyptic visions,
prehistoric animals, sexual orgies, hallucinatory gestalts. There is a great contrast between these and the early, beautiful and often melancholic works
where human figures are only seen in the distance. He painted a fruit tree in
blossom many times during 1877, the last one six months before the presentation of his illness. There is much to suggest that he already had paranoid
delusions at this time. (Photograph: Statens Konstmuseer.)

– that is to say, the autistic withdrawal and lingering in the delusions which
are connected with an archaic picture of the world – also constitutes a
defence against any confrontation with the surrounding world. Progress
may be too quick: a direct emotional response is expected or in other ways
too high an ambition is maintained, which the patient because of his
vulnerability or his lack of cognitive abilities is not able to live up to.

   If the self is too brittle, the person might never find his way out of an
autistic defence. This is what has occurred with primary chronic schizophrenics who retain a certain 'defect' – that is to say, a tendency to be
'eccentric' or in some way different – something which can increase after

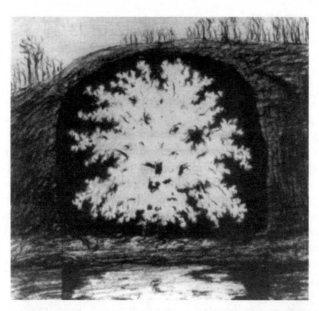

Figure 16.3 Many years later – we do not know when exactly – Hill made the pen drawing called 'Blossoming Fruit Tree in the Mountain'. The picture illustrates how the artist, behind the isolation of his illness, carried within himself the memory of how these pictures once represented the highest form of beauty. The picture can also be seen metaphorically as an indication of how there is always normal psychic life behind the ill facade in schizophrenia. (Photograph: National Museum, Stockholm.)

each episode of psychosis. The degree to which this 'defect state' results from an as yet undiscovered organic/neurobiological change and from the kinds of psychological factors mentioned above is not yet known.

The defensive mechanism can be likened in its function to the stance adopted by someone with a slipped disc. This person has discovered how to attain a relatively pain-free position if he moves in a rigid but distorted manner. Eventually, in cases that have been like this for a long time and with a lack of good physiotherapy, the stance can become cemented by contractures and a healthy bearing becomes more difficult to resume, since the necessary musculature has atrophied or wasted away. Nonetheless the person has reached a relatively painless way of being.

Corresponding mental wasting has been referred to as the *institutionalisation syndrome*. In his or her interaction with the surrounding world, the patient has built up and cemented the self as a chronic person, functioning as an effective protection against pain. Autistic processes provide the most effective way of becoming unreachable both to the outside world and to the healthy part of the self. As a result, delusions and other psychotic thought processes are less impeded and evolve more easily.

'Negative symptoms'

In a specific case, it is difficult to decide what it is within the manifestation of 'chronic negative symptoms' (the dampening of mental functioning, characterised by introversion, apathy, lack of motivation, reduced verbal and motor activity, etc.), that represents woodshedding, or an autistic defence, or the side effects of neuroleptic medication and/or a reactive depression or whatever neurobiological changes that form a basic cognitive disorder. Even if different scales are constructed in order to measure the degree of negative symptoms, it is not easy to differentiate clinically which of the different elements they may be expressing. This approach stresses the fact that the personality's working through of his or her experience of becoming psychotic and thereby risking stigmatisation is a process where the ill person and his environment are working together. In this way, the vulnerability of brain function to psychosis always has psychological, social and functional components in addition to the underlying biological component. This conceptualisation adds to our understanding of the way in which psychological treatment of different kinds are efficacious:

- *Psycho-educational-supportive* treatment seeks to modify this chronic identity by indicating the increased need to work together with those who offer treatment and care. It means that an active learning of new functions, which have been lost during the period of the illness, takes place.
- *Cognitive* therapy supports the healthy part of the self and attempts to decrease the individual's passivity and dependence on psychotic experiences and a depressive picture of the self. This increases the ability to deal with and influence the functional disorders, which result from the illness.
- *Psychoanalytically orientated* (insight-directed) therapy also seeks to reach and to become reconciled with the healthy part of the self which is hidden 'behind' psychotic experiences. Anxiety-provoking feelings and ambivalent relationships can be brought to the surface slowly with the help of the therapist.

These different strategies for treatment (of which therapists are not always consciously aware) indicate the need for having a broad spectrum of methods of treatment, as well as an awareness of what the treatment goals are.

The following case illustrates the process, of self-denigration that I have described being successfully treated by means of psychotherapy. I have not personally followed the patient from the beginning, he lives in a neighbouring country, but I have been able to work with him in a series of interviews with him and with his therapist and through hospital records.

A dialogue with voices

A 22-year-old student, Chris, became ill with vivid auditory hallucinations of a commentating kind and delusions that everything surrounding him was poisoned. The psychosis was triggered by his girlfriend leaving him and the pressure of an examination. Chris was admitted to a rural hospital and was treated with fairly high doses of medication. The effects of this treatment were unsatisfactory. He suffered from side effects and had to be readmitted on several occasions. The diagnosis was chronic paranoid schizophrenia. The voices mostly forbade him to speak. He was now given atypical antipsychotic medication, without any clear improvement.

His condition continued unchanged for several years and everyone considered Chris to be a chronic case. Despite this, a therapist was asked to try to make contact with him. She soon discovered that Chris's lack of talk was not an expression of *the inability* to speak ('negative symptom') but concerned *an active silence* in obedience to his voices. The therapist got him to talk about the voices and what they said. He described, little by little, his many voices, 12 in all. The voices had different characters, while the forbidding aspect was dominant. Chris was able to start naming the voices. As time went on, the therapist also supported him to begin to argue with the voices and to try out defying them, first by beginning to speak and then through slowly starting to take up activities outside the hospital. It took about six months, during which time the medication was lessened and stopped. During the whole of this period of treatment, Chris also continued talking about his difficult childhood, which he now succeeded in disengaging himself from. After a further year he moved back to his home and was able to resume his unfinished education. He has not relapsed and is now able – several years later – to describe his experiences in a balanced and quite open way.

In an interview, I asked him whether he still heard voices. He told me that he did sometimes, and that they became louder when he was more under stress. He remained aware, however, that it was something that was happening in his head and not exterior to him, and he was able to ignore them just as his therapist had taught him. Chris, who had trained as a chemist, tried to describe to me the world of his voices with the help of a drawing. He made two circles that almost covered each other. The one underneath he called 'my self' and the one on top 'the voices'. As long as 'my self' was covered, he experienced the voices as real and was forced to obey them. He lived entirely in their world. When he met with his therapist she got him to question this obedience, to name and to take control over the voices and try to push away 'the voices' from 'my self' (see Figure 16.4). When this happened, the voices became extremely upset and began to shriek and make threats. In spite of being in great agony, Chris defied the voices. After that they lost their intensity, were pacified and disappeared little by little. 'It was as though the voices needed to make me live inside my inner world and to guard me from living in the exterior world with others.'

COMMENTS

In conjunction with an intensive psychotherapy containing both dynamic and cognitive techniques, Chris has recovered completely from his paranoid schizophrenia. A remaining vulnerability factor is his tendency to hear vague voices, which in themselves do not have a psychotic quality: that is, he has no delusional beliefs about their origin. During his illness, the voices forbade conversation – something which could have become an expression of Chris's self-contempt and strict attitude towards himself. This increased his isolation and his feelings of indifference were presumably fuelled by his high medication, which was unable to remove the symptoms. The condition can be seen as an autistic defensive self-denigration which his therapist began to reach in this combined dynamic-cognitive method.

It should be added that this case, with near complete recovery as a result of psychological treatment, does not mean that all schizophrenic patients should be able to regain full function even with optimal treatment. To a certain degree, the patient may have sustained some psychic damage, along with the postulated neurobiological changes, leading to an unavoidable handicap. All the same, rehabilitating and ego supportive steps taken in combination with sensitively prescribed medication can nearly always improve the quality of life for these patients. It is my conviction that many who currently exist in a chronic state with constant medication and without the kind of psychotherapy that could be of help to them should be able to live a full and valuable life.

Summary

I have tried to convey a way of looking at chronic schizophrenia that is grounded in a combination of biological, cognitive and dynamic

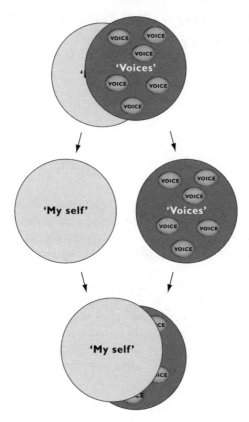

Figure 16.4 Chris's diagram describing his relationship to his voices after therapy. Having been completely under the control of the voices, he is now able to control them himself.

approaches. Chronic psychosis is seen as the individual's way of adjusting to a reality that he or she does not have the ability to negotiate. Different degrees of loss of cognitive capacity and psychological difficulties in coping with life's frustrations add to the maintenance of defences against the confrontation of reality, which characterises psychosis. We do not have enough knowledge about when and how this tendency to remain in a state of psychosis occurs. But these development can be seen in early as well as late-onset episodes.

Chapter 17

Towards a bio-psycho-social model of psychoses

In this chapter I shall gather together some of what I have already said in an attempt to formulate a comprehensive model of psychosis in terms of a psychosomatic disorder. The brain is not normally considered in psychosomatic terms. The brain is the organ in the body that is most rich in neurones and it maintains a constant interaction between a symbol creating mental system and its biological substrate. For this reason, we will neither find one single understanding or explanation of psychosis, nor any other mental phenomena either in a biological or a psychological frame of reference. Such an understanding requires a dialectic point of view, where both systems are given their proper due. But, at the same time, we have to realize how long it will be before we gain more comprehensive knowledge.

A model for the ego's reality integrating function

In his second model of the mind – the structural model – Freud (1923) states that the ego is subject to three categories of demands. It can therefore be threatened by dangers from the exterior world, from the id and the libido, and from the super-ego. The ego controls and organises reality testing: for example, a sense of time, motility and perception as well as the reality of the drives coming from inside the organism. The ego functions include the regulation of the self within social norms as well as the various executive functions, that is to say, the person's actions.

The ego does not 'exist'; it is a theoretical construct[1] and cannot be experienced, as was indicated in Chapter 4. It is defined (according to psychoanalytic theory) solely through its functions. The experiencing part of the personality is known as the self. This self contains the unconscious, the preconscious, and the conscious and is built up from object relations that the person has been able to internalise. Sometimes I use the more usual term, 'personality', in exchange for 'self' in this explanation.

Our representation of reality, which is a part of our conscious self, is constantly created and recreated – constructed – by the ego. The picture of reality can be compared with a biological organism whose cells are constantly being broken down and rebuilt in order to maintain a potential adaptation to the demands of the surrounding internal and external worlds. The ego accomplishes its work as follows:

- The brain registers and scans incoming impulses from the surrounding world.
- It also organises the stimuli which consist of signals (often unconscious) from our inner physiological 'perceptual system'. This leads to experiences of hunger, tiredness, pain, unhappiness, well-being, etc. These two flows of stimuli, from the surrounding world and from the inner world, provide a means by which individuals position themselves within the world.
- The significance, circumstances and meanings of the combining of largely unconscious inner and outer perceptions are interpreted synthetically as

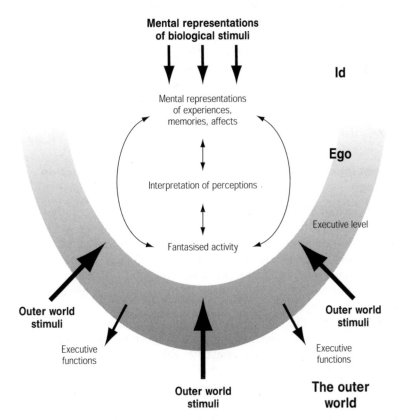

Figure 17.1 The ego's field of action. Mental representations of biological as well as outer stimuli are interpreted through an inner fund of experiences and memories. To a large extent this is an unconscious process. This can result in fantasised actions and thoughts as well as in concrete activities.

a meaningful 'gestalt'.[2] This takes place with the help of the unconscious and conscious memory functions and our inner system of reference, that is to say our symbolic world. The inner representations of objects that we encounter and our experiences include emotional and other associations to those representations. The representational world is recreated throughout our whole personal development and forms a core to our identity as individuals. Both in the *registering* as well as in the *synthetic interpretation*, this *representative* function has an indispensable value for survival and helps to direct our activities.

- Following this the *executive function* come into its own in the shape of a goal-directed activity or through inhibiting a fantasised activity.

Expressed in neurobiological terms, perceptions reach the brain's cortex and are integrated together with other cortical and subcortical stimuli. Connections take place between centres which direct short- and long-term memory functions (among others, the hippocampus) and the prefrontal cortex where normative thinking lies, amongst other functions (see Chapter 6, Figure 6.2). Connections with centres in the brainstem and the limbic system represent affects (pleasure/unpleasure). The executive functions, including the working memory, are activated so that the person's activities and desires are organised with as great an adaptation to reality and security as possible. Every event maintains maximal co-operation between cognitive and affective functions (Ciompi 1997).

Between inner and outer stimuli flows: the scanning function of the ego

Neurophysiological data that have been obtained from studies of how people behave in the face of stimuli from the surrounding world, suggest that the pressure from such stimuli is normally balanced by a counter-pressure from inner stimuli (the body's physiological signals which also include affects), where the ego also has perceptual functions. Neurophysiologically, this confluence takes place in the part of the brainstem that is called the *reticular formation*.

Metaphorically, the ego can be seen as a membrane that is pressed in either of two directions depending on the balance of inner and outer pressures (Figure 17.2). There is a constant registration of impulses stemming from both inside and outside. If the pressure on the 'membrane' is one of the two extremes (that is to say, the pressure is too high or too low on one side), *the ego's ability to assess the situation and to orientate itself will become disturbed* and the excess of impulses from one side will be experienced as coming from the other. The following examples will summarise the different alternatives.

**Internal
stimuli**

**External
stimuli**

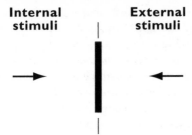

1. Balance between inner and outer pressure (stimuli)

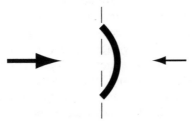

2. Inner (biological) pressure too high

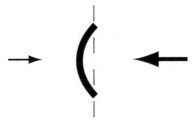

3. External (psychological) pressure too high

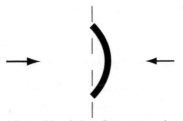

4. External (psychological) pressure too low

Figure 17.2 'The ego "membrane"'. When the 'membrane' between the inner and outer world is forced into only one direction the ego's ability to assess the situation will be reduced and the signals will be misinterpreted.

1   *There is a balance between inner and outer pressures.* The ego is able to interpret correctly the implications of the outer stimuli together with those of the internal representational world.

2   *The biological 'inner' pressure becomes too high.* This happens where there is overactivity in the dopamine or serotonin system or if receptor-active drugs such as amphetamine or LSD-25 influence the brain. This 'state of high pressure' also occurs in lack of sleep, hormonal imbalance, certain brain diseases, etc. (see Chapter 13).

3   *The psychological pressure from the external world becomes too high* in situations of stress. These can include painful experiences, loss or vital 'unresolvable' conflicts (see Chapter 8). A person who has built up a strong tendency to react to stimuli that are threatening because of their symbolic significance, based on early confusional and frightening experiences, will come to perceive specific signals in the surrounding world as dangerous. They trigger anxiety signals which increase the pressure further. In the environment, high levels of criticism and aggression ('high expressed emotions', see p. 84) are a triggering factor for psychosis for the person who has a specific vulnerability. In the same way, another person – because of a lack of cognitive capacity – can find it more difficult to solve problems and he or she can experience acute distress in a situation where taxing demands are made on them and this can result in psychosis.

4   *The pressure of the surrounding world is too low* resulting in inner impulses becoming stronger which leads to misinterpretation and psychosis. This can be the case with intense isolation where external sensory impressions are reduced or where they become very monotonous (sensory deprivation). Perhaps a corresponding mechanism in depression and autism can be imagined. In these solitary conditions the individual can actively shut off outer stimuli. We know from experience that this can constitute a risk factor for psychosis.

Several of the above states can occur together. The ego is functioning at its highest and most complex when it can assess the inner as much as the outer world and integrate the combined demands of both realities. When this is not possible, the self has recourse to regressive solutions.

The self's psychotic construction of reality

Psychosis is created by a paradigm shift in (the construction) of reality – even if, when we look more closely, we can often see a gradual development of psychotic thinking. When psychosis is developing (the prodromal phase) the ego's integrating function has been significantly reduced and the self is in danger of losing its identity and coherence in the face of the threat. This causes extreme anxiety – it has been called 'organismic panic' (Pao

1979) – which emphasises the psycho-physiological character. In order to lessen this panic, the self chooses a 'reparative explanation' from a repertoire of preconscious or unconscious representations on a pre-logical or magic/archaic level. The sense of security or certainty in the self – that is to say, it should not give up or lose a meaningful coherence in the world – becomes more important than does the ability to adjust to reality. The reparative adaptation forms a delusion. The content in psychotic thinking is often not too difficult to interpret, on the level of fantasy, as relating to the person's earlier solution to problematic issues and the situation which was ongoing at the time of the onset of psychosis.

According to psychoanalytic theory, the neurotic's relation to reality is characterised by the repression of pressures/desires from the id and super ego. This diminishes the conflict with the surrounding world in contrast with the dispensing of reality in psychosis. In rare cases, the loss of reality can become so extreme that the borderline for delusional formation is crossed. This condition is linked to more primitive splitting mechanisms, which work in accord with repression and can be seen in certain cases especially in hysterical (dissociative) disorders. The condition has now found a psychotic character while, at the same time, it is significant that it can function in communication with the surrounding world and use symbolic language (see the case of Nina in Chapter 10). Most neuroses (like borderline states) confine themselves to the conventional realm of reality, just as most psychotic reactions do not start off as a deepening neurotic solution to conflict.

Is it possible to influence the psychotic development psychologically?

A question that all theories of psychosis and the treatment of psychosis address is how much is it possible to influence the process: that is to say, why does the broken-down self have to accept the psychotic interpretation? One factor learned from both experimental and clinical experiences of psychosis is that the ways in which the self can react are not fixed.

Psychoses stemming from isolation and sensory deprivation can be fought by active inner counteractive representations, a fact that is confirmed by the descriptions given by many prisoners of how they were able to preserve their ability to think over the course of many years of total isolation under appalling conditions. In his novel *The Days of His Grace* (1968) the writer Eyvind Johnson, who was to become a Nobel Prize winner, describes how a man who sits in the darkness of his prison cell for many years contemplates the bush known as broom. In his imagination, he allows it to grow slowly and to develop, flower by flower:

Twig by twig it grew. Sometimes he would allow the young green shoots to spread over the entire wall opposite, in their most extravagant pattern, before permitting them to bloom. When he had taken a decision, he allowed them to bloom with discrimination, and moved his chains carefully. He was mean with the bush itself; supplying the many flowers one by one, acting the cautious gardener. He put on bud by bud, but with such a lingering hesitation that the blooming developed almost unnoticeably, and the buds swelled without hurry. Later, he commanded them to burst in the same lingering manner, one by one. After lengthy consideration he at last released the most important flowers. They had their definite place in the scheme of things and, like any branch and twig, their own pattern, preserved in memory, in which they must develop each time, at each new blooming. (Johnson 1968)

This literary description bears a great likeness to other survivor stories about extreme enforced isolation, where the person has used different strategies in order to hold on to their contact with reality (Keenan 1992).

Drug-induced psychoses are biologically provoked states but they are also considerably influenced by the psychosocial context around the taking of the drug. The person who takes LSD or other hallucinogenic substances can, after a habit has been formed, either hold on to or resist the resulting delusions from taking charge. Similarly, hallucinations and other perceptual alterations can be held under control and looked at from afar. In other words, there is no *direct* dose–effect connection between the drug and the psychosis.

Many have experienced long periods of lack of sleep where the temptation to interact with the perceptual alteration which can appear can actively be countered to a degree. Many psychotic states develop after a longer or shorter period of lack of sleep.

The person who is about to slide into an acute psychosis can learn to question his experiences and put a stop to his psychosis. A person with *auditory hallucinations* can teach himself to avoid allowing them to take hold and instead actively counteract them by an interpretation that they are hallucinations. Without this ability, the hallucinations will set a course for the development of a psychotic interpretation of the surrounding world – especially when accompanied by mental stress.

One of the most valuable aspects of *psychotherapy* for people with a vulnerability to develop psychosis is that it can teach them to watch for their 'early signs' so that they can act rationally and work against a regression into psychosis. But this demands a very good therapeutic alliance and sometimes many psychotic breakdowns occur before such a capacity is reached. While they are building up, many episodes of psychosis have already had time to reach the paradigm shift and the experience has already become 'a fact'. Influence from others is then avoided as the freshly psychotic ego is already working with its new view of reality.

Antipsychotic medication primarily inhibits receptors rather than psychosis

The division between inner and outer stimuli is significant for the medical view of the work that is to be carried out in the treatment. It is a common misunderstanding that it is the psychotic illusions as such which are being treated with medication rather than the individual's sensitivity to various kinds of stimuli. Psychosis is the final result of the ego's failure to integrate, sort out and order stimuli. One of the possible biological causes for the failing process of integration is the excess of *dopaminergic* (DA)-receptor activity, which is reduced with traditional neuroleptic medication (Healy 1990).

Many of the new generation of antipsychotic medications produce a high degree of inhibition in other neuronal groups, amongst them, *serotonin* receptors. In this way, the extra pyramidal side effects are reduced: for instance, the troublesome Parkinsonian-like symptoms which result from treatment by dopamine receptor inhibitors,. The serotonin receptors are stimulated by drugs such as LSD and mescaline. Therefore the rationale behind antipsychotic medication is that it is directed at conditions that are connected to or reinforced by too high receptor activity.

Conceiving psychosis as an *unmediated expression* of biological dysfunction or imbalance (such as delirium or confusion as a reaction to gross brain disturbance) is, however, not confirmed and a misleading oversimplification. It encourages the idea, now so predominant that treatment with medication is the 'primary' and essential part of the treatment of psychosis. This attitude, which has had deleterious consequences for the actual treatment of psychotic people, in my opinion, is built on an insufficiently careful study of the psychotic process.

Psychosis, as I have claimed earlier, is a direct expression of the ego's inability to maintain a coherent integrating function. The self resolves this lack by means of regressive fantasies and illusions. That this lack of ability to create an all-encompassing, reasonable, objective, meaningful 'gestalt' out of reality can be linked with disturbances in the biological substrate is not the same as saying that psychosis is secondary to biological conditions. What the biological correlation of psychosis is, we do not yet know.

The importance of this reasoning is evident when observing the action of antipsychotic neuroleptics on psychosis. Usually, it takes less than an hour for neuroleptic medication to reach the dopamine receptors. The motor side effects from antipsychotic medication appear quickly as does the subjective experience of alarm and displeasure. Clinical improvement can, on the other hand, appear days, weeks or months later – or not at all. Antipsychotic effects are, statistically speaking, indisputable but (in contrast to the side effects) harder to predict at an individual level. The impact of DA-receptor inhibitors, according to this reasoning, is primarily in creating indifference (not sedation!) rather than being used directly as antipsychotic (Healy 1990; Kapur 2003). Their impact is more like a sort of 'not taking too much notice effect' – for better or for worse. The ego is given the opportunity to build up a more accurate picture of reality than it was able to when subject to the pressure from overactivated DA-receptors. This process may take days or weeks. The 'therapeutic window' is narrow and in terms of the upper effective dose is significantly lower than one had been led to believe earlier (see Chapter 24 for further information). With a good response the ego will now resume its former integrative ability.

Summary

A psychosomatic model has been presented, whereby the ego co-ordinates external stimuli with those from both the inner physiological world and the inner world of representations of memories and experiences. The synthesising interpretation of reality function can suffer if any of the co-ordinating parts is under- or over-functioning.

Under different types of stress, the vulnerable personality will avoid its earlier balanced interpretation of reality and psychotic ideas may appear unchallenged. Up to a point, the individual can learn to control his psychosis and delusions and hold on to a more correct vision of reality. Both the experiential world and psychosis are thus both open to influence by means of the person's conscious thinking and intentions. This is most important to remember when antipsychotic treatment is being discussed. The effects of medication should be discussed in terms of them creating an 'indifference'. This gives the personality an opportunity to gain a 'breathing space' and to retain better control over his or her interpretation of reality.

Part II

In support of recovery

Chapter 18

Traditions of thought in the history of psychiatric ideas

From the history of ideas, there are four traditions which influenced the development of mental illness in the west:

* the oldest is the prehistoric *magical-demonic tradition*
* this was challenged in around 400 BC by *Hippocrates' teaching of the four humours*
* during the same period the *Platonic* study of the *passions* arose
* much later, the *Enlightenment* viewed man in rational scientific terms.

Many people like to think that the representations of life and circumstances devised by philosophers and other theorists come and go as they make room for something newer and wiser. Obviously in a way this is true: knowledge of our outer world and our inner universe increases all the time and progresses onwards. At the same time, these ancient views remain incorporated in our existence. They form a basis for psychiatry as well as for other medical practices. They remain with us for better or for worse even if their concrete manifestations have altered. It is important to be aware of this when trying to understand today's psychiatric perspective. Otherwise, in an eagerness to embrace new technology, it is all too easy to wait for something new instead of developing and altering what we have.

A magical-demonic way of thinking and the need for hope

Magical-demonic thought has followed mankind from pre-history. Illness, similarly, is considered to be something bad which intrudes and takes possession of the person. Such intrusion might reflect punishment by higher powers for the breaking of a taboo or reflect some God-given order. It can also represent our need to control a threatening future and to influence the dictates of nature. Within the community, the doctor is considered to be experienced in the ways of the unseen; yesterday it was the magician/witch, today it is the priest/doctor/therapist. Seances gathered for healings, prayer meetings and exorcism are today's unconcealed expression of this tradition. Even people who perhaps would not admit they believed in God can pray for help and support when in dire need. When our illness appears incurable we are more open to approaching an unconventional practitioner who, often due to their charisma or reputation, offers a promise of healing.

Many studies regarding the effectiveness of different forms of psychotherapy show that the essential aspect of what works and what does not work is the therapist's ability to create a *therapeutic alliance* with the patient (Luborsky *et al.* 1993). The English psychoanalyst Michael Balint (1972) talks about the therapist's 'apostolic function'. It implies that the person who is under treatment feels appreciated and respected and that the therapist encourages an optimistic attitude, which motivates the patient and influences the way he sees things. Of course, this does not mean that the therapist's experience and training do not count, simply that something over and above this is required.

We know very little as to what this extra something is – only that the best psychotherapeutic or medical methods lose much of their potency if the practitioner does not encourage trust in the treatment and hope for improvement. Research into the placebo effect (the effect of medication which does not contain an active ingredient but can still have a curative effect) shows how essential the trust factor is for the full potency of the treatment. More recent neuro-immunological researches also reveal that people who are trusting and have a reasonable hope of surviving cancer, for instance, have a healthier immune system than those who have given up hope (Solomon 1987). People working with those who have developed psychosis know the value of hope even more clearly. It is a great challenge for staff to offer encouragement in order to maintain hope but, at the same time, not to deny reality.

The teachings of the four humours and psycho-pharmacological treatment

During the fourth century BC, Greek philosophers, most notably Hippocrates, developed humoural pathology: a model used to explain the origin of physical and mental illness as a disturbance of the balance of the humours or body fluids These bodily fluids, which were also connected to the four elements in the world, consisted of blood (Latin *sanguis*), phlegm (Greek *phlegma*), the yellow bile (Greek *cholé*) and black bile (Greek *melaina*).

From this early body fluid theory the Greek physician Galen (circa 100 AD) developed his psychology on the four basic temperaments: sanguine, phlegmatic, choleric and melancholic. This intuitive classification differs astonishingly little from modern theories of human temperaments, which often describe similar types. The pathology of humours had a marked impact on the theory and practice of medical art. Through bleeding, applying leeches, sweating, the use of emetics, enemas and diuretics, attempts were made to influence the body's fluids. These were not infrequently detrimental to the patient. The patient could, however, trust the treatment methods as they were sanctioned as being based on 'scientific knowledge and proven experience'. Humoral pathology was abandoned during the 1800s in favour of more concrete, anatomically based forms of treatment.

Within psycho-pharmacology today it is of central importance to consider affective and psychotic disturbances as disturbances in the hypothetical balance between different transmitters and the receptor system in the brain. Alternatives to dopamine and serotonin receptors are currently being sought in the quest for new answers. Thanks to refined methods of research, together with the fact that this approach is strongly backed by the financial support of the pharmaceutical industry, it has a dominant position within the psychiatric profession. Internationally, treatment for psychosis is still often seen as synonymous with antipsychotic medication. The palpable goal or dream of finding the drug that will finally solve the imbalance in man's soul can be discerned. Even Freud (1940) had these visions: 'In the future, perhaps we will be able to learn to influence directly the quantity of energy and its distribution within the mental apparatus with chemical substances. Perhaps this will result in different, still unimagined possibilities for therapy.' Freud has been proved partly right.

Plato's theory of the passions and the psychoanalytic theory of the unconscious

Plato (427–347 BC) also spoke about the effects of a lack of balance, but he referred to its physical and not its mental aspect. He described how sickness in the soul was caused by all too powerful feelings, passions, hate and suffering. The ideal was therefore to reach a balance of mind, to be calm and upright. Health was reflected in self-knowledge and in the avoidance of becoming the slave of passion. *Catharsis*, the cleansing of the soul, freed you from the sickness of becoming filled with feeling. This was the essential aim of classical theatre.

The modern understanding of psychic health and sickness grew during the nineteenth century and was depicted in art, literature and psychiatry. It gained its psychiatric breakthrough with Freud's *Interpretation of Dreams* in 1900. Freud presented a theoretical connection between early repressed feelings and later behavioural disorders and states of anxiety in his teachings regarding the unconscious. As described above, the therapeutic view was seen psychoanalytically as a redistribution of the psychic energies, which was reached through insight and abreaction of the distressing affects, in order to restore psychic balance.

Early psychoanalysis saw its value as one of freeing locked and unconscious feelings by means of catharsis. Eventually it became a way of treating the personality which was locked in by early repressed problems through the talking cure. A marked optimism regarding psychotherapy grew up after World War II and, in psychoanalytically influenced hospitals in the USA, chronic psychotic patients began to be treated with psychoanalysis and without medication. After a wide-ranging follow-up research study (McGlashan 1984) it became devastatingly clear that progress with this often deeply handicapped group of patients was poor or even negative. As a result psychoanalytically oriented treatments in psychosis gained a bad reputation in the medical world, especially in the USA.

In Europe, the development of psychodynamic thinking has taken another direction in that many consider it to be an essential addition to the biological and cognitive explanations of psychosis. Methods of treatment in working with psychosis have come to be much more pragmatic. A fruitful line of development lies in the synthesis of dynamic and cognitive theories, which is today borne out in more and more centres.

The questionings of the Enlightenment and the radical criticism of psychiatry

Thinkers such as Rousseau and Voltaire during the eighteenth century and Marx and Mill in the nineteenth century directed themselves towards mankind's potential in terms of their personal development. The child was seen as an empty page at birth. The new rationality implied a freedom from those explanations that had suggested that psychic illness was the expression of Divine wrath and punishment for past sins as in the theory of the pathology of humours. Philippe Pinel (1745–1826), in the spirit of the age of Enlightenment, described psychic illness in terms of individuals who could be understood and who were in need of sympathy and humanity. Through more simple activities and work – what later came to be called occupational therapy – he wanted to counter the demoralising effects of isolation and unemployment. The development of education during the nineteenth century, Marxism's new eschatology and the later liberalism inherent in Mill's radical view of the freedom of man marked new directions from the traditions of the Enlightenment.

Together with new psychoanalytic directions, sociology and social anthropology gathered a strong foothold, particularly in post-war USA. Rather than the more pessimistic biological theories it was easier to accept a liberal tradition, which complicated and deepened Freud's views. The significance of upbringing and environment overshadowed everything else where it concerned the understanding of the healthy personality and the psychic ill health of the adult.

The 'anti-psychiatry' way of thinking which held sway during the 1960s and 1970s can be seen as a latter-day expression of the attitudes of the Enlightenment. The dominating medical way of seeing things and the total institution were questioned and heckled in a general criticism of authoritarian social models. Psychiatry was forced to take a deep look at itself. De-institutionalisation and anti-medication, as we shall see in the next chapter, became slogans that were supported by the community's economic interests. The flip side of this revolt against authority was contempt for any scientific thinking. A new reductionism was created.

The expression of a dualistic view of humanity, where the physical and mental are seen as separate entities (as opposed to seeing the mental as emanating from the physical like a secretion from a gland), was inherited from many centuries previously. What we have today is a move away from dualism towards monism. We look upon the manifest expression of mental activities, 'the mind', as if it were simultaneous with physical, molecular activities. Different languages describe the same events as different sides of the same coin. One way of looking at it is in the relation between psychoanalysis and neurobiology.[1] 'The unconscious' is no longer solely an area for psychoanalysis but a notion that has just as great a relevance for the biological study of consciousness.

Chapter 19

Attitudes in the twentieth-century treatment of psychosis

At the beginning of the twentieth century, psychiatry was seen by the state as an area for medical responsibility. In about 1900 the number of beds for psychiatric patients in Sweden was 4500: around the same as today's number of psychiatric beds in relation to the population. Thousands of sick people waited for years to be given somewhere to go where they could be treated. Often they lived in miserable conditions in cellars or poorhouses. Around the turn of the twentieth century, a series of new psychiatric hospitals was built with room for up to 1000 or more patients in each. In the 1960s there were 34,000 places in mental hospitals (besides around 5000 for 'retarded people'). This represents 0.5 per cent of the Swedish population, equal to the prevalence of schizophrenia (SOU 1958). Many more were on the waiting list. The effective exclusion of the psychically ill from the community has subsequently been strongly criticised, not least because of the chronic institutionalised state it can generate in patients. However, it is easy to be critical of this lack of outpatient care in retrospect. We must not forget the humanitarian ethos that lay behind the creation of such institutions, which addressed the needs of those who needed care but had been unable to get it.

The hospital system, just as the system in the community, was strictly hierarchical with the head consultant as all-powerful with the protection and support of the state authorities. The hospitals were usually situated outside built-up areas and formed small communities in themselves. Many had their own farms and livestock, which allowed for a high level of self-sufficiency and offered (low-paid) work for the patients. The hospital staff, who during the first decade of the 1900s were still known as servants, were to a large degree serfs, working up to 100 hours a week. They lived in the hospital and even their private lives were monitored. In many hospitals they had to ask permission to leave the premises (Beckman 1984). Those who wanted to get married had to ask the consultant physician for permission. If permission was denied the only alternative was to give up the job. In 1908 'the servants' organised 'The Swedish Hospital Employees Union'. These people had a working-class identity and in the beginning had no formal training. When nurses who came from the 'educated classes' were given access to mental hospitals the level of training was improved. At the same time, conflicts and tensions between the groups were generated which continue to this day.

It was difficult to oversee what occurred on the wards, even if it was laid down that leniency should be exercised. The rights of the patients had still not been given any legal status. The distance between doctors and workers on the wards was wide. If the head consultant wanted to give the patients greater freedom, conflict could arise as a result of the union's desire to protect the staff's working conditions. With this militaristic hierarchy and discipline, it is not surprising that patients too could be subject to the staff's outbursts of anger, favouritism and mob systems, similar to those encountered in any totalitarian state. Nonetheless warm relationships still built up between patients and carers, with the consultant viewed as the enemy. The staff were explicitly told not to hold conversations with the patients about their problems. New staff who talked to their patients or tried to talk to them were soon frozen out by their colleagues. Talk was confined to the few doctors. However, it was expected that the patients should be observed, their behaviour and forms of activity in which they engaged were all to be monitored. As a result supervisory lists with narrow columns were ticked off.

One can divide the methods of treatment that were developed during the 1900s into three groups. The early decades were characterised by a lack of specific methods of treatment. This was succeeded in the 1930s by a huge influx of very powerful forms of treatment that were often very painful and damaging rather than helpful. The latter half of the century has, for better or worse, witnessed the introduction of more specifically orientated medical treatment. Also, advances in social psychiatric and psychotherapeutic directions began to challenge the one-sided dependence on medication. The struggle between succeeding theories has been intense. Today we find that there is a dialogue between these two attitudes. However, aspects other than the patient's needs have an influence on these questions. The huge incomes (and economic investment) in the pharmaceutical industry as well as the politicians' need to offer the kind of treatment which is economically acceptable, if short sighted, dominate development today. The political debate concerning care is in great need of more consumer-orientated research as well as the scientific knowledge that can inform it.

The first decades: guarding and keeping

Up until the 1930s there were no specific methods of treatment of psychosis. According to a widely read psychiatric textbook of the period the priority for the staff was to make sure that the patients were prevented from harming themselves or others. In order to make the need for supervising and care less strenuous, the patients slept in rooms large enough for 10 to 20 people. Those who were admitted to a mental hospital could, with good reason, expect to remain there for a number of years; for many it could mean a lifetime. The head consultant alone decided when they should be allowed to leave. The person who had been admitted to care had, in principle, no say in the matter. It was not until 1929 in Sweden that a law was introduced regarding compulsory committal, which allowed for the patient to be treated of his or her own free will. Those who were institutionalised were disenfranchised until 1946.

In Sweden up until the 1960s remaining in bed was routinely decreed for each new admission for the first week. This was considered to have a calming effect. It was also meant to help the patient to see that he or she was ill and to encourage them to co-operate with the staff. For disturbed patients long periods in a bath were ordered, sometimes for one, two or even many days on end. The bathrooms were difficult for the staff to work in as the patients might throw their excrement about or splash dirty water at them. Therefore, many were wrapped up in sailcloth with one hole for the patient's head and another at the foot end for warm water to be poured in. There are reliable descriptions of how the skin could suffer from these frequent long baths. Inevitably the use of such treatments placed great demands on the professionalism of staff, as they could easily be used to punish provocative patients.

The most frequent forms of medication used were opium-based and long-lasting barbiturates and sedatives such as bromide. Scopolamine and atropine also had a certain calming effect but made the mouth dry and caused constipation.

The era of 'heroic treatments': 1930–1960

In the 1930s substances were introduced all of which, more or less powerfully, directly influenced the functioning of the brain. At the beginning, new hope was engendered in the care of psychosis. Since it depended on the use of medical methods, the psychiatrist's standing was increased and psychiatry became a specialised discipline comparable to others. However, the patients often had to pay an appallingly high price for these treatments.

Inducing fever as a form of treatment

In 1927 the Austrian Julius von Wagner Jauregg was awarded psychiatry's first Nobel Prize for his discovery of the favourable effects that the treatment of malaria had on general paralysis – the late stage of syphilis. The method was used increasingly in the treatment of schizophrenic patients. They were given injections of malaria-infected blood or chemical substances that brought on high fevers. However, it was abandoned because the results were uncertain, the risks were high and the patient's distress was great.

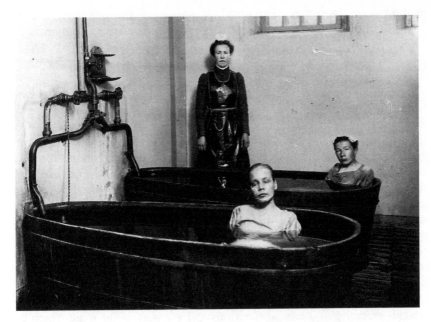

Figure 19.1 Long periods in a bath: Marieberg's Hospital Museum, Sweden.

Insulin coma

At the beginning of the 1930s the Viennese physician Manfred Sakel tried out insulin coma treatment for the first time. Sakel's early reports described up to 80 per cent improvement in patients and as a result of the hope engendered insulin coma soon became a norm for acute schizophrenic patients. The methods meant that the patient was given such a high dose of insulin that the blood sugar levels in the brain sank to such a level that he or she lost consciousness. After around half an hour the patient was awoken and given a glucose solution by means of a nasogastric tube. Going to sleep and waking up was often accompanied by aggression, intense hunger and marked sweating. Sometimes potentially life-threatening episodes of vomiting or epileptic fits were caused by the effect of the low blood glucose on the brain. On occasion the coma would be reversed too late with the result that the patient either died or sustained brain damage. Due to the extremely high level of nourishment contained in the treatment the patients quickly became obese and looked more and more grotesque, which made returning home even more difficult. A course of treatment of this kind entailed 60 to 90 induced comas and if there was no effect it could be repeated several times.

In spite of Sakel's early positive reports, results were not good enough to make such stressful treatment of the brain acceptable. During the 1960s the method was completely abandoned in favour of the new antipsychotic medication.

Lobotomy

The culmination of physical treatment of the brain took place with prefrontal lobotomies. In 1935 the Portuguese Egan Moniz discovered, after experimenting with chimpanzees, that if one cut the connections between the frontal brain and the more deeply situated parts of the brain, chronic agitation and anxiety could be stilled. As a result certain hospitals routinely began to carry out more and more of these operations – at first only on chronic schizophrenic patients, but later with first-episode psychosis patients who did not improve quickly enough. In the ensuing enthusiasm surrounding the success of this treatment insufficient attention was paid to the side effects of the operation – it was simply considered that positive effects outweighed the negative ones. In 1949, Moniz was awarded psychiatry's second and most recent Nobel Prize, which had the effect of further legitimising lobotomy for many years.

The frontal lobe of the brain is, amongst other things, the seat of man's ethical, executive and critical functions and the part of the mind which has developed the most as a result of recent evolution. Moniz's operation involved drilling a hole under local anaesthetic in each temporal bone. Afterwards, a small knife was inserted that was drawn up and down, thereby blindly severing the nerve connections. It was up to the head consultant to decide who should be given the operation, although the doctor had to obtain the family's consent before the procedure. The common complications were personality alteration with indifference and sluggishness. Minor personality alterations were presumably the outcome of all the operations, but because the illness had been dramatic and in itself had created an alteration in the personality there was a tendency to disregard the negative effects. Many were left with persistent incontinence, epilepsy or obesity. Death occurred as a result of haemorrhage or infection.

In the museum of Sidsjön Hospital, in the north of Sweden, appalling descriptions can be found of 131 lobotomies which were carried out between 1946–47 (Eivergård and Jönsson 1993). Only 12 per cent of the treatments are described as having been successful insofar as patients were able to leave the hospital in an 'autonomous condition'. A further 16 per cent were released from hospital still requiring ongoing care. Of the operations 37 per cent resulted in 'improvements in level of care required', 25 per cent did not improve, 4 per cent were made worse, and 5 per cent died. At the beginning of the 1950s approximately 500 patients had been operated on at Sidsjön Hospital. In effect, this consisted of everyone who could be operated on.

Prefrontal lobotomies have now completely disappeared and have been

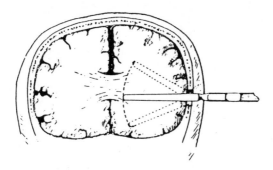

Figure 19.2 The incision in lobotomy: such treatment took place in Frösön in the 1940s (Illustration from *Modern Swedish Care of the Mentally Ill,* Lundquist 1949).

relegated to psychiatry's capacious chamber of horrors. Now, on rare occasions what is known as capsulotomies are carried out in cases of very severe treatment-resistant obsessive compulsive disorder. The operation is done stereotactically and with radiation techniques and is considered to result in less significant personality changes. Psychosis is no longer an indication for such treatment. An essential difference from the earlier attitude towards lobotomy is that, today, the operation is no longer allowed to take place without the patient's consent.

Convulsive treatment: from cardiazol to ECT

At the same time as insulin coma treatment was being used, convulsive treatment was becoming more popular. The indications for it were wider and could include more or less everything from acute schizophrenia to kleptomania. The method was introduced in 1937 by the Hungarian Ladislaus von Meduna who claimed that epilepsy reduced the risk of schizophrenia. Meduna had tried different more or less toxic seizure-inducing preparations before he found *cardiazol*. This produced an epileptic grand mal seizure some minutes after an intravenous injection had been administered. During the time that the seizure developed, and before loss of consciousness, the patient experienced an escalating and very severe anxiety which often meant they had to be held down and forced to accept the subsequent treatments. These were given two to three times a week over a three-week period.

In 1938 the Italian Ugo Cerletti induced seizures by applying an electric shock between the temporal bones, meaning that the patient could be spared from suffering the chemically induced pre-epileptic anxiety. Also, electric shock treatment (or to give its more modern term, *electro-convulsive treatment*, ECT) was often coupled with extreme anticipatory fear in the patients, especially as up to the beginning of the 1950s it was carried out without anaesthetic. The treatment was handed out in the 1940s and 1950s just as if the patients were on a production line. The physician and four or five attendants walked round with a portable apparatus, and gave it to patients who waited in their beds in the hospital wards. Before giving the treatment, two attendants took a firm hold of the patient around the shoulders and arms, a third held the pelvis down and two others held the legs. Serious complications included shoulder dislocation and compression of the vertebrae as a result of the violent epileptic fits. It does not require much imagination to picture the patients' reactions to the screams let out during the seizures of those unlucky companions who were treated ahead of them.[1]

At the beginning, the rule prescribed 20 to 30 treatments and the series could be repeated time and time again in the face of a lack of alternatives. Often ECT was combined with insulin coma or was given in 'block shocks' of two to three treatments in succession. After such treatments many patients displayed an acute confusional syndrome with disorientation and double incontinence; they could only lie in their beds. Eventually they got better, but it was not clear as to whether or to what degree they had sustained permanent brain damage.

During the 1950s a muscle relaxant called *celocurin* was introduced. It was given seconds before the electro-convulsive treatment was applied together with an intravenous narcotic. The procedure was now rendered less unpleasant and the patients were relieved of having to suffer massive cramps. It was also possible to demonstrate that the curative effect did not come either from the electricity or the muscle contractions; rather, it was caused by an epileptic seizure triggered by the electric current in the brain.

Many people have had concerns about the harmful effects of ECT. Administering an electric current that was much too strong or lasted for too long could result in brain damage. The author was one of the first psychiatrists who were given compulsory training in anaesthesiology in order to carry out ECT under narcotic sedation. I experienced the dilemma of being forced to carry out a treatment which I did not believe in at the time. So I decided to refuse. However, I discovered John Stuart Mill's work *On Liberty* (1859) where he argues the importance of giving careful consideration to that which goes against the grain. As a result I read through international literature concerning the effects and risks of ECT. I presented my newly acquired knowledge regarding the evidence-based indications for the treatment at a seminar for psychiatrists and was thereafter able to demand justification and clear indications in the case of each patient who was sent for treatment. From there on the frequency of the use of ECT was reduced to 25 per cent of its previous use in the hospital where I worked.

Today, ECT is usually given with electrodes on only one temple. A normal series consists of around six treatments. Schizophrenia is no longer a common indication. The main indications are severe and untreatable states of depression (or mania) with a high risk of suicide, aggression, homicide or life-threatening dehydration. Catatonic conditions together with post-partum psychoses that do not improve after a reasonable period of time can also be an indication. The treatment in these cases can usually be significantly effective, sometimes life saving.

Sterilisation

Even if sterilisation is not intended as a treatment but rather as a preventative or 'racially hygienic' measure, it must be considered as such. Like lobotomy, sterilisation was carried out without consent. The decision was taken by the doctor, on the advice of the social administrator, or as a result of the family's permission. Indications were usually eugenic, reducing the risk of 'abnormal' genetic inheritance, or social, where the woman – it was less often considered for men – was not able to look after the child. The boundary between mental deficiency and mental illness was vague and subjective. During the 1940s, 200 to 400 sterilisations a year were carried out in Sweden on mentally ill patients, sometimes together with abortion. Compulsory sterilisations were forbidden as a result of a new law in the 1960s.

The last 50 years: neuroleptics, social psychiatry and psychotherapy

'Anti-psychiatry'

The resistant nature of mental illness to treatment encouraged the use of the methods described above. However, the simplistic view of psychosis as a disease of the brain provided further justification for these practices. From this perspective, it is easy to justify methods involving operating on or medicating the diseased organ. The treatment concerns brain pathology with no regard for psychological processes. One was not inclined to listen to the patient's complaints about side effects since the measures taken were considered to be a necessary evil. Furthermore, by definition, the subjective experiences recounted by the patients were not considered reliable. This disregard of subjective experience provides a further explanation as to why there was a systematic and extreme deterioration in the quality of life of many patients in the last 50 years following on from the introduction of neuroleptic treatments.

In his book *Asylums* (1990), the sociologist Erving Goffman describes the destructive influence of the overall institution on people because expression

of the individual's needs was not acceptable and the staff took care of everything that was life sustaining. If the patient was not ill before he or she
entered the hospital, he or she would eventually become so. In *The History
of Madness* (1961), the French writer on the history of ideas, Michel
Foucault, created a historical narrative from the perspective of those who
were mentally ill. He showed the need to identify and keep dissidents, mad
people and criminals apart in order to consolidate one's own normality.
(Naturally this is not, as many wanted to think, an explanation of the occurrence of mental illness. On the other hand, it illustrates the rejecting power
of the concept of mental illness.)

The Scottish psychiatrist Ronald Laing made a breakthrough with his
book *The Divided Self* (1960), and with A. Esterson in *Sanity, Madness and
the Family* (1964). The schizophrenic's symptom was, Laing claims, natural
and understandable in the face of the distorted and false family in which he
or she had been brought up. This simple and one-sided way of looking at
things gained considerable popular acclaim. Over the decades, it caused
some organisations that advocated for the mentally ill to become entrenched
in a negative attitude towards mainstream clinical psychological thinking
and psychiatric methods of treatment of psychosis. Laing and others saw
psychiatry as a sick society's instrument for exerting control and power. His
ideas were animated by an anti-authoritarian ideology which had a strong
influence during these decades.

With his book *L'instituzione negata* (1964) and his slogan 'Destroy the
mental hospitals', the Italian professor of psychiatry Franco Basaglia started
an important transformation of the psychiatric system of healthcare. As a
result of his campaigning the so-called 120 Law was introduced in 1978,
which in principle forbad hospitalisation for mental illness in Italy. He
believed that psychiatry should function outside the institution, working in
the community with patients and their families. Acute psychiatric care
should be offered in ordinary hospitals. Even though the Italian experiment
only went halfway in its resolve and in certain areas failed, these ideas have
had an important influence internationally and have added to the development of methods of care of mental disturbance taking place outside the large
institutions.

Social psychiatry and neuroleptics facilitate the discharge of people from hospital

There is a widespread notion that the increased number of people discharged from mental hospitals was a result of the routine use of the antipsychotic medications which started around 1954–55. However, this is an
oversimplification. In many North European countries deinstitutionalisa-
tion had already started towards the end of the 1940s. It began in Great
Britain but soon spread to other North European countries.

The Norwegian psychiatrist Örnulf Ödegard (1964) studied the frequency of the number of discharged patients with a first-episode psychosis in all the Norwegian mental hospitals before and after the introduction of antipsychotic medicines in 1954. He found that the frequency of patient discharges who had been admitted between 1955 and 1959 had increased minimally after antipsychotic medication had been introduced, in comparison with those who had been admitted between 1948 and 1952. The frequency of discharges for those who had been admitted over the whole of this period was greater than for those who were admitted between 1936 and 1940, a decade earlier. Ödegard suggests that a part of the cause was due to the demand for labour after the war. After analysing the methods of treatment in different hospitals, Ödegard concluded that those hospitals which had already functioned successfully did not show any significant increase in the discharging of patients treated with antipsychotic medication. In hospitals where psychotherapy and occupational therapy were less developed, the discharges increased significantly with the introduction of neuroleptics.

The therapeutic community

During the latter part of the 1940s the English psychiatrist Maxwell Jones and other pioneers introduced the social psychiatric concept[2] of the 'therapeutic community' in several psychiatric hospitals in Great Britain. Group therapy was introduced along with a more democratic staffing structure (Jones 1970). The patients were also given the freedom to take part in making decisions within the community. The need to strengthen and modernise staff training now became a priority. The period spent in hospital should be made use of as a time when the patients could learn more about themselves and about their relationships with others. This would help them to be better prepared when they left.

This social psychiatric attitude spread during the 1950s. Doctors and nurses from many western European countries visited English hospitals, especially the Dingelton, Cassel and Henderson hospitals, in order to gain practical training. Further visits were encouraged, as seeing patients progress made them feel more secure about discharging their own patients from hospital. In co-operation with the social services, institutions for the

Table 19.1 The frequency of those hospitalised with 'functional psychoses' in Norwegian hospitals who were not rehospitalised (Ödegard 1964)

Year of admittance	Per cent permanently discharged
1936–40	53
1948–52	63
1955–59 (treated with neuroleptics)	67

rehabilitation to work were also created, along with other supportive activities. The social psychiatric attitude in western Europe was mainly built on social psychology and group dynamic thinking.

In the USA there is a long tradition of the development of outpatient centres for individual treatment. They introduced easy access to mental health centres, which could help people who could not afford private psychotherapy and in 1963 a law was passed to establish such developments. Federal funding would only be offered to those psychiatric services that gave a comprehensive service to the population, that is to say, assistance for acute cases, outpatient access and day and night care. Patients in psychiatric hospitals still consisted of what was considered to be a second-class group and the methods of treatment were less adapted for them than for those people who sought help for less disabling problems. Admittedly, many were discharged from hospital in order to move into one of the new institutions that grew up in the form of 'halfway houses'. After some decades the number of psychiatric beds in the USA decreased from about 600,000 to around 80,000. Many of the new private residential centres were inadequate. Those who could not afford hospital treatment became homeless. For medication they were referred for more routine treatment in dispensaries.

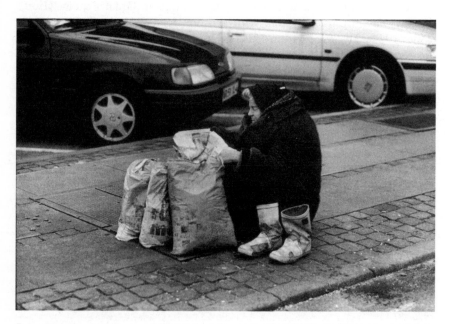

Figure 19.3 'Bag Lady' in the 1990s: in decades to come this will be held as an example of a lack of psychiatric care around the turn of the century. What will the problem be in the next generation? (Photograph: Gregers Nielsen/Bildhuset.)

The new psycho-pharmacology

After the Frenchman Jean Delay published his report in 1952 stating that *chlorpromazine* (Largactil) had a tranquillising effect on patients, it did not take long for the medicine to be introduced on a worldwide basis. The patients' disorganised behaviour disappeared and the levels of violence and anxiety seen in inpatients decreased, which allowed most of them to be discharged to some form of community care. Other compounds (also known as neuroleptics or antipsychotics) that had similar effects to chlorpromazine, and were often chemically similar, were quickly developed (see Chapter 24).

In the same decade it was discovered that *lithium,* in a simple salt solution, decreased the severity of manic-depressive fluctuations. A variety of anti-depressants was developed, one of the most commonly prescribed being imipramine (Tofranil). This is one of the *tricyclic* group of antidepressants that were used for a number of disorders, most notably depression. A new group of sedatives was introduced, the benzodiazepines, which were found to be safer treatments for anxiety and insomnia. Leading brands include Librium and Valium which are still used today.

When the cure is worse than the condition

Suddenly psychiatry had a growing arsenal of specific and useful treatments. This allowed for the withdrawal of the drastic methods of treatment described above. The historical dream, based on anatomical pathology and of explaining and hence treating mental illness according to a medical model, seemed close at hand. At first neuroleptics were used with a certain caution, but soon the doses were increased, sometimes in an uncontrolled fashion. It was possible to show that regular medication reduced the relapse rate.

Injectable long-acting 'depot' medication was developed so that patients could be given medication by means of intramuscular injections every two to four weeks without becoming dependent on them. The Parkinson's disease-like side effects were very marked, for example, muscle stiffness, tremor and a subjective experience of discomfort, but these could be countered to a degree by means of other medications. However, these in turn produced new side effects. The general principles of the treatment of psychosis were as follows: high dose neuroleptics, in tablet or depot form, coupled with medication for Parkinsonian side effects. Patients were advised to continue this for at least two years. Those who were diagnosed as schizophrenic had to follow this treatment for life, which meant that treatment with neuroleptics became a new instrument of control not just of the mental illness but of the patients themselves.

During the last decade of the twentieth century, thanks to new research methods available such as the PET-imaging technique, it became possible to demonstrate that the antipsychotic effect was already reached at just a tenth of the doses routinely prescribed. The side effects were not an unwanted but necessary evil: rather they indicated that the dose was too high. Issues that patients and their families had been complaining about for years were suddenly taken more seriously. In many places in the world these substances began to be used in much lower and more reasonable doses. The USA and eastern bloc countries are still an exception; the same is true of the developing countries but there people also suffer from a lack of neuroleptics.

Psychoanalysis and psychotherapy

The 1950s were also a turning point in the place of psychoanalysis in the treatment of psychosis. Psychoanalytic training institutions grew significantly during the 1960s and 1970s throughout the western world and psychoanalysis began to be accepted in academic institutions in many places. The American psychoanalyst and researcher Otto Kernberg (b. 1928) played an important role in the academic adaptation of psychoanalysis, synthesising the English object relations school with American ego psychology (see Chapter 4). In psychiatric and psychological training in the USA psychoanalysis became a dominant theory and those who wanted to have a psychiatric career usually went through personal psychoanalysis. Increasingly, psychoanalytically orientated treatment was given to people with schizophrenia, although this occurred mainly outside the public sector. The psychotherapeutic and pharmacological-medical treatments of psychosis were practised in competition with each other instead of as an integrated whole. This was something that damaged both patients and the development of psychological theory.

The only kind of care available to those who did not have private insurance cover was in crowded and dilapidated mental hospitals. The effects of psychoanalytic psychotherapy were overestimated, creating clinical stagnation and increasing frustration. The insurance companies, who were disinclined to pay for long and expensive psychoanalytic treatment where there was no curative effect to justify the expense, withdrew most funding towards the end of the 1980s. Internationally an increasing interest in the development of psychopharmacology was seen together with more behavioural orientated short-term treatment.

Democratisation and public control

We can now remember or read about injustices from the recent past secure in the feeling that today's situation is more humane, but those who were then responsible for care were no different or less humane than we are now. The need for curative treatment was just as strong and the suffering of those who are ill still constitutes an urgent challenge. Within the medical profession there will always be new and promising methods, which will be accepted for a time. It is important to remember that all the methods mentioned in this book did appear to have some therapeutic efficacy in certain patients. We must be aware of the frailty and limitations of our current perspectives, no matter how humanitarian this might seem.

Ethical and humane psychiatric care arises not just out of internally determined professional standards, but also from external organisational, cultural and political factors. That conditions have now changed for the better in many ways is due largely to the intensive process of democratisation and the official regulation of psychiatry. However, it is a vulnerable system and can break down quickly with just a few changes in attitude and external conditions. For this reason I will outline some historical lessons which I see as essential for the understanding of how the dehumanisation of psychiatric treatment in the name of medical science was able to proceed. I would also like to emphasise the risk that such problems might return, and where this potential lies in current trends:

- A dominating medical model of illness encourages the attitude that expertise rests only with psychiatrists, and so only they can make valid criticisms of methods which may in fact be repressive or inhumane. Ethical standards may be lowered when certain practices receive medical sanction (Milgram 1958).
- Much academic and practical knowledge was derived from institutionalised patients. The textbooks were based on studying patients who had been ill for a relatively long period of time. By then, psychiatric illness had become entrenched and harder to influence. Without recognising the external factors that link institutionalisation and chronic illness, drastic methods of treatment become easier to justify.
- Those who were originally admitted to a mental hospital did not possess full jurisdiction over their own lives. After a while they were placed under guardianship and lost their rights of citizenship. The view of mentally ill people as second-class citizens without democratic rights increases the risk of dehumanisation. In the name of medicine and in the pursuit of science it then becomes easier to permit experimentation and ambiguity over indications for treatment.
- Client and family organisations have been active in and essential to the process of reducing the loss of rights within psychiatric care. The organisational and judicial processes in relation to enforced hospitalisation can appear bureaucratic and time consuming for those who work within psychiatry. Often it is difficult, as well, for the patient's representative to argue against psychiatric expertise, even though it is known that this has the potential to be misleading or might not be centred on the patient's best interests. Rather, without the powerful and constant presence of democratic vigilance and insight, psychiatric treatment can easily turn into an instrument for arbitrary control and oppression.

Chapter 20

The requirements, demands and organisation of treatment for psychosis

Many aspects of contemporary western treatment of psychosis are counterproductive with regard to maximising the recovery of the patient: that is to say, care and treatment are more conducive to the organisation of the care of the sick rather than the needs of the patient. When psychiatry eventually took over the care of the mentally sick during the nineteenth century, many people worked with great humanitarian inspiration in order to offer the same opportunity for treatment and care as available to those who suffered from physical illness. Mental asylums were created with large facilities for their care organised by medically qualified staff. Psychiatric care was relatively insulated from the rest of the community. This made it hard to obtain help quickly when it was needed, and once detained it was even harder to escape from the treatment. The result was that slowly but surely the number of people in care increased. During the middle of the twentieth century, psychiatric clinics attached to hospitals began to take over the role of the mental hospital. This marked a humanitarian reform in that the isolation of psychiatry was countered.

Today, we can see that it is time for new reforms that specifically concentrate on the specialised care of those with psychosis. Neither the medical nor psychosocial resources currently provided produce the results that are desired and that are possible. For professionals, the population and the people who make the decisions it is essential to look at the problem through the eyes of the patients. So, let us now look at acute inpatient psychiatric care from this point of view.

On being admitted to an emergency psychiatric ward – through a patient's eyes

When a patient with psychosis is admitted to an acute ward it is often under compulsory section. To be placed suddenly in a situation of total helplessness is felt by most people to be a shocking experience, which may haunt them for a long time after recovery. These experiences must not be taken any less seriously because of the fact that a few patients have a more positive reaction to their first episode of care. Often this can happen to a sensitive person in their early twenties. When he or she has been searched for illicit drugs, and after belts and other objects that might be used for the purposes of suicide have been removed, the patient is given a bed. Often people who have been on the wards for some time will harass the newcomer, wanting cigarettes or money. Fellow patients mumble or talk to themselves or walk up and down the corridors, while others may sit staring in front of them.

Many patients have described their experiences on an acute psychiatric ward as a hell from which they feared they never would escape. Their fear of becoming chronically mentally ill is increased and further reinforced by the fact that nobody appears to treat them as others had done outside the hospital. They see people around them in whom they recognise their own fears of mental illness – such fears are naturally rife too in those who are ill. Night time can be even more terrifying when fellow patients can be heard crying, overwhelmed with bewilderment and anxiety. Many experience total abandonment when they are more or less forced into receiving injections after they have said they do not want any medication. One can be afraid of being poisoned or damaged in some other way by medication and feel oneself to be fully justified in refusing. Distressing side effects may confirm their fears and encourage a greater antipathy towards medication. Many patients get worse following admission and protect themselves in ways that only result in a further loss of contact with reality. In this environment everything seems to point to an expectation that they should go mad.

Every day the patient encounters around fifty or so different faces. The staff changes from day to day. Often they come to work in their everyday clothes. If they do not have a badge showing their name and job title – something which occurs frequently on many wards – it can be impossible to know if they are members of staff or patients. All too often the staff can be found in the kitchen, the office or around the exit to the department rather than remaining with the patients, who feel imprisoned within their illness. Family and friends who visit are confused by the difficulty they have in finding someone to explain to them what is happening or by the lack of privacy and of having somewhere to talk.

The intended curative effect of medication is countered by this kind of environment with the unfortunate consequence that the treatment must last longer and use higher doses. As a result the motivation to continue treatment after the patient has left the hospital is very low. The environment on this kind of ward can be said to be as counterproductive as giving penicillin to an infected child who is living in slum conditions without also making sure that the environment is made hygienic.

Many might find this description of an acute psychiatric ward at the end of the twentieth century unfair and exaggerated. While there have been improvements in psychiatric clinics and hospitals during my 40 years in the profession, in my experience the atmosphere described above still pervades many departments. The staff often maintain a surprising loyalty towards their place of work in the face of criticism. It is easy to lose objectivity in such an environment. These conditions are defended by rationalisations: for example, that the patients do not know what is best for them or that the necessary changes would be too costly. Both arguments are equally false. Questions about staff solidarity and security can dominate union debates.

Counterproductive aspects of current hospital care

- Around half of all the people with a first-episode psychosis have had their symptoms for six months or more and many of them have sought help without their condition being diagnosed. As a result an important opportunity for treatment has already been lost and the psychotic episode will tend to last longer than necessary.
- The acute psychiatric ward that provides the normal resources for treatment of an acute episode is often incompatible with the needs of the patient. For example, architecturally they have been constructed on the intern medical approach of the 1800s and this structure has remained essentially unchanged over the last hundred years. Isolation, rest, medication and control were the central themes that originally motivated their design. This has been accentuated by union demands and the requirements for security on a regimented basis: searches, locked doors, refusal of 'permission' or 'freedom of movement' before the consultant has decreed it. The patient's autonomy is consequently strictly reduced or non-existent.
- The dehumanising process of admission, stripping away so many of the things which give us our sense of identity, can affect the integrity of the patient's ego. This exacerbates the degree of psychotic behaviour. The ward indirectly begins to evolve a punitive content. This is seldom something which the staff is conscious of, but is one which the patient is strongly aware of.
- The psychiatric wards are too large. They are intimidating places with a mixture of acutely disturbed and chronically ill patients displaying anxiety provoking and sometimes aggressive behaviour. New patients often try to protect themselves by withdrawing into themselves and it therefore becomes more difficult to engage with them. The need for control and restriction required by a few very ill and unpredictable patients determines the overall setting and further adversely reduces the potential for other patients to recover.
- Many research studies indicate that psychotic patients are best looked after in a ward which is calm, friendly with a clear agenda, ordered and with a low level of aggression (Friis 1986). This reasonable attitude, which ought to be obvious without the need for research, is entirely

consistent with the psychotic patient's greater sensitivity to stress and their 'thin skin' in relation to external influences.

- Treatment with neuroleptics is often introduced immediately, without ensuring their necessity. Due to the fact that the patient frequently gets worse when he is first admitted, and due to the demand for a swift patient turnover, the initial dose given is often much too high and the doses are increased too fast. Side effects result of a painful and sometimes frightening kind and the patient's trust in the medicines, especially in neuroleptics, is undermined. As a result, the potential for co-operation ('compliance')[1] after the patient has left is markedly decreased.

- A dialogue is replaced by interview and assessment of symptoms. The family is not actively involved in the treatment but instead receives (if they are lucky) 'information' regarding the diagnosis, treatment and prognosis. The patient's depersonalisation is increased by a tendency to identify the patient solely by their illness. Both the patient and family learn to pay heed to the nature and degree of psychotic symptoms when assessing recovery while the patient's personal resources are neglected and eventually forgotten. This can add an iatrogenic (caused by the treatment) psychosocial handicap to an emerging neuropsychological functional disability.

- A principle of discontinuity is unintentionally built into the chain of care that these patients move along. After a night spent in an emergency ward the patient is transferred to the acute ward, and then from there to attending the outpatients department or moving to the ward for long-term patients. The rehabilitation team will then take over and finally psychiatry will delegate their responsibility when he or she is transferred to the auspices of social services. With each move the relationships that may have developed are lost and the knowledge acquired about the patient's personality and resources is seldom passed on. The information that follows the patient becomes reduced to more and more stereotyped descriptions of symptoms and a list of prescriptions.

A functioning care organisation

How should good and rational care of patients with psychosis look? How should it be honed to the needs of the patients? There are two goals in the treatment of psychosis. The first is to replace the psychotic way of thinking with a non-psychotic way: that is, the function of the ego is reinstalled. The other is that the consequences of any potential neuropsychological functional disability should be minimised.

Any such organisation designed from a psychological point of view should be able to accomplish clinical work which is important and difficult; what is simple and obvious needs little organisational structure. Work with people with psychosis is one of the most complex and difficult challenges for

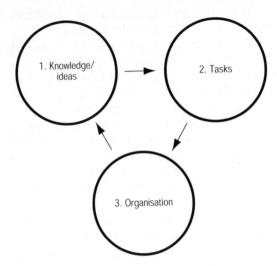

Figure 20.1 The relationship between proficiency, assignments and organisation.

psychiatric care providers. New information and research findings appear in quick succession. For this reason, if we want to have a functioning organisation, we must first concentrate on the knowledge that we have about the nature of psychosis and its treatment. Then it will be possible to formulate the work that has to be done. Only then is it possible to design such an organisation rationally. The final organisation should be able to develop and change in order to accommodate new challenges and scientific knowledge.

The nature and treatment of acute psychosis

This section summarises the key points about the nature of psychosis along with the situation and needs of those affected. This lays the groundwork for the discussions in the following chapters about how wards treating psychosis should be organised. This is the present state of our integrated knowledge – in future decades we may have new experiences which will in turn direct us to a new way of thinking.

1   First-episode psychosis is a serious disorder. In around a third of cases it will resolve with current treatment methods without the patient needing long-term follow-up. Nonetheless, the mental trauma of having been so ill is often serious. In the other cases a chronic relapsing and remitting psychotic illness develops and for more than a third of cases, to a greater or lesser degree, a chronic cognitive disability develops.

2 In first-episode psychosis it is essential to investigate and exclude organic causes such as brain disease, hormonal disturbances, toxic substances, etc. In addition, patients with chronic mental illness suffer from a higher level of undiagnosed medical conditions.

3 The longer the duration of untreated psychosis (DUP), the more entrenched the psychotic thought processes become, resulting in greater social isolation and exclusion.

4 The first five years are especially important for prognosis. During this period the sense of exclusion can become more or less intense. It is a good prognostic sign if an individual can learn to recognise his 'relapse signature' – that is the symptoms which are early indicators of relapse. This allows the individual to compensate for his vulnerability and the residual features of the illness.

5 Although we still lack the research which will clearly confirm the claim, it seems quite clear that early, goal-orientated work improves the prognosis. All the same, many forms of treatment are double edged. Antipsychotic medication lessens the incidence of relapse in the majority, but the side effects diminish the quality of life. Psychotherapy is essential if it is adapted to the phase of the illness, to the person's resources and to their external circumstances; otherwise it is meaningless and even negative in its effects.

6 The vulnerability-stress theory emphasises the psychotic individual's strong sensitivity to stimuli of both an emotional and cognitive nature. Scientifically speaking, this is best illustrated in the research on expressed emotion, where it was shown that relapse occurs more frequently in situations where there is a high level of criticism and hostility as well as with emotional overinvolvement. Other research suggests that these factors are just as relevant in psychiatric wards. With increased stress, such as more insecurity, overwhelming demands and emotional provocations, the vulnerable individual withdraws into himself, thereby increasing his tendency to splitting and psychotic thought processes.

7 There is no evidence that parents are the cause of schizophrenia. However, there is evidence that in both early and later childhood difficulties in the home may accentuate a biological vulnerability to developing schizophrenia. Many schizophrenic people have had a childhood that would be considered to be quite 'normal'.

8 The family can act as a protective resource by lessening the effects of the patient's vulnerability However, the gradual development of psychosis can generate anxious, overprotective and even aggressive responses, which may arise out of worsening dysfunctional structures. Sometimes a family member might become 'overinvolved' with the illness – totally taken up with this person's life – something which can be damaging for all concerned (see Chapter 27).

9   In some families, one or more members may have personality problems that may result in indistinct boundaries between family members and the use of powerful primitive defence mechanisms such as projective identification. The resulting family dynamics further complicate the patient's development of self-reliance. Presumably this reflects complex mixtures of genetic and psychological inheritance.

10   The individual with a chronic psychotic illness appears to live in an unresolvable conflict between the need for reassurance and the difficulty of dealing with it when it is given. This *need–fear dilemma* is characteristic of psychosis, independently of whether it primarily reflects a biological or psychological vulnerability. The staff must be made aware of this dilemma, which is an accentuation of an existential condition that at some point and to some degree occurs in everybody's life.

11   The acute psychotic episode has, like somatic damage, an inherent capacity to cure itself. This capacity can be disturbed if the psychosocial environment is fraught with negative stimuli with the result that further psychotic processes occur. At the other extreme it can also be disturbed by all too demanding expectations on the part of the people providing treatment.

12   Some acute psychoses resolve themselves relatively quickly without medication. In most cases, however, a low dose of antipsychotic medication will be found helpful in the recovery process. Such medication is generally necessary in cases of more long-lasting schizophrenic illness.

13   Benzodiazepines, the new generation of hypnotic medications, can have beneficial effects on anxiety and sleep disturbance in patients with an incipient or acute psychosis. Judicious prescribing can reduce the need for, or at least the total dose of, neuroleptic medication.

14   The psychological trauma of the illness itself, along with the experience of other people's reaction (including medical staff), can result in post-psychotic depression. Sometimes what appear to be 'negative symptoms' can be a side effect resulting from over-medication with antipsychotics.

15   Suicide is as significant a risk in acute onset of psychosis as it is in later stages of schizophrenic conditions. The risk is highest in the first five years of the illness, especially at times of acute psychosis and after discharge from hospital.

In the next chapter I address the issues of treatment and care needs of patients with psychosis. I describe some alternative approaches to service organisation and delivery and discuss their evidence base.

Chapter 21

The assessment and treatment of patients with an acute psychotic episode

When someone with symptoms of psychosis or someone close to them first seeks psychiatric assistance, the symptoms may have been manifest for years. There may have been contact with primary care or social services, who may not have identified that there is a mental health problem, or have been unable to engage with them. Usually, a situation is reached where the person feels himself to be overwhelmingly controlled by a frightening world and is increasingly suspicious of other people's attempts to help. It is when the diagnosis of psychosis is made for the first time that assistance can become more adapted to the person's specific needs. (From this description one realises that we do not know how often psychoses resolve without having been diagnosed because some may simply never present for help.) The aim of intervention is to optimise the treatment of psychosis. The doctor's underlying aim during the initial contact is also to gain a preliminary understanding of the nature of the psychosis – both medically and psychologically.

After the 1970s and 1980s, with the closing of large institutions, care of all forms of mental illness became decentralised. However, many practitioners began to experience the need for a subspecialisation of the work involved in treatment. The first such group to be delineated was the long-term psychotic patients. It quickly became evident that they needed the kind of support and care that all too often differed from what was on offer to those with personality disorders or with acute mental illness. Since then other areas of subspecialisation have developed (for example, neuropsychiatry, forensic psychiatry and substance misuse). With all these competing for influence it is unrealistic to expect the general psychiatric worker to keep abreast of recent developments in the rapidly expanding body of knowledge on treatment of psychosis.

The need-adapted care of psychosis

The Finnish psychiatrist Yrjö Alanen has emphasised the importance of developing a 'need-adapted' care of psychosis (Alanen *et al.* 1991; Alanen 1997). According to Alanen, the need for psychotherapeutic consideration is central. Specific methods such as medication, family therapy, individual therapy, etc. should be adjusted to the patient's needs. The assessment of these needs can by guided by the phase of the patient's illness. I agree with this attitude and would like to summarise and expand the following points (regardless of whether they concern the first episode or a relapse):

- provision of immediate help
- crisis intervention
- continuity and accessibility
- a lowest optimal neuroleptic dose
- suitable night-time care.

Providing immediate help

As soon as someone seeks or needs help for psychotic symptoms, he or she should be able to contact a specially qualified member of staff. Preferably this should occur within a day. The sufferer often exists in a threatening and bizarre world where there is no one to trust, not even his carers. The carer can become another threat to be avoided. The first few meetings, which ideally take place in the home, should address diagnostic issues whilst attempting to develop a therapeutic relationship. It may be possible to find some degree of awareness of illness even in the most defended patient. This denial may result in part from fears of detention and institutionalisation. If the home visit can be arranged at short notice, the family can often deal with the crisis in such a way that the patient need not have an emergency department assessment and may well avoid the need for hospital admission. If this does happen, early involvement from a member of the psychosis team can limit unnecessary and potentially traumatising emergency interventions.

Crisis intervention: family meetings and formulating the problem

Meeting with the family

The family should be engaged with the treatment right from the beginning if possible. Many first-episode patients do not live with their families. They may not have contact with their original family or may refuse to make contact with them. In such cases the work that has to be done has to take place on an individual basis. In spite of this, I would strongly emphasise the family's role in this kind of treatment. I have experienced how easy it is to allow the importance of the family to be lost sight of. The importance of a family contact is well documented and again in my experience including the family at the earliest possible stage can enhance the social network and hence the healing process.

If the patient consents, contact can be made with the family. The family members needed in order to understand the situation – parents, siblings, partner, children – may be invited to a consultation with the patient. This meeting constitutes an open invitation and does not include any kind of 'therapy'. The aim is to allow everyone to express their point of view in relation to what has occurred and to help lessen anxieties and maximise communication with and between the relevant members of the family. The family members have often felt themselves to be living on the edge of a volcano. They do not understand what is going on. Outbursts occur when no one is expecting it and the shock, anxiety and sadness in relation to what is happening have exhausted everyone, resulting in sleep disturbance and other stressful reactions.

During a first-episode psychosis there is a great risk that contact with and understanding within the family break down completely and that a process of exclusion is set in motion or becomes fixed. By engaging the family it is easier to get to know what the problems are and what resources are available. It offers the possibility of understanding both the sufferer's and the family's needs for support in the future.

The team should try to meet with the patient and as many of the members of the family as possible. Careful attention should be paid to the setting. For example, if the meeting takes place at the centre where the psychosis team is based it is important that the room used is big enough to accommodate everyone comfortably; it also helps if coffee or other refreshments can be offered. Sometimes one member of the team might support the patient during the meeting whilst another attends to the rest of the family. Several hours might have to be set aside for these preliminary meetings (see Andersen 1990).

A first home visit (case study submitted by psychologist Sonja Levander)

A man telephoned, at the suggestion of his GP, because he was worried about his son. Since the previous summer, his son Steven frequently isolated himself in his room in the basement of the family house and had really not wanted to have any relationships with either his family (mother and father) or others, including his girlfriend – 'a Persian aristocrat' – whom he saw now and again. Sometimes he would come up to eat but avoided all attempts made by his family to involve him in conversation or any form of activity. He had not worked since the spring when his job at a library had finished. Lately he had begun to play the saxophone again – until two years ago he had been a saxophonist in quite a famous band – but now he played loudly, especially at night. His father worried because his son never seemed to go to sleep. When the duty nurse offered to visit the family at their home, the father was horrified. He only wanted a little advice. Was there nothing that could be done medically?

The father wanted to hang up and suggested he might ring later at a more convenient time, which he did the following day. He and his wife were now quite worried since Steven had lit a fire in the garden during the night and was constantly running in and out of the house. They didn't know what they should do, but found it absolutely impossible to tell Steven that they had contacted a psychiatrist. The nurse tried to show the father that it might be easier for them not to have to carry the difficulties with Steven by themselves and suggested that he and his wife might come and talk to someone on the team. They couldn't do this since they were unable to leave Steven. They feared that he might burn the house down. After a while the father agreed to come by himself, providing he could come at once. Steven seemed to be asleep down in the basement.

The father arrived by taxi and was worried and anxious when he met the team doctor. He explained that Steven had lived away from home for two years after his school finals. Amongst other things he had spent one year in America where he had played the saxophone, but seemed to have got involved with 'bad company' there. He might have taken drugs as well, but as far as his father knew he was not currently using drugs. In answer to the direct question as to whether there was something that they could help with, he burst into tears and said that he felt he had lost Steven when he travelled to the USA and that he and his wife were in fact now frightened of him. They didn't know what to think. The doctor explained that it was not so unusual for people seeking help to feel this way and suggested that they should all go back to Steven's home together.

When they arrived home they sat in the living room, with the mother sitting on a chair in the doorway. She pointed to the hall and the stairs to the basement and made gestures suggesting that they should not speak too loudly. The doctor suggested that it would be a good idea to call Steven so that he could see who had come to visit. The mother called her son who came halfway up the staircase, where he remained. The doctor explained that she had come when his parents had called to say that they were worried about him; they didn't know how they could help him.

'I don't need any help.'

'But there is something which is making your parents so worried and you yourself don't seem to be able to sleep properly.'

'I don't need much sleep and I need to practise for a performance.'

'But everyone needs to sleep and especially if they have to work.'

'No, it is not demanding, only stimulating.'

'Is there nothing that can be done to make the practising easier for you?'

'No. Yes. I have a backache.'

COMMENTS

The above case study presents a fairly typical account of the kind of difficulties that are met with during a first home visit to a person who is really about to enter a psychosis. The family is paralysed by their fear that they might do something wrong. It is possible to sense, too, Steven's fear of being trapped and his fear of being ill at the same time as being afraid of what was happening in his inner world. Perhaps his backache could present an opening for a closer contact with him? It transpired, however, that he shied away from contact although further attempts were made. Instead the police brought him in some days later in a fully developed psychosis.

The formulation of the problem

When talking to the family, one asks about their different experiences of what has occurred before and during the development of the psychosis, and they are asked to describe what they think the actual problem might be. The acute psychosis is reframed as a reaction to a crisis in a vulnerable person and the experiences of the rest of the family members are taken into account. The dramatic reaction generated by the psychosis is defused in this way. It also constitutes a less confrontational way of challenging the psychotic person's misunderstanding of reality. It may help them to listen to and eventually take in what others say.

Furthermore, there is a need to make clear and yet flexible plans for the immediate future, using whatever resources are available: for example, the potential for a close and ongoing contact. The 'contact staff' who are detailed to work with the family (there are usually two) should ideally cover for each other and in this way maintain the continuity. Without being able to make any definite predictions, a sense of hope for the future has to be instilled. Daily contact may need to be offered during the early stages.

It should be pointed out that home visits in families with an acute psychotic member are often very challenging, generating anxiety, and testing the tolerance and creativity of the carer. Usually it is necessary to work individually to support the patient along with the meetings with the family. Whatever approaches are combined, it is essential that the overall plan should have structure and clarity. Talking with and listening to the patient should be a priority. Naturally the doctor's medical and diagnostic job must be combined with these other needs in a carefully thought out manner.

From my own experience and from the experience of many others, it is often helpful to work with a so-called *family map* (or *genogram*) during the acute phase. The map, which is really an extended medical history, can be sketched out during the first meetings with the family after the patient has been admitted. It can be looked at as an indirect illustration of the vulnerability-stress model. The idea is to get a concrete picture of the family's emotional environment, with regard to important events, illnesses, mental problems, deaths and catastrophes. It should first centre on the patient's siblings, then the parents and their siblings, and eventually the paternal and maternal grandparents (Figure 21.1).

A family map helps to give a visual retrospective coherence to the family's emotional situation. Experience repeatedly shows how drawing a family map during the first meetings lessens the patient's psychotic behaviour temporarily and helps the family members co-operate and listen to each other – something which members of the family may not have experienced for a long time. Both professionals and carers may worry that talking about problems in the family will only worry the sufferer and worsen the psychosis. However, providing that each individual's point of view is respected in the family meetings, this is seldom the case. After the first phase of the illness (see p. 52) the need for family meetings is less evident and they should take place only when some of the family members or carers ask for a meeting.

Continuity and accessibility

My experience is that the first meetings are central to the establishment of a co-operative relationship with both the patient and the family. One of the risks of transferring a patient's care to an inpatient ward, rehabilitation service or day hospital is that these relationships, which are a valuable resource, may be lost. Such relationships are central to the healing process. If the patient remains in the community it is important that both the patient and relatives can contact the team during the day in the event of a crisis. Nighttime telephone contact should be available so that patients who have already been assessed can be managed at home, as far as possible. In many clinics, arrangements are made to visit acute patients at home during the night. With this ease of access it is easier to prevent or treat a relapse in good time.

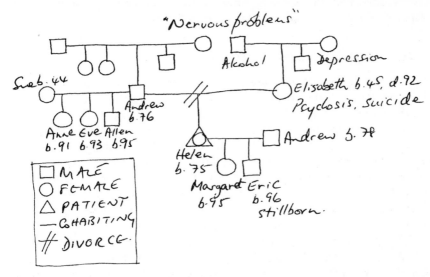

Figure 21.1 An example of a family map (genogram). This was drawn with the help of the patient and relatives during one of the first meetings. It started with the patient (Helen) and her husband and children. Next her parents and siblings were placed in the genogram and then her grandparents. Important events were noted such as deaths or mental illness. This kind of map helps to create an understanding for the patient's psychological and social background as well as special vulnerability factors. It also makes it possible to see the relationships more clearly for the patient herself as well as for everyone else involved. In this case the stillbirth of Helen's son clearly became central as the triggering experience. The patient's vulnerability can be understood against the background of her mother's depression and psychosis.

In principle the same group of individuals that met with the patient and family at the beginning should continue to look after them. This continuity remains important even when long-term treatment is needed. Most relapses occur in the first five years. Consequently this is the time when the need for accessible professional help and support is greatest.

A lowest optimal neuroleptic dose

During the first week one should aim to deal with the patient's anxiety and difficulties in sleeping. Apart from talking with the patient this is best accomplished with hypnotic medications such as benzodiazepines. If the psychotic symptoms are disturbing or indicate a significant level of risk, a low dose neuroleptic can be used. The dose should be increased slowly to help avoid side effects. It can be an art to motivate the patient to try medication. It may help to remind the patient of his own description of his problems:

for example, that 'the thinking process isn't functioning as it should'. These aspects are more fully illustrated in Chapter 24.

Suitable night-time care

Experience shows that, in acute wards, great importance should be given to the need for trust, understanding and a low level of stimulation. Ideally the patient should remain at home in a familiar environment in order to address these needs. However, sometimes this environment can be inappropriate. Relatives can be too worried or become overinvolved, making constant suggestions or questions, which heighten the emotional level (expressed emotion) instead of decreasing it. If the patient lives alone, the home can become very dilapidated or messy after a period of illness. Finally, experiences of persecution, delusions and hallucinations can make it impossible to live at home, if the home has become the focus of their fears.

If the patient needs to come in for care and treatment it is best for them to go to a special crisis home for people with acute psychosis. Unfortunately few of these exist, but experience shows them to be very useful. They are often established in urban houses or flats. It is important that it should be neither too big, impersonal, disturbing or crowded, nor contain too many chronically ill patients. Each patient should have one or two key workers or therapists, who can also maintain contact with the family. Admission to this kind of home usually stabilises the situation.

With these supportive resources it is possible to provide 24-hour care for most acutely psychotic patients. Such care is not primarily adapted for the most disturbed patients but is suitable for the majority of psychotic patients. One must ensure, as part of one's assessment, that the patient is capable of responding well to the relative openness, negotiability and freedom from restraint of such crisis homes. Suicide and violent behaviour seldom take place in these environments (Cullberg et al. 2000). Ideally one should keep the staff numbers relatively low, something which often reduces tension in a crisis of this kind. However, it must be possible to offer extra staff support in crisis situations. Patients who are acutely suicidal or whose psychosis has resulted in unmanageable aggression need to be cared for on an acute psychiatric ward until these problems have resolved. Here they can still maintain an ongoing relationship with their allocated workers from the psychosis team. The crisis home facilities are often not suitable for patients with prominent manic symptoms.

Diagnostic formulation and investigations

The psychiatric management should include a preliminary formulation of the nature and degree of the psychosis. The capacity of the patient and their social network to contain any disturbed behaviour resulting from the psychosis should also be assessed. Decisions have to be made about the need for hospitalisation and medication. Furthermore, a preliminary assessment should be made about any underlying cause(s) or triggers: whether there are elements of affective illness, physical illness or substance misuse. Any diagnosis should be provisional as this allows for the broad variation in initial presentation and helps prevent therapeutic nihilism.

A physical examination should not be recommended before it is felt to be acceptable to the patient. In some cases the patient can refuse – and then it is a question of compromise and a need to think about what the situation really demands. After all, a physical examination may often be postponed unless there is overriding evidence of a physical cause.

EEG, CT or MRI of the brain should also not be carried out until a good relationship has been fostered with the patient. However, in cases where there might well be organic problems, it must take place early on and then it is essential to encourage the patient to co-operate. The reason for carrying out these relatively troublesome and expensive examinations is that in around 10 per cent of cases of first-episode psychosis there are significant findings in the brain. These are more often than not negligible, but may be relevant to treatment. My experience is that patients, with few exceptions, appreciate careful investigations and react positively when they find that nothing pathological has been discovered.

Neuropsychological investigations (for example, WAIS-R)[1] should preferably be done once the psychosis has resolved, or at least stabilised. These tests give information regarding cognitive deficits, which sometimes make the psychotic processes more understandable. They can also help plan rehabilitation.

A subspecialist team for first-episode psychosis

During recent decades international research and experiences have been collated. The consensus is that it is beneficial to provide people suffering from a first-episode psychosis with a containing environment with longer term continuity of care. The necessity for continuity of care is a high priority for this group because of the high risk of relapse and developing functional disabilities. Research suggests that caring for both chronically ill and first-episode patients together can create additional problems. The chronically ill patients are often better able to express their needs, overshadowing the needs of the first-episode patients. With a sustained period of contact with first-episode patients the level of support needed can be continually reassessed and knowledge regarding their resources and those of their families can be more firmly established. I now present a few projects which differ in their organisation but have the same central aim of keeping their patients' needs a priority. They have all been evaluated scientifically.

The Soteria projects

The Soteria projects ('soteria' is Greek for someone who rescues – a saviour) were first developed in California in the 1970s (Mosher *et al.* 1995). Under the leadership of the psychiatrist Loren Mosher, patients with acute psychosis were treated primarily with humanist and psychotherapeutic methods of working. Only half of the staff had psychiatric training; the rest were employed on the basis of the merits of their personalities. Neuroleptics were prescribed only as a last resort. Many of the ideas were formed as a result of the contemporary anti-psychiatric vogue. This is one of the reasons why the Soteria movement was viewed with scepticism by the psychiatric establishment. The enterprise was evaluated in comparison with a control group, which was treated in a conventional psychiatric ward. The result showed that 67 per cent of the Soteria patients were successfully treated without the use of neuroleptics during the first six weeks compared to 0 per cent of the control groups of patients. The outcome between the approaches did not differ in spite of this. A comparison between the subjective experiences of the different forms of treatment has not been done, but one imagines the difference would be considerable.

In the mid-1980s the psychiatrist Luc Ciompi of Switzerland started the Soteria Bern project (Ciompi *et al.* 1992). This was based on his theoretical considerations about psycho-biological vulnerability and psychic overstimulation in schizophrenia and on his studies of factors which influence long-term prognosis. Treatment was organised according to the stress-vulnerability model. Patients were cared for in a villa where there was a low-stimulus environment. Patients were in groups of six and the staff were selected more for their personal qualities than for their professional qualifications. They worked long shifts in order to maximise continuity during the first period when the psychosis was still dominant. The use of neuroleptics was minimal. Treatment took place in close co-operation with the families and in three phases with increasing demands being made on the patients actively to participate at each phase. This project has been carefully compared with randomised control groups. The initial results were very good with 63 per cent of the patients who had been discharged in a good or very good mental condition, virtually or completely asymptomatic. At two years follow-up, the results were closer to those of the control group's which received high quality traditional care. One likely explanation for this is that it had not been possible to continue providing such a high level of contact after discharge from hospital. Another explanation is that the two- to three-year period following the initial phase of illness that was studied represents a further risk period, and that this must be treated with just as intensive an involvement as with the first period. Today there are several similar Soteria homes in Europe and a review has been recently published (Ciompi and Hoffman 2004).

EPPIC

Another model is the EPPIC (Early Psychosis Prevention and Intervention Centre) under the directorship of the psychiatrist Pat McGorry and the psychologist Jane Edwards in Australia (McGorry *et al.* 1996). Here they have set up a project in an area of Melbourne, with 800,000 inhabitants. They receive referrals for those who have a first-episode psychosis and follow the patients for, at most, 18 months. They provide care and treatment for the acutely ill in the form of home visits, family education and support, low dose pharmacological treatment, systematic cognitive-behavioural psychotherapy and where necessary admission to hospital. Evaluation of this project has shown very good results. After a year the severity of symptoms was reduced and quality of life was improved. The main weakness of the study design was the use of a historical control group. As yet there have not been any long-term prospective randomised controlled follow-up studies.

The essential thing is not to look for a single model for first-episode psychosis patients but to focus on providing as much support as local resources permit. Within EPPIC a combined research and treatment project for young people with early signs of psychotic illness has also been carried out (see Chapter 26 for further elaboration.)

The Parachute project

The Swedish Parachute project (the metaphor is meant to suggest a soft landing following psychosis) was started in 1996 as a two-year, multi-centre project with 17 participating clinics (Cullberg *et al.* 2002). It examined the development of the organisation of care as well as research. The catchment area was 1.6 million inhabitants, that is one-sixth of the population of Sweden. The project studied all identified cases of first-episode psychosis in patients aged between 18 and 45. Individuals who had brain damage or current history of severe alcohol and substance misuse were excluded. The treatment was 'need adjusted', which was defined according to the criteria delineated at the beginning of this chapter.

The Parachute project's principles for treatment of first-episode psychosis

1 Early intervention (< 24 hours).
2 Crisis and psychotherapeutic orientation.
3 Family meetings.
4 Continuity and accessibility to the first-episode service for five years.

---

5 Lowest effective antipsychotic medication. Initial treatment without neuroleptics when possible.

6 Therapeutic inpatient milieu (personal, low stimulus, non-institutional).

During the two-year period 253 patients met the criteria for first-episode psychotic illness according to DSM-IV. Those with a non-congruent affective psychosis were also included. Less than a third refused to take part in the research or could not be followed up after one year. This left 175 participating patients. These have now been followed up for five years studying numerous clinical, social, psychological and biological parameters.

A comparative study using a historical control group made up of first-onset patients cared for between 1991 and 1992 from three of the clinics has been completed (Svedberg *et al.* 2001). The prospective (contemporaneous and followed from the beginning) comparison group from a high quality psychiatric clinic is still not finished. The three-year results confirm expectations (Cullberg *et al.* 2005). The group treated using first-episode principles shows symptomatic improvement compared to the historical control group which shows a similar response to the prospective control group. However, the treatment group shows less functional disability, in spite of less antipsychotic medication (with very few on depot medication) and less inpatient care. As a result, the mean total direct cost of care was considerably lower for the Parachute patients.

Several clinics that took part in the Parachute project have not been able to provide the level of care stipulated, especially with crisis home care. However, even taking this into account one can conclude that intensive psychosocial treatment can be used in acute psychosis. It lowers the dose of neuroleptic medication required, lowers the need for depot and improves levels of function. The clinics did not receive any extra economic resources for this reorganisation of care.

The OPUS trial

This project is ongoing in Copenhagen. Methodologically it is superior as it is a randomised multi-centre trial of integrated versus standard treatment for 547 first-episode psychosis patients (Nordentoft *et al.* 2004). The approach to treatment is similar in many ways to that of the Parachute project, and to the EPPIC project. The results of integrated treatment are significantly better than with standard treatment, in terms of symptomatic improvement, with fewer inpatient days per patient and better satisfaction with treatment.

With the results of these projects in mind it seems unethical and also uneconomical to continue the traditional care system for first-episode patients (and potentially for all patients with psychosis).

The late phase of psychosis: supporting the healthy part of the personality

In the late phase of psychosis the patients have become less disturbed by their delusions and hallucinations. Alternatively these symptoms dwindle and may slowly disappear. 'Islands of sanity' become more marked (see further Chapter 5 regarding the different phases of psychosis). Attempts should be made to contact the 'healthy part' of the patient's personality in order to strengthen and support its functioning. To do this the carer must assume that the patient has a potential for healthy functioning that coexists with the psychotic part – even if this is in no way apparent. Delusions and hallucinations should be challenged respectfully and seriously, rather than flippantly or dismissively. Often the patient is being treated with neuroleptics. If the psychotic symptoms remain although the dose is adequate, a change to another atypical neuroleptic might be appropriate; otherwise a careful increase of the dose should be tried. All this has to be done in close co-operation with the patient as far as is possible.

If the patient can accept the existence of his psychosis it will help him or her to identify when a relapse is approaching. Ideally, the patients themselves should be helped to reflect on what has happened rather than supported in dismissing their psychotic experiences ('sealing over'), and later denying the intervention that occurred as a result of their psychotic experiences. Many patients who have just recovered from a psychotic episode find being challenged by their carers about their delusions and hallucinations too provocative. This reinforces the tendency to 'seal over' and hence deny any future vulnerability. It is often valuable to go back to the formulation of the problem that was offered by the patient during the first phase of illness in order to see what has happened and how they have changed.

The *depression* that one often sees when the psychosis begins to resolve is at least in part an understandable reaction to the fact of the illness and the painful experiences that go with it. Many patients and relatives who have experienced an acute psychotic episode have the impression that it represents the first expression of a chronic mental illness. It is important to talk this through and to emphasise the positive aspects of the prognosis as well as the potential for compensating for their vulnerability. It is also important that the family participates in making plans for the future (with the patient's consent).

The recovery phase: to strengthen the ego and reduce vulnerability

When the patient is free from psychosis

For the patient who appears to have recovered completely it is important to rebuild contact with his pre-existing social network. Joint meetings with members of the family or work colleagues can be helpful at this point.

Most of those who have had one psychotic episode are likely to have at least one relapse. For this reason it is also important to go through early signs of relapse and to discuss methods of preventing it in an informative and educational way. Sometimes several relapses have to occur before the patient begins to accept their illness or that he or she might be able to influence its development. Many develop a clearer understanding of their psychotic illness when it is explained in terms of a specific vulnerability (see Chapters 6 and 7). It is also possible to explore what triggered the psychosis (Chapter 8), which may in turn be linked to the identified vulnerabilities. Comparisons with other types of illness can be useful. A high level of vulnerability to psychosis can be compared to the increased vulnerability to infections seen in immune deficiencies. This non-judgemental approach can help replace denial, guilt and blame with a more realistic explanation, which in turn may increase the patient's sense of control. It then becomes easier rationally to discuss the things that can be done to reduce vulnerability: medication, psychological help, adapted living conditions, and the ability to detect early signs of illness.

The psychological support given varies according to the patient's needs and the care resources available. Group discussions with other patients who have experienced a first-episode psychosis encourages some people to face their vulnerability and enables them to discuss their experiences of stigmatisation and exclusion.

It is now also important to decide if and for how long regular medication should be recommended. For patients in early stages of relapse, it is of immediate importance. The dose should not be so high that it disturbs the ability to function or produces side effects and obviously not so low that it has no impact at all. The experience of many workers in this field suggests that low doses of a neuroleptic – perhaps the equivalent of 2 mg haloperidol – can have a long-term preventative effect. In patients with good insight and a strong network it is often possible to use even lower doses. Sometimes it is only necessary to prescribe medication when there are signs of a relapse.

With certain patients an ongoing but unresolved problem of separation or other developmental issues have triggered or contributed to the psychosis. Readjustment becomes more difficult and increases the risk of relapse. In this situation it is of great importance that patients are offered an appropriate form of psychotherapy. It is possible, too, to see recurrent depressive crises in the late phase of the episode where the patient may need both psychotherapeutic as well as pharmacological treatment.

Many patients who have been through an acute psychosis have had early traumatic experiences which have contributed to their vulnerability. Depending on the strength of the patient's personality and motivation (as well as on the clinic's resources) psychotherapy may be indicated. The patient can take possession of his life history for the first time. The (non-psychotic) experience of coherence may also be significant for the healing process.

The essential thing, in my experience, is not which school of thought the therapist belongs to. The decisive factor is the quality of the patient–therapist relationship. It should encourage re-engagement and a sense of hope balanced against an awareness of the level of vulnerability and functional disability. This must be informed by their expertise and knowledge in weighing psycho-pharmacological benefits against risks. Therapists who work with patients with psychosis tend to become more like each other in their psychotherapeutic attitude and understanding of insight. They need to have realistic goals and a high degree of flexibility.

Early co-operation with employment centres, insurance and social services

Many first-episode psychotic patients will have had a long period of social difficulties in their studies or problems at work. As soon as the clinical situation allows for it, it is important to find out how they have functioned at school, at work and with friends. Many patients who may appear 'well' from a psychiatric perspective do not have enough training or education, or are too sensitive to compete on the open employment market. So it is important to support the patient early on in their contact with different rehabilitation organisations, and to make sure that the social services attend to the improvement of living conditions, etc. It is valuable to encourage study or vocational training during long-term illness in order to help protect people from being pensioned off at an early age with the ensuing loss of self-confidence.

Persistent psychotic symptoms

Around a third of people who have become ill for the first time do not recover after six months or longer and continue to suffer from persistent delusions or hallucinations – or vestiges of them. In these cases the prescription of medication should have been reviewed, and appropriately adjusted or supplemented. A decision has to be made as to whether a specific psychological treatment for the remaining symptoms is indicated. In these cases techniques which depend on cognitive-behavioural therapy (CBT) can reduce hallucinations, delusions and depressive symptoms resulting in an increased social adjustment for many patients (see Chapter 25). This kind of therapy can be carried out by ordinary members of staff with appropriate training and supervision.

Chapter 22

Psychosis and suicide

From a metaphorical and literal perspective a psychotic episode is the killing of the self – one's own self is put out of the running. It is not unusual for the person who has experienced a psychotic episode to say afterwards, 'If I hadn't become psychotic then I would have killed myself.' The experience of an insoluble or disturbing life situation could have been too powerful. There are also many dynamic similarities between the thought of death and psychosis. Losing one's life and losing one's mind both entail relinquishing one's personal identity. However, there are also many important differences, amongst others that the suicidal person often shows an pre-existing inclination for suicidal thoughts. It may be that a 'suicidal process' has developed even before the psychosis.

Incidence

There is hardly any research about how often suicide occurs during the development of a psychosis. On the other hand there are many studies of the incidence of suicide during the course of a schizophrenic illness. The most reliable figures suggest that between 8 and 12 per cent of all those with schizophrenia eventually commit suicide. This means that schizophrenia, together with bipolar illnesses and alcohol abuse, is one of the psychiatric conditions with the highest mortality. It is probable that those psychoses with more marked affective traits – especially schizophreniform, schizo-affective and affective psychoses – have an even higher suicide risk than schizophrenia. In these cases we see a combination of psychosis and acute affective problems that result in the defences against suicidal impulses being weakened even more.

'Almost an execution'

Three years earlier Helen had suffered a long-term depressive psych-osis (described in more detail in Chapter 25, p. 288). She was forcibly medicated for six months without effect. However, by moving to another ward and receiving intensive psychotherapy Helen made a full recovery.

Several years later she showed signs of relapse after having worked 'day and night' to complete an important report for her work. When it was finished she shut herself in her house and did not answer the telephone. Since I had treated her before, I was alerted by the parents. I went directly to the patient's home and was able to let myself in with the mother's key. Helen had extensive bruising round her neck after trying to hang herself – the hook had come away from the ceiling. The extent of her delusions was unclear, but she exhibited profound hopelessness saying that she was not worth admitting to hospital. (It subsequently transpired that she had visited a police station the previous evening saying that she wanted to give herself up as she 'understood' that they wished to interrogate her because she was a criminal.) Because of the high risk of suicide she was admitted compulsorily. Despite being kept under close watch she succeeded in slipping away from the ward and hanged herself from a tree.

COMMENTS

Helen's severe psychotic depression developed very quickly, over a period of a few days after a longer period of great stress and poor sleep. Her overall mental state had previously been very good. She had responded well to psychotherapy and had changed the way she lived to suit her own wishes. This relapse was triggered by work-related stress. Terrifying memories of the previous long-term compulsory treatment returned during her inevitable compulsory admission. She had psychotic ideas about her own guilt and badness. Her suicide almost had the character of an execution in which she did not even grant herself a 'stay' in order to contact her psychiatrist for help. Her grandmother had spent most of her life in a mental hospital and so there must have been a genetic vulnerability in this talented patient. This case also shows the incredible power that can drive a suicidal wish.

Suicidality during the development of psychosis

During the prodromal phase the person senses diffuse rumblings in the personality as harbingers of a possible catastrophe. They feel that their inner resources are insufficient to control the situation. In such a situation a depressive anxiety along with feelings of hopelessness can lead to desperate suicidal acts – perhaps as a final paradoxical attempt to gain control. The diagnosis can become clear as consciousness is regained after a suicide attempt with medication or poison, if delusions – which may be denied later on – emerge.

Plastic surgery on a normal nose

A young man was admitted after a serious suicide attempt: an overdose of sleeping tablets. Some months earlier he had had plastic surgery to his nose which he thought was bulbous and unsightly. According to the surgeon's notes there was nothing remarkable about his nose, but he had not wanted to go against the patient's wish. After the operation the patient was dissatisfied with how it had turned out. He said that his ears also looked strange. This time he was refused an operation and this appeared to be the trigger for his suicide attempt. Waking up in the intensive care unit he told the consultant psychiatrist how gangs were looking for him. He said that he had kept out of their way for the past six months to avoid being attacked by them. He believed that this was because they suspected him of being homosexual, which he was not. This was part of the reason he had wanted to change his appearance. When reassessed a few days later the patient appeared bemused by these ideas and it was not possible to elicit any symptoms of either psychosis or depression. He was discharged at his own request. Two months later his sister reported that he had committed suicide. She said that his behaviour had become increasingly strange towards the end. He had not wanted to go out and had said that he was being persecuted.

COMMENTS

It is not unusual for patients to reveal important information relating to their psychosis when regaining consciousness. This may be due to the effects of the anaesthetic. Later they may deny all knowledge and even feel that they were duped into making these revelations. It thus becomes a difficult balancing act between the therapist's need to know more and the patient's legitimate demand for privacy and integrity. The psychiatrist suspected that this patient was in the prodromal phase of a psychotic episode but did not think that he could do any more as the patient refused to let him meet his family and outwardly seemed to be in full control.

During the early stages of the psychosis, up until its peak, suicidal acts are less common. However, they can result from command auditory hallucinations. One or more voices may urge the person to jump from a balcony or run into a busy road; these experiences may be so intense that it is virtually impossible to resist. Self-immolation (setting fire to oneself) in psychosis may be a form of self-punishment, or a self-sacrifice for mankind, or result from some kind of religious delusional self-identification (for example, that one is Christ; see the case study in Chapter 15, p. 176). A depressive component is often found in these psychoses (see also the case description of Szandor in Chapter 10).

Giving up his resistance

Peter, a 20-year-old very talented artist, was admitted to hospital with features of a schizophrenic illness after having spent the previous year abroad living a miserable destitute existence. His father had found him when he received reports that his son was acting strangely and had arranged for psychiatric help. Initially Peter refused to co-operate in any way and adopted a sneering and rather arrogant attitude towards staff and fellow patients. He was even less inclined to take medication. However, it gradually emerged that he suffered from auditory hallucinations and believed that experiments were being conducted upon him. A great deal of effort was made to establish contact and motivate him to try medication. After more than a month he told staff that he would be prepared to take medicine if the female house physician with whom he had spoken the most was the one to administer it. He now appeared to be extra calm and had even trimmed his hair and beard. The doctor in question was not on duty that particular day and it was decided that she would see Peter the following day. The same night Peter hanged himself with a rope he had made out of towels. Everyone was staggered and deeply shaken. Great effort was put into trying to understand why Peter had taken his life in this situation. The interpretation that felt the most plausible was that when he abandoned his defensive attitude by finally asking for help he came into contact with his weak and dependent side that he had previously kept at a distance through his superior attitude. He was unable to tolerate this side of himself and this awoke an even deeper hopelessness.

Another kind of risk arises in the later stages of a psychotic illness. Insight into the illness can result in a catastrophic reaction because the ideas which had dominated the patient's life for the preceding weeks or months have turned out to be false. The overall meaning and perhaps grandiose feeling of being chosen which the psychosis had given to one's life become untenable. The paranoid system collapses resulting in feelings of shame, exposure and humiliation at what one has said and done in front of friends, relatives and work colleagues. There may be feelings of guilt about things one has done under the influence of the psychosis, perhaps reinforced by a hypomanic lack of judgement, which can also feel crushing. In addition one is forced to face the problems that had preceded and perhaps contributed to or triggered the psychosis. These had been concealed by the illness, and their re-emergence may make suicide feel like a natural way out. Clearly it is of major importance that post-psychotic depression is identified by psychiatric staff and treated appropriately (see Chapter 21).

Another risk during the recovery phase is that the side effects of high-dose neuroleptic medication are so distressing that they can drive the person to suicide. Many descriptions in the literature depict how side effects of neuro-leptic medication such as akathisia (psychological or muscular restless-ness) or dysphoria (a state of mental unease) can be incorrectly perceived by staff as residual symptoms of the illness. Further increases in medication can result in increasing desperation which in turn leads to suicide. Inevitably such suicides will be under-reported as some cases will be viewed as resulting from untreated psychotic symptoms.

Suicidal acts among patients suffering from schizophrenia

Many, perhaps most, who have suffered from schizophrenia over a long period will have had thoughts about taking their own life at some point. In these cases the social and psychological consequences of their illness often awaken existential issues in the ill person that drive him or her to suicide. Patients with paranoid symptoms in particular run this risk whilst suicidal ideas and acts are more unusual in those with autistic/negative symptoms.

I have recently led a study looking at suicide attempts in schizophrenia. During interviews with the control group (people with schizophrenia who had never attempted suicide) it emerged that all of these patients had had serious suicidal thoughts or plans but had not put them into action. This illustrates how strongly suicidal thoughts are linked to schizophrenia (Stefenson and Cullberg 2005). In another qualitative study, this time of accounts from care staff and relatives of individuals who had taken their own life after a long period of schizophrenic illness, it emerged that many of the patients had clearly expressed feelings of loss and hopelessness with regard to important aspects of their personal lives: family, parenthood and professional activities (Stefenson and Cullberg 1995).

Many committed suicide in a phase when they had few symptoms and outwardly appeared to be functioning well. However, they had also expressed a fear of relapsing, saying that they would not be able to endure being ill again. In some cases it seemed that suicide had been triggered by the early signs of a relapse.

In all the cases a major life event had occurred in the period leading up to the suicide. A unifying feature of these life events was some kind of separation experience. The death of a relative or loss of someone close (including a psychiatric worker) acted as significant crisis triggering factors in these high-risk individuals whose social network was already weakened.

Ursula was 35 years old when she took her own life with an overdose of antidepressant medication. She had been diagnosed with schizophrenia 16 years earlier and had had a number of relapses. Prior to falling ill for the first time she had had a good social life with friends and many interests. After her first psychosis Ursula married and had a daughter. When she wanted to breastfeed the baby it was agreed that she would stop medication. A short time later she fell ill again, developing hallucinations and delusions. The following years were characterised by alternating periods of relapse and remission. Without medication she easily relapsed; with medication she was fatigued and suffered neuro-muscular side effects. Her husband eventually filed for divorce and Ursula, who lost custody of her daughter, was only awarded visiting rights. After this she often expressed her despair at not being allowed to look after her daughter. She became increasingly obsessed with how she could regain custody. Four days before her suicide she wrote a well-formulated letter to her ex-husband (who had not stopped supporting her). She described how since the divorce she had felt that her life was a failure. She wished to return to the time when her daughter had just been born. She did not mention anything about wanting to take her own life. However, she had indicated this in a conversation with a female friend.

The other theme that emerged in this study concerned failing to achieve an independent life: for example, being unable to cope with attempts at rehabilitation or being afraid at the prospect of starting a new job. Three women committed suicide within three months of having moved back to their parental home. All of them had spoken of this in terms of a personal failure.

The suicidal acts of schizophrenics can occur at any time during the course of the illness. The first year of illness is usually considered to be the most high risk. Suicides related to psychotic symptoms are more unpredictable than those which occur in the later phase of the illness. These can often be understood in terms of difficulties in adjusting to reality. The methods used are often more lethal than those usually seen in psychiatry (e.g. hanging, jumping from a great height). Relatives and friends may have become accustomed to and worn out by disturbed behaviour. As a result they may not notice the warning signs in advance, or not realise their true significance. The high risk of suicide in psychotic patients means that it is essential that all mental health professionals regularly review their caseload for evidence of increased risk. Key workers must receive continuing supervision and support in their professional work as part of this process.

Working with patients at high risk of suicide – ethical problems

There is a group of high-risk patients with a relapsing and remitting illness where the non-psychotic periods are filled with depressive despair and thoughts of suicide. Relatives and the staff on the ward frequently experience the understandable and very unsettling anxiety that the patient will commit suicide. Often they see no solution apart from increasing the dose of medication or using depot injection as ways of 'insuring' against suicide. However, this can have a paradoxical effect if the psychotic symptoms are already fully controlled. The danger then is that quality of life is worsened by the sedating effects of higher doses of antipsychotics. This sedation may be interpreted as a positive response to treatment. From the patient's point of view it is an undesirable side effect, and at these higher doses there may also be one of the many unpleasant side effects. The resulting subjective distress (which may be masked by sedation) in such a situation can increase the risk of suicide.

There is a poorly defined group of personality disordered patients who have a vulnerability to psychosis which is exacerbated by a number of factors such as relationship difficulties, substance misuse or lack of social success. They have often been subjected to traumatic events during their early childhood or later in life. In the face of adversity and disappointment suicide attempts can often occur. For others with this kind of a debilitating functional disturbance, life can feel meaningless with the wasted years leading to despair and suicide.

The treatment of these patients is complex and challenging. Short-term risks must be weighed against long-term benefits. There are serious ethical dilemmas that have implications for practice. These ethical problems cannot be resolved with simple rules of thumb but must always be kept in mind within the ward: for example:

- where there is a conflict between the professionals' need to protect the patient and the patient's need to make their own decisions
- the risk that humanitarian protectiveness develops into paternalism or into a destructive power struggle with the patient
- carers and professionals are at risk of 'burn out' (demoralisation and lack of motivation) as a result of working with a patient who repeatedly creates high levels of anxiety in them

- when individual therapists or workers become reluctant to take on or care for high-risk patients – in this situation support and supervision are essential
- the object of psychiatry is not to prevent suicide at any cost, rather to reduce the risks whilst providing treatment and care.

The number of deaths from suicide amongst patients with psychosis has, as mentioned earlier, been around 10 per cent during the first five to ten years. These are usually people who have not had access to psychotherapy or to help with mourning for the life that they had hoped for before they became ill. We have to keep in mind this underlying high but 'normal' suicide rate when making considered judgements about risks. Indifference and a 'so what?' mentality have to be avoided, as does paternalism, partly by offering the patients the best that is possible in terms of treatment, and partly by being aware of the restrictions inherent in psychiatric practice which can inadvertently take too much responsibility for the life of the patient. With 'need-adapted treatment' (see Chapter 21) the risk for suicide seems to be considerably reduced (Cullberg *et al.* 2002).

What does it mean to 'do the best you can'?

'If you have done your best, you have the right to fail' is a maxim that is supportive of the member of staff who looks after a patient who might commit suicide. 'Doing one's best' also means that the head of the clinical team takes responsibility for making sure that the necessary psychotherapeutic treatment and supervision are available, in addition to general psychiatric treatment and knowledge.

There are some patients who become destructive whether they live with their families, on their own or on a psychiatric ward. Such patients can benefit greatly from a residential home that is run along psychotherapeutic lines, reducing their destructive acting out and so their risk of suicide. This partly protected environment can promote the process of long-term recovery and rehabilitation into the community. The patient can be supported in this kind of environment whilst slowly being helped to take responsibility for his day-to-day life (see Chapter 14 for more details about the critical periods of psychosis and the possibilities for recovery).

A splitting process often occurs in a staff group when one or more patients appear suicidal. Some support a strict supervisory, paternalistic attitude whereas others wish to promote the patient's autonomy. The not unreasonable expectation that these apparently contradictory aspects can coexist then becomes more difficult as members of the team blame each other for their coldness or naivety. The staff group now becomes the outer arena where the patient's inner struggle takes place. It means that the staff must be given competent supervision, so that it is possible for them to see how destructive the interactions have become within the group. It is helpful to understand that they are often a reflection of the patient's disturbance. A key distinction is whether these positions are taken unconsciously or as a result of a reflective process within the group. In the latter situation it is easier to cope with the uncertainty of the situation and the anxiety that ensues.

Any medical interventions such as antidepressants or sedatives need to be well judged and perceived as positively therapeutic by the patient as well as the staff. It is important to be able to distinguish between medical interventions for therapeutic purposes and those which are designed to relieve one's own anxieties or those of other staff. These patients are often prescribed several medications at the same time, which may have an effect on different receptors. This makes their overall effect more difficult to assess and it may well be negative as a result of increased risk of side effects.

The same kind of consideration needs to be given to the question of compulsory treatment and supervision. A patient who is acutely suicidal needs some degree of supervision to prevent them harming themselves, but at the same time it is essential to be aware that the suicidal behaviour can become a tool in a desperate struggle between the patient and the treating team. This is further complicated by the fact that these situations are not mutually exclusive: the patient can be suicidal and may be caught up in a struggle with the treating team.

It is painful when a patient who has been dominated by the drive to ruin his life or to commit suicide, in spite of the attempts that many people have made to stop him, finally succeeds. Many capable staff abandon psychiatry for this reason. Such tragedies should not lead us to believe that there is no point in working psychologically with suicidal patients who have a vulnerability to psychosis. In fact I have seen the most persuasive cases of psychotherapeutic success with a number of personality disordered patients with a vulnerability to psychosis. But the emotional and short-term economic costs for all concerned with these treatments are usually high. However, these short-term economic costs are small in comparison with the expenditure that has to be made on a chronically ill patient. This is no different to the costs of lifesaving work that has to be carried out with physically ill people.

The emotional needs of the staff – the importance of protection against 'burn out'

The relationships between patients, staff and the institution as a whole are very complex. Staff who work with psychotic patients or people with psychiatric functional disabilities for a large part of the day may well become demoralised and unmotivated by their work. This results from the daily exposure to the patients' psychotic thinking and primitive impulses and consequent destructive behaviour. Individual staff's commitment to therapeutic work is frustrated by these phenomena. Staff in this position need support and supervision, and additional opportunities such as further train-ing and possibilities of work in other areas.

In the traditional psychiatric ward the exhaustion that results from work-ing with psychotic patients is overcome with a variety of defensive approaches, which often become a feature of the institution. These include increasingly 'distancing' of oneself from the patients (for example, excessive paperwork, or using only a 'symptom' oriented medical model which avoids addressing emotional issues). These processes reduce the empathic compon-ent and the intensity of the staff–patient relationship. This has a number of effects. Most importantly it reduces the potential for doing psychological work, and so has a detrimental impact on treatment outcome. The reduced level of involvement requires less emotional effort by staff and less organised supervision for them. It also makes it easier for them to leave their jobs.

It is clear that at a conscious or unconscious level this process of 'dis-tancing' appears to give many short-term benefits for the individual staff member and the institution. However, in the longer term it has a negative impact on staff morale as their work becomes disengaged and mechanical. Recruitment and retention suffer, and supervision becomes reactive (to cri-ses) rather than reflective and proactive (not just thinking about patients when they are in crisis). In this sense these ways of working can be viewed as institutional defences.

Chapter 23

People with long-term psychosis in the community

Within traditional Swedish psychiatric treatment, people with debilitating chronic psychosis were placed in remote residential care homes. These residential homes were complemented with 'family care' for those patients who made least fuss. That implies a kind of boarding condition in the country without any expectations of meaningful activities. In the past, these methods of care represented a necessary and humanitarian need for security, food, space and attention for those patients who could not look after themselves. Today they express an outdated and counterproductive psychiatric attitude. It strengthens the identity of being a 'chronic' patient and inhibits the natural tendency towards healing which depends on appropriate stimulation and self-reliance assisted by specific methods of treatment.

During the last decade fewer patients have been placed in such homes. The overwhelming tendency is to support as many people as possible in their own homes and those who cannot manage should be accommodated in protected homes and group homes offering different levels of assistance, where they will get both support and stimulation through meaningful occupation. Unfortunately, this goal has not yet been reached in many places. New slum areas consisting of homeless former patients have arisen. The social isolation of the former mental hospital may have been replaced by rented accommodation, which is no less isolated. This lack, which is the result of ignorance in the community coupled with a lack of co-operation between psychiatry and social services, cannot be accepted as an argument for the return to mental hospitals which is taking place in many western countries today. A far better alternative would be to learn from good examples. Here I will mention only a few examples as they all work on similar principles. An early milestone in the move towards integrating within the community those who have a functional disability was the Wisconsin project.

The Wisconsin project

While the Italian psychiatrist Franco Basaglia and his circle were changing Italian psychiatry in a near revolutionary way to the sound of loud trumpeting in the 1970s, a more reformative development was taking place in certain places in the USA and in many other places in the world. In Wisconsin, USA, the psychiatrist Leonard Stein and the psychologist Mary Ann Test started a social-psychiatry orientated enterprise within an area which included 350,000 inhabitants (Stein and Test 1980). They showed that with certain methods taken from the dominant hospital care system, many more patients could live at home, many were able to work, and the quality of their lives improved. The resources freed for this were reinvested in mobile open ward teams and acute ward facilities offering a 24-hour service. For years after patients had been discharged from hospital, due to the lack of effective social services, the mobile team had to continue their supportive work by finding employment for people and then help those with functional disabilities to adjust to their workplace. They also found accommodation and support with self-care training and economic planning over and above the specific psychiatric work needed for the control of symptoms and the prevention of suicide. The principles behind the Wisconsin project, which should still be valid with any form of work with people with mental disabilities, are simple:

1   *An assertive attitude* should be maintained in relation to people whose functional disabilities lie in their lack of motivation and tendency to withdraw. A persistent attitude towards those clients[1] who do not keep their appointments; energy spent on the work of motivation and a calm tolerance has shown that most clients, sometimes against all odds, were able to follow through with the programme.

2   *The programme is directed towards every client's individual needs* and level of functioning. Each person is assigned two contact people who are in charge of the programme and who can ensure continuity.

3   *The training takes place in the home or at work.* People with functional disabilities can learn to cook or clean at a rehabilitation centre but they are often unable to transfer their learning to their home. To learn to do these things in a training centre is not the same as being able to function in an open workplace. Also, relatives and work mates often have to be encouraged to help with the teaching.

4   *It is important to build on a person's experiences and on their strengths* rather than to focus persistently on the symptoms of the illness. The patient should not be given too much support since this can lead to an increase in passivity.

5   A vital part of the work consists in *maintaining the client's role as a responsible citizen.* Emphasis is placed on the fact that people live in the

community because it is their right and not because the community allows it. Many past patients have learned that their illness is an excuse for any kind of behaviour. This attitude should not be encouraged; rather they should be encouraged to prize good behaviour. Bad behaviour carries the same consequences as it does for others in the community. Obviously, this does not apply to people with acute psychosis, which is why a clinical assessment in acute cases is necessary in order to decide what is most appropriate.

6   The possibility of a *24-hour support system* has reduced the need for inpatient wards significantly. Co-operation between the mobile team and the routine functions of psychiatry services ensures support.

Stein and Test have also shown that the very beneficial results which have been achieved with this work collapsed during some years when resources were withdrawn and so it was necessary to start again with many of the clients. An important outcome learnt was that many people who are functionally disabled by their mental health must be supported for their entire lives in order to prevent the handicap from becoming too great. The Wisconsin resources were significantly lower in comparison with Swedish resources. On the other hand, they have a more accessible employment market making it easier to find work opportunities.

From the principle of care for the ill to the principle of normalisation

During the great reform in psychiatry that occurred in Sweden in 1994, responsibility for the long-term rehabilitation and normalisation process was to be taken over by the local communities for those people when psychiatry felt it had done what it could in its treatment of acutely psychotic patients and where their home and work problems were a priority (Sou 1992). At the same time, the equivalent economic resources were transferred from the county councils to the communities in order to build up support and services for the long-term mentally ill who were functionally handicapped. Their number has been assessed at around 40,000 out of 9 million inhabitants in Sweden, half of whom have a significant handicap. This well-intended reform has stumbled ahead, especially in large cities. Here communities have still not taken full responsibility for creating single or communal protective places for living with the necessary supportive resources. Protected places of employment where people could enjoy the value of being part of the working community and which would help to decrease the need for treatment – and other care contributions – are still glaringly absent. There are many reasons for this:

•   Among community services and local politicians there is a dire lack of knowledge interlaced with negative and prejudiced attitudes against this group of people. Therefore, it is not surprising to find resources are given priority in more familiar fields.

- The social services' contribution easily becomes split off together with unmotivated and psychiatrically ignorant staff who quickly withdraw in the face of difficulties.
- In many cases, psychiatric services transferred patients to the community without making sure that their disabilities are taken into account or even assessing what sort of functional disabilities they might have. Psychiatry also withdrew from their opportunities to inform the social services about how to understand and work with psychiatric clients. When these people suffer a relapse into acute psychosis and need intensified support and sensitive help with medication, psychiatric staff must also be available to assess what is needed and be prepared to visit them at home or admit them to hospital. This should be done in co-operation with staff from social services. Otherwise the situation escalates and worried and disturbed neighbours end up calling in the police. The admission to hospital and eviction from home which then follows might have been avoided with an attentive and more immediate psychiatric service which was available on a 24-hour basis.

Personal ombudsman (representative)

In Sweden the establishment of a personal ombudsman represents an important aspect of reform in psychiatry. Every person who belongs to LSS (deriving from the laws that give the right for support and service for those who have the kind of handicap which hinders social functioning) is entitled to have a personal representative. The reform has as yet only been carried out on a trial basis but the results have been very positive in reducing hospital care and increasing quality of life. A personal representative is the 'advocate' for his or her client's interests in the community and makes sure that effective co-operation takes place between the different people involved. The personal representative should not help the client with food or cleaning which is something the social services are expected to do. The need for someone to keep an eye on the disabled person's rights have become indisputable.

Supported accommodation

Some people do not manage to live by themselves in spite of the contributions made by social services because their handicap is too severe or has become entrenched through long-term institutionalisation. A place has to be found for them in a group home with staff who are available during part of the day or, in certain cases, on a 24-hour basis.

If the person living in this type of accommodation has a history of substance misuse and becomes difficult to maintain, special accommodation that cares for such patients having problems from psychosis may be necessary. Another factor is brain injury, which adds to the difficulties and can mean increased problems with controlling impulses leading to such disturbing behaviour that isolation becomes necessary.

When a person is unable to care for themselves at home

The disabilities of certain people with schizophrenia may manifest in a marked lack of ability to maintain order and hygiene in the home. Old food lies festering in the refrigerator or is left scattered about, rubbish piles up, and the toilet becomes blocked. Some people who have not been helped for a long period of time find themselves having to wade through dust, old newspapers, clothes and other rubbish in order to get around their home. Personal hygiene is often neglected.

Regular meals are neglected and a repetitive menu or lack of food causes malnutrition. Many only go out when it is dark and shop as quickly as possible. Others will not eat ordinary food but choose an alternative such as cornflakes or flour in water. Cooking is much too difficult. The psychotic illness becomes accentuated by the neglect of nutritional needs. The fridge door may be left open, the electric cooker not turned off, cigarettes are left burning leading to serious fire risk.

Relationships with neighbours can become tense. During the times when the person is mentally unwell and may look unusually strange or frightening, neighbours understandably become afraid, especially for their children. Fears can be increased if the person begins to shout abusive insults, wanders about talking to himself, bangs on the walls or on the radiators due to beliefs about being spied on. This behaviour is a sign of loneliness. It provides an overt reflection that the level of care is too low and/or the person is perhaps in need of further medication. Yet it may lead to the neighbours demanding that the landlord evicts the tenant. When matters have escalated to this degree it is usually useless to try to influence the situation by psychological means. A short period in hospital can be followed by some kind of contact with the neighbours and community support. The problem with living close to a very disturbed person with schizophrenia should not be minimalised. The neighbours may need support and advice as to how they should conduct themselves. Simple information explaining the nature of the disability can be vital, as can the offer of access to telephone contact with someone should the problems continue. If the situation is hard to influence it is a sign that the level of care may need to be increased, either with a daily visit from a contact person or by transferring the person to sheltered housing.

Reactions of local residents to a new residential home

Often when a new residential care home is opened the neighbours become extremely concerned (Palmblad and Cullberg 1990). Petitions initiated by one or two active families may begin to circulate. Some neighbours may find it hard to resist adding their signatures to the list, but for many it is an expression of strong feelings and bitterness. The landlord and local council are drawn in and often the home is prevented from opening. It is important, for this reason, to send out information to the nearest residents whom it might concern in advance. They should be invited to a local informative meeting where those responsible can give a detailed explanation about the nature of the people who would be living in the residential home. The primary concerns that the neighbours express are fears that their children would be open to sexual violation and that illicit drugs might be introduced to their area. Another common worry is that the mentally ill will cause disturbances and anxieties are ventilated regarding the decrease in the value of property caused by the care home.

It is important to listen respectfully to these misgivings which are expressed by people who feel their investment in their homes is now threatened by the authorities. It is also noticeable that there is a powerful and irrational fear of madness latent in many people who unconsciously have the belief that it can be 'catching'. Information should be given explaining that the people concerned are not dangerous, describing the kinds of disabilities that they might have, and reassuring them that there is no danger of alcohol or narcotics. Sometimes it may be necessary to hold several meetings and to provide a telephone point of a contact who can deal with questions or complaints.

The problem of substance misuse – a dual diagnosis

Substance misuse is a severe problem for many people who suffer from mental disabilities. Usually it concerns simple forms of addiction with less impact on mental health such as tobacco or sweets. Misuse can, of course, take a more serious form: heavy alcohol consumption or smoking marijuana, for example, are relatively common in big towns. In certain inner city areas about half the patients diagnosed with schizophrenia have been found to have a problem with alcohol misuse or other drugs. The reasons for the misuse are manifold:

- Functional disability creates isolation and a lowered social competence which in itself increases the risk for patients finding themselves in circles where drugs are used and where there is a degree of social tolerance.
- Neuroleptic medication has the effect of subduing the sense of pleasure by inhibiting dopamine receptors. This effect can be counteracted by means of both nicotine and alcohol. With a radically lowered neuroleptic

dose and by changing to atypical neuroleptics this risk should be low-ered. (Drugs such as marijuana and amphetamines can trigger psychoses through the increase in stimulation and can constitute an additional risk if they are used by people who are on the edge of psychosis.)

- A common side effect with the new neuroleptics is that they increase appetite. This can create strong cravings for sweets, which can really only be reversed by means of a change of prescription. Otherwise obesity often results, which further decreases self-confidence.
- Self-medication with illicit drugs and alcohol is a well-recognised and dangerous consequence of anxiety and disturbances experienced in untreated psychosis.

It is important to be vigilant for substance misuse on acute psychiatric wards. Medication to combat side effects and a lower dose of the neuroleptic may go some way to prevent it from happening. Misuse will be a continuing problem as long as those who are functionally disabled through poor mental health find their way into joining other groups of people who are underprivileged.

Chapter 24

Pharmacological treatment of psychosis

The French researchers Delay and Deniker discovered in 1952 that *chlorpromazine* (Largactil) was not only useful as a pharmacological method of controlling temperature in operations where the organism was frozen (hibernating), but that it also had antipsychotic effects. This caused fresh optimism among those caring for people with schizophrenia. Little by little, a number of new substances were synthesised which had similar effects. Those who discovered them called the group of compounds neuroleptics (Greek *lepsis*, to grip hold of). Today antipsychotic medication is the usual term. During recent decades research has begun to show the sites and mechanisms of action of these medications in the brain. New compounds have been developed that have subtly different target sites and mechanisms of action for producing their antipsychotic effect. These substances are now called atypical neuroleptics.

Receptor pharmacology

The human brain contains around 100,000,000,000 nerve cells or *neurones* that maintain contact with each other by means of their offshoots (dendrites).

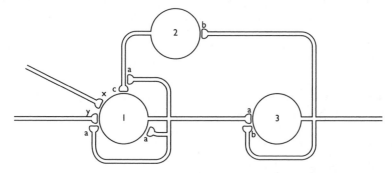

Figure 24.1 Schematic picture of a neural network. This shows how the nerve impulses are conveyed by means of synapses (a, b, c, x, y) and how the feedback loops take place.

In the places of contact, the *synapses*, the signal is transmitted by means of a chemical process from one neuron to the other. A process takes place whereby a certain *transmitter*, usually a molecule synthesised from an amino acid or several amino acids temporarily unite with a *receptor molecule* releasing the signal, which stimulates the receptive ('post-synaptic') neuron. The transmitter may be reabsorbed and reused, or broken down. One hundred transmitters are known today and have been identified and at least 300 receptors. Their sites in the brain, their genetic equivalence or what pharmacological and physiological functions they fulfil are still insufficiently mapped out. Some of the receptors that are of especial interest to the psychiatry of psychosis are as follows:

1   *Dopamine receptors.* According to current knowledge, these have five subtypes: dopamine D1–D5. The dopamine system emanates from the accumulation of cell nuclei in the middle brain. It is involved in the modulation of motor behaviour in the *striatum*. Connections are made to the *limbic* system which modulates sensual experiences and to the cortical, primarily the prefrontal areas which control cognitive processes. The dopamine system is central in the brain's *motivation and reward system* and regulates our mood. Amphetamine and cocaine increase the release of dopamine in the brain, while the classic neuroleptics block the action of released dopamine.

2   *The serotonin system.* This has different types of receptors and also proceeds from the middle brain and is projected through various routes both to the *limbic* and *cortical* areas. The hallucinogenic substances mescaline and LSD-25 stimulate serotonin functioning while, for example, clozapine restrains them. (Many of the modern antidepressive preparations block the reuptake of serotonin in the receptors where this transmitter substance accumulates.)

3   *The GABA-receptor system.* This is an important inhibiting receptor which is spread over a large part of the central nervous system. Amongst other things, the *amygdala* in the temporal lobes is rich in GABA receptors. The amygdala is central for emotions, learning, reactions to fear, etc. These receptors are amongst others stimulated by benzodiazepines, which subdue anxiety and relax muscle tension.

Certainly many other receptor systems are significant for the psychiatry of psychosis. The 'classic' neuroleptics interact with many of these and have, as a result, multifaceted and sometimes undesired effects.

Antipsychotic medication

By means of positron emission tomographic (PET) studies, where the radioactivity of marked molecules which attach themselves to specific receptors in

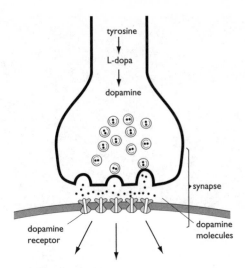

Figure 24.2 Schematic picture of a dopamine-receptor synapse. In the pre-synaptic part synthesis storing and breaking down of the dopamine molecules occurs. These are received by specific receptors in the following neuron and the signal continues on to the next synapse. The dopamine molecules then leave the receptor and there is a reuptake by the pre-synaptic neuron.

the brain is registered, it has been possible to show that the so-called classic neuroleptics – for example, chlorpromazine (Largactil) and haloperidol (Haldol) – bind with dopamine D2-receptors. They thereby inhibit the release of dopamine. After a threshold dose, within a few hours the immediate pharmacological effects are a decrease in emotional activity, extra-pyramidal muscular co-ordination disturbance as well as hormonal disturbances. Clinicians view these as undesirable side effects. How the antipsychotic effect, which appears much later, arises and can be understood is less clear. For several conventional as well as atypical antipsychotics it has, however, been shown, that a blockade of the D2-receptor (with an antipsychotic effect) can be achieved with doses that do not cause neuromuscular side effects (Figure 24.3).

Since the side effects prevent many patients from using conventional neuroleptics, intensive searches for substances that have other receptor functions have been carried out. The so-called atypical neuroleptics which also bind and inhibit serotonin receptors have been synthesised. Although they produce very few extra-pyramidal symptoms, this does not mean that they are without side effects.

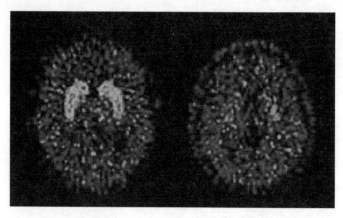

Figure 24.3 PET-scans of the brain in horizontal projection. The left-hand image shows D2-receptors (unmedicated) specifically located in the deep cerebral nuclei, termed *corpus striatum*. They are visualised through the radioactive substance IIc-raclopride, which specifically binds to D2-receptors. The right-hand image shows the same individual after a dose of 6 mg Risperidone. Here the receptors are blocked by the medication. The light parts in the images mark high D2-activity (modified from S. Nyberg and L. Farde).

Neuroleptics that block dopamine

The original chlorpromazine (Largactil) is a phenothiazine preparation like most of the early neuroleptics. Other phenothiazines are thioridazine (Melleril), levomepromazine (Nozinan) and other low-potency preparations. These are used less and less frequently today because the side effects are difficult to deal with. Since they influence many receptor systems at once they are considered 'dirty drugs'. Beside the antipsychotic effect, their sedative and subduing effects are marked.

At an early stage preparations were discovered that were also antagonistic to dopamine but had a different molecular appearance and could be given in lower doses so hence had a high potency. Haloperidol (Haldol), fluphenazine (Siqualone, Moditen), perphenazine (Trilafon, Fentazin), flupenthixol (Fluanxol) and zuclopenthixol (Cisordinol, Clopixol) are common high-potency preparations.

Serotonin blocking atypical neuroleptics

Clozapine (Clozaril) was the first atypical neuroleptic preparation. It is a low-potency preparation which was shown to have beneficial effects on many long-term schizophrenic patients who were treatment resistant. The effects are primarily due to the powerful inhibition of serotonin receptors.

For that reason it does not result in the usual extra-pyramidal side effects, that is to say, Parkinson's disease-like muscular symptoms (see below). However, it does produce other side effects which reduce its usefulness. Weight gain is a very common problem that may necessitate a change in medication. Fatigue and heart palpitations can also cause problems in many patients. Another important drawback is the risk of a toxic bone marrow reaction with a serious decrease in the number of white blood cells (agranulocytosis). Although this is relatively unusual it can be detected early by careful blood monitoring to prevent serious illness.

Risperidone (Risperdal) is a high-potency preparation, which binds both with dopamine and serotonin receptors. Extra-pyramidal symptoms are, therefore, less significant than with haloperidol. The doses of risperidone and haloperidol are comparable. The pattern of side effects is similar but less marked.

Olanzapine (Zyprexa) does not give extra-pyramidal side effects either. Weight increase is often marked – the preparation shares this effect with clozapine – and often causes tiredness. Unrelated to the weight gain, olanzapine (like clozapine) also has a tendency to evoke Type II diabetes.

Ziprasidone (Zeldox) is a newly released substance in the medium-potency range. Its side effects are described as mild.

Quetiapine (Seroquel) is also a new low-potency preparation with insignificant extra-pyramidal and weight gain side effects. Besides the high cost, no negative aspects are known as yet. However, these always tend to appear after a few years' use.

Frequently it is claimed that atypical neuroleptics have a better effect on negative symptoms (apathy, lack of will, loss of speech) than the typical ones, but this is not necessarily so. In several controlled studies their effects have been compared with haloperidol. The haloperidol doses have been too high – 15 mg a day or more – and thus the comparisons with the new substances are 'unfair'. Many of the so-called negative symptoms with haloperidol would have been side effects as a result of an over-medication.

Methods of administration

Conventional neuroleptics come in tablet and liquid form as well as by injection. They are also given in depot injections. This means that the drug is slowly released from the injection site in the muscle and can be helpful for patients who find it difficult to take their medication regularly. The effect of injections can last as long as three to six months after administration even if they are recommended to be given at intervals of two to four weeks. Most of the atypical neuroleptics still lack depot forms. (See Table 24.1.)

Table 24.1 Effects and dose relationships of common neuroleptics (3 = strong, 2 = moderate, 1 = weak)

PREPARATION	Antipsychotic	Sedative	EPS	Autonomous side effects	Depot preparations	Dose relation
Chlorpromazine (Largactil)	3	3	1	3	D	50
Fluphenazine (Siqualone, Moditen)	3	1	3	1	D	5
Flupenthixol (Fluanxol)	3	1	2	1	D	1
Haloperidol (Haldol)	3	1	3	1	D	1
Perphenazine (Trilafon, Fentazin)	3	1	2	1	D	5
Zuclopenthixol (Cisordinol, Clopixol)	3	2	2	2	D	5
Clozapine (Leponex, Clozaril)	3	3	1	3	–	50
Olanzapine (Zyprexa)	3	1	1	3	–	5
Risperidone (Risperdal)	3	1	1	1	D: slow release not oil based	1
Ziprasidone (Zeldox)	3	2	1	3	–	10–15
Quetiapine (Seroquel)	3	2	1	3	–	50

Dose–effect studies

In contrast to treatment with antidepressant drugs, neuroleptic treatments show no clear relationship between the serum level of the medicine and its therapeutic effect. On the other hand, what can be seen is whether the substance appears in the blood or not: that is to say, if the patient has taken the medicine, and if the amount in plasma is significantly low or high in comparison to the ordinary dose. This will indicate whether the person is a rapid as opposed to a slow 'metaboliser' of the substance. The slower the metabolism, associated with genetic circumstances, the higher the serum levels which influence the receptors. In around 5 per cent of cases side effects appear with low doses due to slow metabolism. Around 1 to 2 per cent have a rapid metabolism and need higher doses than the standard ones.

In those cases with no treatment effect, although the plasma concentration is sufficient, a change to an atypical neuroleptic is indicated. Alternatively, if the situation allows, the risk of slowly lowering the dose can be taken to see if the symptoms change. Paradoxically, relatively often an improvement takes place. There is an increase in vitality, which in turn brings about a greater receptivity to psychological methods of treatment. Today most guidelines recommend use of atypicals as the first line, and clozapine after two different trials of other medications.

A more reliable way of gauging the relationship between dose and effect is through checking the receptor binding by means of PET camera examinations (Nyberg et al. 1999; Sedvall and Farde 1995). As a result of this technique it has been shown that the recommended doses of neuroleptics have been high to start with and are often counterproductive because of side effects (Farde et al. 1992).

A maximal antipsychotic effect is found at a 70 to 80 per cent saturation of dopamine D2-receptors. This is equivalent to a dose of 2–4 mg haloperidol or risperidone a day. The antipsychotic effect is not increased with a higher dose. On the other hand, extra-pyramidal and other side effects occur at a saturation level of 80 per cent. In British and North American literature doses which are five to ten times as high as the optimal dose have been recommended until recently. A series of clinical studies primarily with first-episode onset of illness shows that treatment with low doses is quite acceptable and the therapeutic effects are presumably better than with the usual dose (Kopala et al. 1996, 1997; McEvoy et al. 1991).

Not all patients with schizophrenia will be free of psychosis in spite of treatment with neuroleptics. Some will respond better with an atypical preparation but even then some remain ill. The effect has been compared between those who have been prescribed neuroleptics and those who have not, in controlled placebo studies. The overall net effect was found to be around 20 to 40 per cent better with neuroleptics than without. This is to say that there is a statistically improved effect with regard to relapse rates.

Even if neuroleptics are an indispensable necessity in the current treatment of psychosis, it is important to recognise the limits and negative aspects of these substances as well.

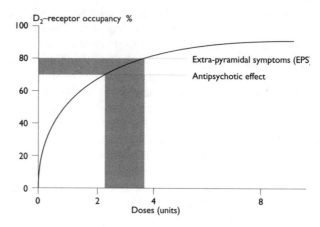

Figure 24.4 Dose levels for antipsychotic treatment against extra-pyramidal symptoms with classic antipsychotic medication. Because of the hyperbolic form of the curve for the D2-receptors, which are occupied by the antipsychotic medication at a certain dose, the interval indicates a fairly narrow area for optimal treatment. This interval ('the therapeutic window') lies between 2 and 4 mg haloperidol or risperidone in most cases. However, in around 5 per cent the metabolism of the medication is slow which increases the side effects and requires a lower dose. A few, 1 to 2 per cent, have a more rapid metabolism and so require a higher dose (Dahl and Sjöqvist 1997).

Direct effects of neuroleptics

Subduing the mind – neuroleptic induced deficit syndrome (NID)

The neuroleptic group was separated from sedative preparations because their psychotropic qualities were not comparable with the ones that are found in sedative pharmaceuticals. A sense of not being well, emotional emptiness, difficulties in getting down to anything and difficulty in planning ahead are the most usual consequences of neuroleptics when they are given to healthy people in a trial, with doses equivalent to a few mg haloperidol. Around a third report experiences of bewilderment, difficulty in doing things and sometimes sleep disturbances. The effects can remain for several days after a single dose (Healy and Farquhar 1998). In these cases a subdued feeling and a lack of initiative arises which are negative experiences and distinct from the effect of sedation seen with, for example, benzodiazepines. This condition has been called a neuroleptic induced deficit syndrome (NID; Lewander 1994). Certain neuroleptics have, in parallel with the subduing effect, more sedative effects.

Patients who have used neuroleptics for a longer period of time are less likely to experience side effects on low doses. They also need higher doses for the same treatment effects.

Muscular extra-pyramidal symptoms (EPS)

- *Parkinson-like symptoms* with muscular stiffness, 'cog-wheel phenomenon' (a jerky resistance is felt when bending and stretching the elbow) and a tendency to tremulousness.
- *Akinesia*, that is to say, lowered motor activity.
- *Akathisia* is an uncomfortable inner sense of anxiety that forces the individual to keep moving and walking about in a characteristic way. Inexperienced staff can misinterpret akathisia for a psychotic disturbance and so increase neuroleptic medication. It can be so distressing as to result in desperation followed by suicide.
- *Acute dystonia* can occur even after a moderate dosage, especially in young men treated for the first time. It is a painful and frightening condition with cramps in the throat, the tongue and the eyes, or in the musculature used for swallowing. An injection of an anticholinergic medication rapidly relieves the condition.
- *Tardive dyskinesia (TD)* is a side effect that appears, in particular, after a longer period of using low-dose neuroleptics. Compulsive grimacing, swallowing or circular movements of the tongue, where the tongue is stuck outside the mouth are unpleasant for those in the environment of the patient and create difficulties in social adjustment. The condition occurs in 10 to 40 per cent of those who have been on treatment for several years, and it often emerges after doses are lowered. TD is dose dependent which means that it is less likely to occur with lower doses. Also atypical neuroleptics seem to cause less TD than traditional antipsychotics. In TD certain extra-pyramidal (muscle co-ordinating) centres in the brain have been sensitised by the use of neuroleptics, so that functioning has been altered. Symptoms usually disappear if the dose is increased but it is often hard to deal with when coming off medication is desired. If the condition permits, total termination of neuroleptic treatment leads to the condition gradually subsiding in most patients, but not in all.

Increase in weight, autonomic and hormonal side effects

Many neuroleptics cause an increase of the hormone prolactin, which can, amongst other things, cause the production of breast milk. Feelings of hunger and a marked increase in weight are other troublesome side effects. This is particularly noticeable with clozapine and olanzapine treatment and can lead to cessation of this medication. Autonomic disturbances such as heart palpitations, sweating or increased salivation occur, depending on which receptor is affected.

The antipsychotic effect: does the inhibition of receptors provide a psychological 'breathing space'?

In Chapter 17 I pointed out that we do not know any biological correlate to the concept of psychosis. Psychosis is only defined in phenomenological and psychological terms. The non-psychotic experience of reality is a product of the conscious ego's continual ongoing work of integrating inner perceptions with the exterior ones. Thanks to our early experiences (memories) we create from this a meaningful integrated 'gestalt' of our inner and outer reality. It is an indispensable requirement for survival that this should be somewhat correctly interpreted – at least in the long run. By this I mean that the essential understanding of the phenomena in the surrounding world, an agreement as to the reasons for what happens and for people's attitudes, needs to be shared between people who inhabit the same cultural group. Due to its survival value we can assume that there is a powerful genetic background to this integrating function of the ego.

Our sense of reality is constantly under attack. We fantasise in our waking lives and we dream when we sleep. Both these activities contain psychological qualities but are differentiated by the ease with which they can be interrupted. When we are psychologically under stress or threat, or when our brain capacity is disturbed, this integrating function of the ego suffers. We can no longer restrain regressive threatening fantasies or wishful dreams from providing dominating private explanations to events, which we would normally desist from entertaining. At the same time we know that a person with a tendency to break into psychosis can, up to a certain point, retain a critical, non-psychotic state of mind with concentration and mental training. With mental work the risk of giving oneself over to fantasies can be pushed away, so that they do not resolve into an uncontrollable psychosis. This is the rationale behind much of psychotherapeutic success in these cases.

As I have mentioned, after an injection with neuroleptics the side effects (which strictly speaking are the immediate pharmacological effects of the drug) occur within an hour. The desired antipsychotic effect is, on the other hand, difficult to predict in specific cases and usually takes days or weeks to be achieved – if at all. We know today that for up to 50 per cent of all who become ill with a first-episode onset of psychosis neuroleptics are not necessary, if the optimal psychosocial requirements are satisfied (Cullberg 1997). There is a strong 'natural' tendency to recover from psychoses that can, however, be supported by the careful prescription of antipsychotics.

It does not seem likely that we will find an explanation, which is entirely pharmacological for the fact that the antipsychotic effect occurs so much later than the other clinical effects. That psychological processes can be thought of as integrating with pharmacological ones can be shown. (The same reasoning may be applied to antidepressant medications.)

Psychosis, according to learning theory, can be seen as a condition of mental overactivity, resulting in the more than usual domination in thinking of such processes as fantasies, memories and thoughts (Miller 1987). The dopamine system is a reward system enhancing motivation and learning, irrespective of whether that which is learned is correct or not. Dopamine antagonists (such as antipsychotics) reduce the tendency to develop conditioned reflexes in research animals. From this perspective, if antipsychotics prevent the new learning of psychotic fantasies in human beings, then these fantasies cannot have such new learning effects and a psychological 'breathing space' will be formed that offers greater potential for the recovery of a normal way of thinking.

From the phenomenological standpoint we can see that antipsychotics do not produce peace of mind so much as indifference (Healy 1989). This indifference implies that emotional stimuli (from the environment or from inner fantasies) are not so engaged and so do not awaken conflicts. The ego's critical and reality testing capacity gains an increased ability to function and illusions can be avoided more easily. If one thinks in terms of the psychosis as exclusively and primarily a biological disturbance in the functioning of the brain,[1] it is natural to treat every patient who has a psychotic symptom with medication immediately and to continue with the medication for a longer period and to assume that this treatment will be effective without bothering so much with psychosocial treatments.

However, it is important to see that antipsychotics, through a series of interactive psychological processes, not only combat delusions or hallucinations but also result in clinical consequences, whether we look at the situation from a dynamic point of view or from the standpoint of learning theory. As I have stated earlier, a number of episodes of acute psychoses disappear over a reasonable period of time without antipsychotic treatment. For this reason it is sensible to hold back treatment for one or two weeks if the situation allows for it. Antipsychotics should then be given initially, optimally in a low dose that does not produce side effects, to avoid future difficulties. The inhibition of receptors should be given time to have its effect on the ego functions, together with psychosocial support, before increasing the dose. When the psychosis has disappeared after a long treatment, the medication should be stopped gradually over a period of weeks or months. It has been shown that if the removal of antipsychotics takes place abruptly it increases the risk of relapse, presumably because the receptors are disturbed by the sudden change. If the risk of relapse is significant it is necessary to try to increase the patient's motivation in favour of long-term treatment.

This reasoning is valid regarding the treatment of psychosis. In cases of mania or other destructive exaltation, with strong aggression or agitation, naturally the fact that the medication has a specific subduing effect can motivate a greater increase in the dose.

The treatment of extra-pyramidal symptoms (EPS)

1   With moderate EPS the first measure to be taken is to reduce the neuroleptic dose. If this does not prove to be enough, an anticholinergic substance such as biperiden (Akineton) or orphenadrine (Disipal) should be prescribed in tablet form.

2   With acute dystonia an intramuscular injection of procyclidine (5–10 mg) is necessary. Relief is immediate.

3   With modern antipsychotic treatment in low doses, EPS is usually a relatively minor problem. It is important to see that the anticholinergic ('anti-Parkinsonian') preparations also have cognitive side effects, amongst others producing difficulty with concentration. Still, all too many, mainly older long-term patients are kept on a much too high neuroleptic medication where the side effects have been inadequately counteracted with powerful anti-Parkinsonian drugs. The desperate experience of empty existence and loss of motivation that the treatment, together with the underlying illness, brings about is very often compensated for by cannabis misuse and/or heavy drinking. Overall there is an increased risk of misuse of most substances.

Sedating and sleep-inducing drugs

In order to restrain a desire to prescribe neuroleptics too quickly, it helps to be generous with sedating medication in the early stages of a psychosis. The painful and disturbing problem for patients with an acute psychosis is primarily the anxiety. Every acutely psychotic person also has difficulty in sleeping which worsens the psychosis. For this reason regulating sleep is of great importance. Anxiety and sleep problems often respond well to benzodiazepines which can be given in normal doses but certain acutely psychotic patients need a significantly higher dose. This can have the result that antipsychotic treatment never has to be used. Unfortunately, benzodiazepines do not have any significant antipsychotic effect, which is why a psychosis that does not disappear after one or two weeks normally must be treated with antipsychotics. As an alternative medication for sleep, zopiclone (Zimovane 7.5 mg) or zolpidem (Stilnoct 10 mg) can be prescribed.

Patients with psychosis are presumably no less likely than others to develop abstinence symptoms and dependency after a period of taking benzodiazepines and similar preparations. This is why it is important to limit prescribing or to reduce the dose as soon as possible. Of course this has especial relevance for people who are known to have a history of substance abuse.

Antidepressant medication and treatment with lithium

The treatment of depression

Depressive symptoms are usually seen in those who are recovering from a psychosis. As discussed in Chapter 14, it is often related to reactions to the experience of the psychosis. Both the experience of 'having gone mad' and of having had to be kept in a psychiatric ward by force undermine most people's self-confidence. These understandable reactions should primarily be treated psycho-therapeutically. Other causes of depression-like reactions may result from overprescription of neuroleptics.

After a longer period when it becomes clear that a disability has developed in a schizophrenic illness, or when the losses in life that occur unavoidably in connection with the illness begin to be apparent, many succumb to long drawn-out depressive illnesses which are known to have a high risk for suicide. In these situations an antidepressant medication can decrease the symptoms in combination with psychological support. Naturally people with schizophrenia as well as everybody else have to face depression that occurs for other reasons, where medication is also indicated.

There is no reason why neuroleptics should not be combined with anti-depressant medications. However, there are clinical observations which suggest that antidepressant medication can lower the threshold for psychosis in certain patients. This has not been confirmed in scientific studies as yet.

Lithium treatment

With recurrent schizo-affective psychoses as with other psychoses that are characterised by affective oscillations (for example, frequently recurring brief psychoses) treatment with lithium often brings with it an improved prognosis. Lithium is prescribed in a simple salt compound. Its working mechanisms are largely unknown. The serotonin system is dampened by lithium, and there are also effects on the intracellular signal transmission. Its main area of use is in the recurrent bipolar (manic) condition. Treatment with lithium results in a clear reduction of the frequency of relapse or makes relapse easier to deal with. Unfortunately, depot treatment is still not available and so medication must be given several times a day. Lithium treatment demands a definite motivation on the part of the patient who needs blood tests to monitor the serum level of the lithium. Initially this may be done weekly during the first months until the levels are stable and then subsequently at less frequent intervals.

Lithium has a limited range of effective (or therapeutic) levels. If the concentration is too high side effects such as dizziness, tremor and diarrhoea may occur. Very high levels may cause kidney failure and coma. Certain people may develop pimples on the skin and increase in weight. These side effects can sometimes become so unpleasant that the treatment has to be stopped. About a quarter of patients complain about a subjective effect, that life appears less colourful than before and less meaningful; not least artists can suffer from this. In these cases it is important to discuss whether the risks involved in stopping the medication should be taken and compensated for with more frequent contact over some years. Members of the family must be included and advised as to how to react in good time if they notice that the symptoms are returning. The treatment should continue for several years before making a decision to stop. Many patients – and their relatives – prefer that the treatment should be continued for life rather than risk a relapse. Today there are alternatives (mainly used as anti-epileptics) to lithium treatment. Valproic acid is claimed to be about as effective. Carbamazepine often needs dosage increase after some time.

Summary of directives for the pharmacological treatment of psychosis

1 Where symptoms are primarily those of anxiety, benzodiazepines are prescribed to begin with.
2 Sleep problems should be dealt with as quickly as possible.
3 Do not expect the effect of neuroleptic treatment over the first days after treatment has started.
4 If the psychosis is hard to endure and destructive, the treatment with neuroleptics should be introduced earlier.
5 To begin with, use a low dose of neuroleptics. In the case of patients being treated for the first time 0.5–1 mg of haloperidol equivalents should be prescribed once or twice a day.
6 For those patients who have been treated with neuroleptics on previous occasions, sometimes a higher dose is required to begin with.
7 If EPS occur, try to reduce the dose first and then prescribe an atypical neuroleptic.
8 Depot preparation is only an alternative in the case of long-term psychoses and where the patient cannot manage treatment in the form of tablets.
9 Do not use several neuroleptics simultaneously.
10 When the patient is free from psychosis, a slow reduction or replacement of neuroleptics should be attempted.
11 If the patient does not respond to the treatment within one to two months in spite of an increase in the dosage, the serum concentration should be checked. If this is satisfactory a change should be made to (another) atypical neuroleptic. If there is still no response try reducing the dose to nothing to see if the symptoms change.
12 Older patients often require significantly lower or minimal doses.

13 After neuroleptics have been used for many years, an attempt to phase them out should be made very slowly, perhaps over a period of six months to a year.

14 In the case of frequent recurrence of psychoses with affective traits, lithium should be tried.

15 'Negotiate' with the patient and let him or her have a say in the treatment. After a number of relapses most people learn to handle the neuroleptics.

16 Be the patient's consultant, not his guardian. If the patient does not have the ability to co-operate at all and a destructive situation is likely to develop, the medication must be administered by force. It should take place 'kindly but firmly' and with a clear explanation to the patient as to why it must happen.

Chapter 25

Psychological treatments of psychosis

Many schizophrenic people regain their health without medical treatment. The diagnosis of schizophrenia is not in itself an immediate reason to have recourse to medication [. . .] To be able to manage the treatment of the schizophrenic person without medication is a special art – but it is often to the patient's benefit.

Manfred Bleuler, *Lehrbuch der Psychiatrie*, 1979

Few questions have proved as controversial regarding the treatment of psychosis as that of the place of the psychotherapist. Even though this question has been an active concern of mine throughout my career as a psychiatrist, I am still not ready to answer it comprehensively. Authoritative claims as to the most effective or ineffective method of treatment are not lacking. As always when it concerns psychotherapy, we have to ask ourselves which psychotic patient should be treated, and in which phase of the illness should the treatment take place. Also what goal can be aimed at and who should carry out the treatment? These questions primarily indicate that it concerns the ability to develop a containing therapeutic relationship. Technical and theoretical knowledge are important tools but must be subordinated to the ability to maintain an empathic understanding of the patient's dilemma of turning away from at the same time as needing contact.

I will discuss scientific studies that take up the dynamic versus the cognitive methods of treatment and then give a summary assessment on the basis of my own experience. At the same time I should like to stress that this book does not primarily aim to provide a handbook concerning treatment in practice.

The psychoanalytical tradition

Two case histories were very important in encouraging hope for cure with psychoanalytic treatment in schizophrenic conditions. The Swiss psychoanalyst Marie-Anne Sechehaye published *La réalisation symbolique* in 1947. Here she describes the treatment of Renée, a very ill, deeply regressed psychotic girl being cared for in hospital, who regained her health slowly with therapy which centred on symbolically satisfying her deeply frustrated needs for her mother's love. Renée, who was adopted by her analyst after the treatment, eventually became a prominent academic. The German edition of the book includes the patient's diary.

In 1964 Hannah Green documented in the form of a novel her dramatic treatment with the psychoanalyst Frieda Fromm-Reichmann in *I Never Promised You a Rose Garden*. It was a bestseller and has been made into a film. In a study of her journal followed by her further personal follow-up 30 years after her treatment was over, the researchers were able to surmise that her original diagnosis was schizophrenia according to DSM-III, but the picture of her illness was considered unusual and affective (McGlashan and Keats 1989). Green later had a successful career as a writer and did not need any psychiatric help following her psychotherapy. In both treatments, which were carried out without neuroleptics, the patient's creative ability to draw and paint periodically played an important role.

During the relatively long periods during which the therapies took place, the patients' youth, their high intelligence, episodes of powerful regression, delusions and self-destructiveness all played a role. Both belonged to a socially privileged group. Since then, many similar expositions have been published which offer powerful evidence that success would not have occurred without such an intense and long-lasting treatment. In Sweden the psychotherapist Barbro Sandin has become known for her similarly strong personally structured method of working. Even the description of her method (Sandin 1986) has been filled out with an autobiographical presentation of one of her patients (Jonsson 1986). I have followed up this person who was originally diagnosed with schizophrenia according to DSM-III criteria, and the seven other formerly schizophrenic patients who were successfully treated and who were accessible, with hospital record studies and interviews with the patients and their therapists (Cullberg and Levander 1991). The recovery is clearly connected to the psychotherapy, which in most cases put a stop to an entrenched chronic process (see further Chapter 16, p. 188).

Systematic studies of the effect of psychoanalytic orientated therapies

It was a shock for psychoanalytically orientated psychotherapy when Thomas McGlashan, research leader at Chestnut Lodge, published a detailed follow-up of the patients who had been treated at this hospital in 1984. Out of over 100 patients with chronic schizophrenia (DSM-III), only a tenth could be considered wholly restored to health. The rest lived with differing degrees of handicap and dependency in spite of the long and intensive psychotherapy that they had been through – even if improved and often with a better quality of life. The following year a study in Boston was published where psychoanalysis and supportive psychotherapy of schizophrenic patients were compared (Gunderson *et al.* 1984). The outcome favoured supportive therapy. However, those patients who had therapists who, prior to the treatment, had been considered to have the best dynamic understanding, had the best outcome (Glass *et al.* 1989). Even if the results must be considered with care – barely half of the patients could be followed up – it was quite clear that the notion of psychotherapy with schizophrenia had to be rethought.

Table 25.1 Systematic studies of psychodynamic treatments of psychosis/schizophrenia

Author	Method	Results	Remarks
May *et al.* (1968)	Randomised study of four groups of first-episode patients who were given either neuroleptics, psychotherapy, combination of these, or no treatment.	Combination neuroleptics plus psychotherapy was the most effective. Psychotherapy only no more effective than no treatment.	Low psychotherapeutic competence. Psychotherapeutic methods inadequate according to modern standards. Only inpatient care.
Karon *et al.* (1972)	Randomised study of three groups, each consisting of 12 acutely ill schizophrenic patients given either dynamic psychotherapy, psychotherapy + medication or standardised treatment.	Psychotherapy without medication group significantly better than the other groups after two years.	Unclear diagnostic criteria, small groups, control group not quite comparable.
Sjöström (1985)	14 DSM-III schizophrenic long-term inpatients were given long-term dynamic psychotherapy. Matched comparison group given standard treatment.	Psychotherapy group significantly better results after six years – much less neuroleptic medication.	Control group matched but not randomised with experimental group. Treatment conducted or supervised by a formally untrained but gifted therapist.
McGlashan (1984)	163 chronic DSM-III schizophrenic inpatients were given intensive psychoanalytic psychotherapy 4–5 times/week.	14 per cent much better or recovered.	Primarily a chronic group. No systematic social rehabilitation. No efforts to integrate neuroleptic medication.

Gunderson et al. (1984)	95 first-episode DSM-III patients with schizophrenia were given either psychoanalytic insight-oriented psychotherapy or supportive dynamic psychotherapy.	Supportive dynamic psychotherapy somewhat better effects. Dynamically best regarded therapists got better results.	Drop-out rate over 50 per cent.
Stone (1986)	72 DSM-III patients with schizophrenia were given psychoanalytic psychotherapy during a mean of 12 months.	10 per cent recovered, 20 per cent low symptomatic, > 50 per cent residual symptoms, 20 per cent committed suicide.	Brief treatment periods, unclear treatment protocols.
Cullberg (1991)	A case finding study of Swedish DSM-III fully remitted schizophrenic patients treated with long-term dynamic psychotherapy. They were compared with 10 non-recovered patients with the same type of psychotherapy.	Eight cases of permanent recovery were found. There were differences between the groups, most notably persistent auditory hallucinations in those who did not recover, and evidence of early personality difficulties in those who did recover.	Seven of the eight recovered patients were treated by therapists, which were supervised by the same therapist as in Sjöström (1985), indicating the importance of selection and technique.

These studies are difficult to compare. In the earliest studies the diagnostic criteria are unclear. Certain studies have been carried out with people who have become ill for the first time for a brief period; in other cases the illness continued for several years. The competence of the therapists together with the intensity of the treatment fluctuated. The drop-out rate in the follow-up studies was very high in many cases. Furthermore, the ward environment's therapeutic or anti-therapeutic effects have not been controlled for.

Classical psychoanalytically orientated treatment, as it was carried out in many private hospitals in the USA, is not suitable for the needs of schizophrenic patients. We now know that the psychoanalytic scenario, can be counter-therapeutic because of its relatively impersonal approach, non-directive conversations, lack of contact with the network around the patient or those involved in their rehabilitation, along with a low interest in relieving the patient's symptoms with medication. This strict method of working, which may be suitable for certain people with personality disorders, has now been abandoned when treating psychosis.

After having treated patients with psychoses for many years with different kinds of psychoanalytical and cognitive methods, and having been in a position to closely follow the work of many colleagues, my experience is as follows. The relatively large group of patients with affective traits in their psychoses – that is to say, acute schizophreniform or depressive psychoses along with those who have a brief psychotic episode – usually find psychodynamically orientated therapy, often in combination with family work and medication, very useful. By the expression 'psychodynamically orientated' I am referring to the method that increases the psychological understanding in a patient of the relationship between their psychosis and any specific vulnerabilities that they may have. This kind of psychotherapy seeks to identify sources of stress in the patient's everyday life that may trigger another episode. It does not primarily mean that the therapist interprets unconscious conflicts in the patient or offers symbolic explanations of different aspects of the psychosis. The essential factor is that a realistic view of internal and external experiences is restored and that the ability for insight into the self is deepened. I would like to make the further claim that every patient who has suffered an acute psychotic episode for the first time should be assessed for brief psychotherapy in order to increase their understanding of their present situation and how they came to react with psychosis. Naturally a cognitive as much as a dynamically trained therapist can respond to this need. I am unable to support this clinical experience with controlled research, as there are no such studies to date.

However, with the long-term 'Kraepelinian' schizophrenic condition, with a psychic withdrawal, ongoing auditory hallucinations and/or disorganised behaviour, I have never seen any progress with dynamic methods.

Amongst those who have propounded psychoanalytic theories of metapsychological formulations of schizophenia are Wilfred Bion (1967) and Donald Meltzer (1992). Up to now, this has been more of a theoretical development than one of ordinary clinical meaning. The most important expositions of current formulations of modern integrative psychoanalytic tradition are Michael Robbins (1993), Murray Jackson (1994) and Yrjö Alanen (1997). Their views are based on object relations theory (see Chapter 4), often in combination with family work, and take account of psychological as well as biological vulnerability factors, where the aims of the treatment must be related to the patient's psychological vulnerability.

An important feature of dynamic thinking is that man is a creator of meanings. Consequently symptoms are conceived of as meaningful, even if dysfunctional. This is equally relevant whether the individual's vulnerability is grounded in an organic disturbance or not. At present the treatment methods are widening and becoming more practical and clinically useful.

The cognitive-behavioural therapeutic tradition (CBT)

The indication that verbal therapies with psychotic symptoms are effective and satisfying for the patient should provoke thought for those who are only able to see psychotic thinking as a quasi-epileptic activity.

(Birchwood 1999)

In the latter part of the twentieth century a powerful cognitive-behavioural therapeutic tradition has sprung up which stands out against the psycho-analytic way of thinking. To view the symptoms, apart from their origins, as expressing a non-functional way of thinking and behaving is central. In the treatment, the patient is invited to note his way of thinking and acting (and in recent years, all the more, his feelings). Systematic methods for change are suggested on the basis of the patient's own account. From the beginning CBT, based on assessing the symptoms before and after the treatment in controlled studies, has gained a relatively high acceptance from psychiatry. During the last two decades these methods have developed strongly not least within the area of schizophrenia. A competitive situation has been avoided with pharmacological forms of treatment.

Simply stated, there have been two main areas within CBT. One consists of a definitive departure from all psychoanalytic aspects regarding unconscious intentions, the significance of early childhood development, etc. The more recent direction, inspired by amongst others Aaron Becks's and John Bowlby's work, expresses a more dynamic way of thinking where the meaning of symbols and of unconscious motivation is not denied (Perris 1988; Fowler *et al.* 1995).

In comparison with the psychoanalytic methods CBT is more active. It is a very systematic and supportive way of working with people to help identify their dysfunctional (psychotic, depressive, etc.) thought processes and in finding ways of changing them. Without denying the importance of the transference (and the countertransference) an attempt is made to create a relaxed and secure therapeutic situation which is open and clear and where the patient is treated as an active co-worker as much as possible.

Areas of interest

Recent clinical research by Jackson *et al.* (1999) has identified three areas of dysfunction that respond to CBT, which has had an important effect on clinical practice:

* the capacity for problem solving and functional thinking
* delusions and hallucinations
* negative effects on the self.

Support in rational thinking and problem solving is a traditional area for CBT. Such support has also been used in the families with young people in a prodromal phase in order to enable family members to contain some of the stress which they encounter (Falloon et al. 1985). The method is also valuable for non-pharmacological treatment of the depression or anxiety often seen with psychosis.

The CBT methods are often influenced by dynamic thinking as the therapeutic relationship may facilitate the understanding of the meaning of delusions in relation to personality and the circumstances of life (Fowler et al. 1998). The systematic, persistent and inoffensive questioning of the patient's delusions, which may be understood as a defence mechanism, differs from the traditional dynamic treatment. An attempt is also made to strengthen the positive view of the self. The delusions can often be hard to dislodge, but a series of cases does show that this method is productive (see the case description of Chris in Chapter 16).

The third cognitive area of interest focuses on the influence that the illness has on the self and its capacity to adapt. This is more clearly influenced by dynamic thinking. The Swedish psychiatrist Carlo Perris has had an international influence using Aaron Beck's psychotherapeutic theories and the psychoanalyst John Bowlby's theories of attachment and separation in early childhood. The person's early attachment to parental figures and their capacity to separate without trauma is complicated if biological vulnerability factors are present. Moreover, these biological vulnerabilities make the individual more sensitive to disturbances in early relationships (Bowlby 1969–80).

The Americans John Strauss and Gerard Hogarty (Hogarty et al. 1997), like the Australian Patrick McGorry (1999), are important in revitalising this tradition of the significance of the self, stressing how a passive identification of illness adds to the 'construction' of a chronic identity (see Chapter 16). They have published carefully tested psychotherapy models adjusted to the individual's phase of illness. Hogarty points out that not only early psychotherapeutic contributions but also those which take place between the second and third years are very important for future adaptation. This has not been dealt with in other studies but corroborates what Manfred Bleuler and others have said about the experience of the first five years after the onset of the illness being decisive.

In summary, CBT has significantly beneficial effects in unselected psychosis groups even if some patients are not appropriate for the treatment. With regard to the overall effectiveness of the treatment and to the question as to which way the statistical improvements have a clinical relevance, it is still too early to say. However, it can be stated that staff working in units for the treatment of psychosis should have both medical and psychotherapeutic training.

Table 25.2 Controlled studies of cognitive-behavioural therapy vs other psychosocial interventions in patients with schizophrenia

Author	Method	Result	Comments
Drury *et al.* (1996)	40 acutely psychotic patients given CBT or supportive treatment.	CBT gives a significantly better reduction of positive symptoms and shorter period for recovery.	33 per cent not appropriate for CBT.
Hogarty *et al.* (1997)	151 patients with schizophrenia given 'personal therapy', family therapy or supportive therapy.	'Personal therapy' reduces relapse by twice as much during three years compared to other methods.	Only productive with patients with family. Less effective in the socio-economically deprived.
Kuipers *et al.* (1998)	60 patients with chronic treatment resistant schizophrenia given CBT or social support.	Only CBT-group significantly improved. At 18 months follow-up 65 per cent CBT improved against 17 per cent in the control group.	Neuroleptic doses not reported. Symptom gains 'paid for' treatment costs.
Tarrier *et al.* (1999)	70 patients with chronic treatment resistant schizophrenia given CBT, support and advice or conventional treatment.	CBT treatment superior at end. Effects remained less clear after 12 months follow-up. Supportive treatment better than routine treatment.	Rigorous method. Neuroleptic doses not controlled. No effect on frequency of relapse. Socio-economic deprivation reduced the effect of treatment.

Towards a synthesis of dynamic psychology and cognitive methods

I have become aware how those experienced therapists with either a dynamic or CBT training show an increasing similarity in their approach to their work. They actively and supportively create contact and trust, which means being alert to change from closeness to distance according to the patient's signals. A concrete and supportive attitude with a strong cognitive aspect dominates from the start. Among dynamic therapists this is often expressed as the formulation of the problem. In this book I emphasise the important aspects of the patient's own formulation of his or her problem. By asking the patient to explain in their own words how he or she understands the problem which led to their making contact with psychiatry, one is not just asking for information. If the patient experiences it as a meaningful question, one can be certain that he or she, as best they can, will try to mobilise their thinking and ability to express themselves: that is, the very abilities which are disturbed by the psychotic mechanism. Nothing incites the striving for an understandable formulation so much as an interested, listening and knowledgeable partnership.

Helen – an interrupted separation

Helen, who was 31 years old, had a responsible job in a big organisation. She was remarkably gifted but lacked self-assertion. Ten years previously, when she was employed abroad as an au pair, she became depressed and experienced suicidal impulses. For eight years she had lived with her partner, a man she felt was using her and who also threatened her physically. Inspired by a girlfriend's recent separation, she wanted to leave home but did not have enough energy to take the final decision. Exhausting nightly quarrels over a six-month period eventually made Helen give up her resolve. She reacted with an almost complete lack of sleep over a month. At work, she increasing felt that she was being watched, that her colleagues were experimenting on her and that events were being arranged in such a way that she might break down and resign. She did not suffer hallucinations. She locked herself into her home. Her partner called the police and she was admitted by force to a psychiatric clinic. From the beginning, her depression dominated the picture and there was an overhanging threat of suicide. Antidepressive medication had no effect. Little by little the paranoid picture revealed itself and Helen experienced the whole hospital as a police organisation which wanted to accuse her of a crime that she had not committed. The staff and the patients were undercover agents. When she refused to try the antipsychotic medication Helen was offered the choice between depot neuroleptics and ECT. She 'chose' the depot neuroleptics but essentially was treated by compulsion in this way for three months. However, the medication had no effect on the delusions but produced a marked apathy. Now, for the first time, she was referred to the clinic's department for first-episode psychosis.

After this Helen returned to her successful career. She found her own apartment, moved away from her boyfriend and felt that she had rediscovered the pleasure of living. Since she still needed further psychotherapy she was referred to a private psychotherapist.

COMMENTS

Helen's diagnosis was depressive psychosis. If she had been received with a psychotherapeutic understanding from her first contact with services the development of her illness would presumably have been less complicated. The treatment was now directed towards building up a new trust and to lessen the traumatic effects of the initial compulsory treatment. Her paranoid delusions could be systematically scrutinised and examined. Clarification of the conflicts in her life, which had triggered the psychotic crisis, gave Helen a markedly increased self-understanding. All the same, her personal vulnerability remained and she wanted further psychotherapy. However, as a result of a period of overwork and sleeplessness several years later, she fell quickly into a deepening depression again. The end was tragic (this was considered in Chapter 22, p. 248).

The earlier competitiveness between the schools of therapy should by now have become a dwindling history. Instead we should expect a broad specialisation of psychological treatments for schizophrenia and other psychoses. The dynamic knowledge of psychological processes in general and psychotic conditions in particular, according to the different needs of the patients in different phases of the illness, should be combined with cognitive techniques and an empirical attitude. Obviously, some therapists (as some patients) will be personally more inclined towards a dynamic way of understanding and others towards a more cognitive one. The essential factor is our insight that the one method is not enough and that they often act complementarily.

'Personal therapy'

An expression for this attitude is the 'personal therapy' which the Hogarty group in Pittsburgh, USA, developed especially for patients with schizophrenic disabilities (Hogarty et al. 1995). It takes place in three phases where the first is to support the patient in becoming aware of the illness, combined with a sense of hope. The vulnerability-stress notion is introduced and the therapist makes a 'contract' with the patient in relation to how he or she is going to cope with the future in order to reduce the risk of a relapse.

The second phase concerns the development towards a greater awareness of thoughts and feelings, a kind of basic training in how to be reflective about oneself. Relaxation techniques are also taught. This phase takes place over around a year but can vary a great deal.

The patients who manage to reach this goal enter phase three. This is about teaching the patient to see the connection between events in the world outside and their inner feelings. Special attempts are made to teach the patient to deal with critical remarks and to resolve conflicts. To do this, special protocols are kept and homework is given.

A three-year follow-up of the 151 patients with schizophrenia or schizo-affective illness first treated in this way revealed that those who lived with their families had the most positive effect from the treatment, while those who lived alone often relapsed. Possibly they were less able to make use of the therapy because of their social deprivation. Naturally, it is not possible to follow these recovery phases closely. Patients are often hard to motivate, they drop out of treatment easily, suddenly get worse or demand other solutions for other reasons. Modern psychotherapeutic work with long-term psychotic patients is often built up around similar ideas.

Robert Liberman's social skills training

This method is directed especially towards those patients who have developed a cognitive functional disorder. It is designed to complement other contributions: dynamic or cognitive psychotherapy, medication or rehabilitation. The method has become very popular in many countries. Emphasis is placed on the patient creating their own goals. A positive and supportive approach is combined with attempts to measure the results. The method has been developed further to teach about medication, how to reduce the risk of relapse, control of symptoms, resolving conflicts, everyday behaviour, and so on. The treatment is offered individually or in a group of four to eight people with two group leaders. A great emphasis is put on activating the members and on engaging them in the work. Homework, role playing and video are used as methods to enhance insight. Controlled studies have been done which show an increase in overall ability to live an independent life although there is no clear indication that symptoms decrease (Liberman *et al.* 1998).

Residential homes offering psychotherapeutic care

In Chapters 14 and 16 I touched on the need for a period of time in a protected environment which could encourage a recovery process and support the work towards personal development. In practice problems result from new hospital admissions which for many are experienced as counter-productive to supporting long-term recovery. The home environment may be inappropriate – not least because the family may not be able to deal with the stress in the longer term. Unsupported single accomodation combined with medical and social care is often insufficient to prevent further relapse. Homelessness may often result, especially when the support of friends and relatives has been exhausted. Substance misuse and suicide are serious risks in this phase.

An important resource for young adults who have not fully recovered their psychosis is therefore a therapeutic environment where they can be given psychological treatments. Certain homes are more psychodynamically orientated and others are more centred on cognitive treatment. Both types have been evaluated scientifically and function well for this group of patients (Werbart 1997; Svensson 1999). When identifying a home it is important to match the patient to the abilities of the staff, their potential level of engagement and the internal structure of the home.

Art therapy

A way of increasing the opportunities for offering psychotherapy is by means of allowing the patients to paint pictures and then to talk about them. Many psychotic patients have a capacity to express their predicament creatively and feel relieved when they can paint. To be able to talk about the contents of the pictures without too much of an interpretive stance can often complement the verbal therapeutic work.

Knowledge of the body and physiotherapy

Long-term psychotic patients' relationship with their bodies, its boundaries, needs and care are often problematic. In the last decades in Sweden physiotherapists have become increasingly important in the care of psychotic patients, not least by helping them to find an increased experience of their inner representation of their bodies. It includes conscious or unconscious memories of joy and pleasure as well as of suffering and vulnerability, all of which are closely bound up with the body. Many patients with psychosis, above all those with personality disorders, have been the victims of abuse of one kind or another when they were young. Others have for unknown reasons, perhaps genetic, a disturbed perception of their bodies with indistinct boundaries. Sometimes patients with schizophrenia do not know what they are wearing, if their shoes fit, if their shirt is turned the right way out or if their trousers need hitching up with a belt. Many don't bother to protect themselves from dirt or avoid spilling food. These problems may be worsened by or even result from institutionalisation. Education about the body improves the ability to integrate the body in the total experience of the self: to learn to 'stand, feet firmly planted on the ground'.

Family meetings, family therapy and psycho-education

Family meetings

If possible, the family should be included in the treatment of every patient who has become ill for the first time. This has been emphasised many times in this book. The family's interest will vary depending on the stage of the illness. During the acute phase there is often a need for the family members to share and formulate their understanding of their history. This may focus on the family's problems, as well as their strengths and supportive capacities and how the psychosis might be understood at that moment in time in the family's history. For this reason the closest relatives may be invited to a series of joint meetings with the patient (if this is possible and the patient does not refuse) and two experienced therapists. This can take place and be helped by making a 'family map', which is drawn by the family members under the supervision of the therapists. There are different ways of doing this (Figure 21.1, Chapter 21, p. 239 illustrates one such model).

Family therapy

The family meetings are not designed as treatment but are meant to be more informative and to create an opportunity for contact. To be treated without feeling the need for it would be experienced as a violation by most people. On the other hand, if the therapist observes the tensions within the family which are hindering recovery, it makes sense to take up the problems and offer family meetings in order to discuss and work through the problems. A supportive approach that avoids scapegoating and provocation promotes engagement and disclosure of sensitive information.

Even family therapy is enmeshed with its underlying theory. A traditional psychoanalytic approach, in spite of many attempts to accommodate this, is all too likely to reinforce the feelings of guilt which many parents with mentally ill children harbour towards themselves or the other parent. Thus that model has largely been given up.

Systemic models may be more useful in understanding family tensions. Here the family is seen as a dynamic system, where everyone is interdependent on each other. The personalities of the different members and personal strategies in their lives influence all the others who will behave differently. If anyone becomes ill the others can withdraw concretely or emotionally or alternatively have recourse to strong dependencies or alliances. The systemic model also shows how exclusion can become entrenched, and how the risk of relapse in a vulnerable person can be increased or decreased by other people's attitudes. In a naturalistic follow-up study Lehtinen (1993) examined first-episode psychosis patients regarding the risk of relapse. One group had been treated with the systemic model and another with crisis orientated family therapy. No difference was found between the groups during the first year. During the following four years the group that had systemic treatment had a markedly lowered rate of relapse.

Appropriately selected families can be offered sessions aimed at reducing their level of emotional expression (EE, see Chapter 7). Leff et al. (1985) have shown how systematic work to lower the EE level has resulted in reduced relapse rates (see Figure 7.1, Chapter 7, p. 85). Gerald Hogarty and his group (1991) have also shown how family treatment clearly reduces

Table 25.3 Effects of family intervention (Hogarty *et al.* 1991)

Type of treatment	No. of patients	Per cent relapse Year 1	Per cent relapse Year 2
Family treatment + neuroleptics	21	19	20
Social training + neuroleptics	20	20	50
Family treatment + social training + neuroleptics	20	0	25
Only neuroleptics (control group)	29	38	62

the frequency of relapse in comparison with simply prescribing neuroleptics (see Table 25.3).

The effect size of family intervention is no less than the effect of neuroleptics. Information on different aspects of schizophrenia and their treatment are included in this supportive information. The central message is that schizophrenia is a disease affecting the brain. This can help counter the belief that the parents are in some way to blame, and so reduce feelings of guilt. Modifying dysfunctional interactions within the family system can further reduce vulnerability to relapse (Kuipers *et al.* 1992). Clear guidance is given on how to approach this.

Psycho-education

Where there is a low threshold for relapse or incomplete recovery, various models have been developed to help the family cope. The aim is to increase knowledge about psychotic illnesses, their causes, treatment and prognosis. This takes place in a short series of lectures combined with group discussions. A number of families are invited to participate. This is very similar to what takes place in the Liberman method of social skills training. The relatives can also be invited individually. All these approaches are not simply educative, but also enable the identification of new problems and potential solutions. In families where one or more of the members have significant personality disorder the communications can be very difficult to understand. In this situation a systemic psychotherapeutic approach may be useful.

There are now methods available that work along with systematic lectures, group discussions and individual family conversations. These support the family in developing a way of living with the patient which aids communication and stabilises the emotional climate. The background to this is the knowledge that relapses are reduced by lowering hostile communication in those families who openly express their criticisms and irritations. Often these problems are indicative of the degree to which the family is distressed by the situation and that the members need help and support in order to be able to change. Contact with support groups can be decisively helpful. In Great Britain, Rethink (formerly the National Schizophrenia Fellowship) is one example. Sister organisations exist in other countries that can influence both government and mental health services and ultimately the quality of life of the mentally ill.

Chapter 26

Preventing psychosis

The following areas of prevention are central:

- *primary prevention* – to forestall the occurrence of an illness
- *secondary prevention* – to shorten the duration of illness and ensure treatment effective and
- *tertiary prevention* – to prevent or reduce further manifestations of the illness, that is to say, rehabilitation.

In serious and disabling psychotic illnesses the preventative aspect of every phase of the illness is of the utmost importance.

Primary prevention

To forestall the occurrence of the illness

In order to make prevention effective it is necessary to know the causes of the illness. Schizophrenia and other psychoses are a very heterogeneous group where both the background factors and possible preventive contributions vary a great deal. The essential genetic factor can lie in a vulnerability, which can be an asset or a handicap. Personality traits that may be partly genetically determined may reinforce an introverted thinking which may be a risk factor for psychosis. On the other side, in combination with an artistic ability, these traits may strengthen creative gifts. A specific gene has not been linked to the illness and it is hard to believe that one specific gene or a few genes can explain most aspects of psychosis. In Tienari's (1991) study of high-risk individuals he found fewer children with psychoses in families with a low degree of conflicts. This means that the expression of a genetic vulnerability (phenotype) can be influenced positively by a supportive family network. (However, Tienari did not take account of other risk factors such as prenatal and perinatal damage in his study.) A preventative but perhaps somewhat idealistic step would be to support the parents of vulnerable children in providing as good an environment for their development as possible, perhaps with easy access to advice, improvements in schooling, etc.

Prenatal and perinatal stress increase the risk for schizophrenia significantly – especially when there are family disturbances. Unfortunately this factual observation has not yet been explained in specific terms (i.e. a causal pathway identified). An unfortunate consequence of the increased survival rate of very premature babies (with the associated risk of minor brain injury) may be an increase in their subsequent risk for developing psychosis. Naturally, one would assume that better health for the mother and antenatal care would have a beneficial effect on this. An intensification of the psychological support for parents at risk should also improve the future prognosis. However, since the incidence of schizophrenia is so low, the impact of such intensity of psychological perinatal care on incidence would be difficult to evaluate.

Overall, programmes that concern primary prevention do not play an essential role today. Secondary prevention is much more important.

Secondary prevention

To obtain effective assistance early on during the onset of the illness

The first signs of serious mental illness have been considered and it is important to reach the person before the symptoms have become all too marked and ingrained as often the process of exclusion has set in. Figure 14.1 (p. 159) shows a model for a psychotic illness from the premorbid phase to the prodromal phase where early symptoms make themselves felt.

In some cases it is never possible to know if non-specific symptoms are signs of a looming psychosis or not. An examination revealed that when a questionnaire was given to secondary school children where symptoms corresponding to DSM-III's prodromal symptoms for schizophrenia were asked for, nearly half of them qualified for this diagnosis (Yung and McGorry 1996). This suggests that the method of formulating such a questionnaire is not acceptable, partly because it is necessary to have a much narrower set of characteristics in order to be minimally precise in seeking out prodromal symptoms. The prodromal characteristics according to DSM-III have now been abandoned.

So it is primarily not until brief psychosis-like symptoms occur that one can be in a position to talk about a high risk. This 'duration of untreated psychosis' (DUP) or 'at risk state' implies increased isolation for the person who has been experiencing the symptoms. His or her thinking becomes all the more rooted in misunderstandings and mistrust. The ability to work or study suffers badly. About half of all first-episode psychotic patients have a

DUP which is longer than one month and these people would probably gain very much with an intensified early psychiatric intervention. Many major research projects focus on how to identify such individuals early, how to decide if they are at a high risk for developing psychosis, and if so how it should be prevented (Figure 26.1).

In an Australian project (Yung *et al.* 1996), the 'at risk state' has been defined as:

- 'diluted' or subclinical psychotic symptoms – corresponding to schizo-typal personality traits
- brief, transient psychotic symptoms, perhaps in combination with drug abuse or under another form of stress
- decrease in the ability to study or work is a serious indication together with the other signs
- occurrence of psychosis in other members of the family.

Of the first 20 young people who were referred to this Australian project a third developed a psychosis within six months. A system of treatment was then created where young people who were identified as high risk were randomly allocated to two groups. One group was offered psychotherapy and if necessary a low dose of neuroleptic. The other group was followed

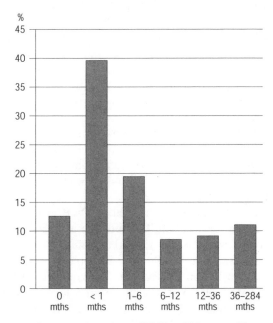

Figure 26.1 Duration of untreated psychosis (DUP) in 208 cases of first-onset psychosis in the Parachute project (Cullberg *et al.* 2002).

up without any specific treatment. The preliminary results showed that the young people who received treatment were less open to psychotic breakdown. Later results are less conclusive.

A large project in Stavanger, a city on the Norwegian west coast, has set out to make the people in a large area aware of early signs of psychosis by intensive media coverage (Larsen et al. 1998). Similarly, large areas around Oslo and in Denmark have been compared to see if it is possible to shorten the period of untreated psychosis, and also to reduce the incidence of schizophrenia by means of media-generated messages. The first goal has been achieved, but for the later one it is still too early to judge.

Ethical aspects

If a person can be saved from developing schizophrenia it is worth the work that has been contributed – both from humanitarian and economic points of view. It is still too early to say in which way early intervention may best do this. The period after puberty up until 25 years old is often filled with problems such as depression and uncertainties over identity. Many need psychotherapeutic support but it must be supplied without increasing the risk of developing psychosis. In trial projects that study the prevention of psychosis it can be hard for the staff to control their worry about the risk of psychosis, even when young people and their families are motivated to seek out treatment. Experience tells us that these young people are anxious about losing their sense of integration and so are often inclined to withdraw from such therapeutic contact. False positives, that is misidentifying those with 'normal' developmental crises, are a major concern in this area of work. Those identified as at risk may become stigmatised and distressed unnecessarily. By the very nature of preventative work it is not possible to identify these people or to know in which cases the development of psychosis has been prevented.

Another ethical problem is that it is not yet proven that treatment with neuroleptics is without risk in these early cases. It is possible that neuroleptics and the new antipsychotics may have a permanent effect on the receptor systems. The indication for their use in prevention of psychosis must therefore be considered very seriously.

For these reasons I believe that we should not begin widespread early detection or screening projects until we possess a greater degree of knowledge from scientific research. On the other hand, this does not apply to improving interventions for people who become ill with a first-episode psychosis. It is evident that in places where optimal services for first-episode psychosis patients are established, the patients ask for help at a much earlier point in their illness. Thus the DUP period will be 'automatically' shortened.

Early intervention with first-episode psychosis

The principles in these cases have already been described in this book. Today it seems to be a well-established fact that there are great advantages in providing special intervention facilities for first-episode psychotic patients where they can find help without feeling stigmatised (McGorry and Jackson 1999). The therapeutic environment of psychiatric units and clinics must also be developed to optimise care for these patients.

Tertiary prevention

To reduce the disability derived from the psychotic illness

Tertiary prevention is intimately bound up with secondary preventive contributions. It is especially important to optimise access and contact between the patient and services during the first five years after a first-episode psychosis. After that period there is a lower risk for relapse. The sooner patients can better learn to counteract their illness and recognise the nature of their disabilities, the less likely it will be that social exclusion will follow. That is, patients who show signs of not recovering completely early on must learn to understand and handle the recurrence of the illness as well as their disabilities. Their relatives need to be included and become a party to this process.

As independent a life as possible and the opportunity for employment or a meaningful activity for those who are unable to compete in the open employment market is no less important than medication and other treatment. Finally, the mentally disabled must also forge a social life with other people in order to improve their quality of life, despite any residual handicap.

Chapter 27

On being a relative

Carers and the immediate support network

The problem of dependent bonds is different during various stages of the development of the psychotic illness, and naturally different for the relatives, depending on whether one is a parent, sibling, or child to the patient.

The adult relative or sibling

For a parent the first phase of the illness is dominated by a sense of impotence – of not having any influence on the frightening and destructive events, and also by the pain of not understanding what is going on. One asks: Is the strange behaviour a sign of laziness or of a bad upbringing? How tough should one be? There are often different views as to why the situation has occurred. The allocation of blame for the illness or the problems that result create conflicts and increase tensions between those living at home.

When it is no longer possible to turn a blind eye towards the symptoms of psychosis, the impact of events can become shocking. A relative is sometimes forced to call in the police and can later be blamed for this. The family is in an acute state of crisis and the need for experienced support is great. What has happened and what will happen? Is there any hope? Are there any understandable reasons for the breakdown? Often psychiatric representatives offer meagre information and no one seems to take an interest or responsibility. The painful interaction with the ill member of the family is an added burden. How should one react? How shall I talk to my son? Many find that the only thing that happens is that medicine is prescribed.

If the psychosis does not go away completely or the condition is treated with high doses of medication for years, the fear that the illness may become chronic are intensified. This phase is often filled with the search for alternative forms of help, possibly prompted by bitterness toward psychiatry. This bitterness may result in the patient or family feeling unsupported, unassisted and misunderstood, thus left carrying too much responsibility. The damage done to family life is often serious by this stage and the relationships between the members of the family are neglected. One of the parents often assumes responsibility where the spouse and/or the other children feel themselves to be overlooked.

After a couple of years the hope for recovery may have dwindled, or if a more or less traumatic relapse has occurred, a sense of sorrow or bitterness characterises the next stage. There is sadness over the loss that has occurred, that one of the family has changed so much, and bitterness over the lack of understanding that they have been met with. It is at this stage that most people make contact with some organisation for relatives, which can be decisive for the future course of events. The sorrow sooner or later will be healed – at least on the surface – in an acceptance of the situation.

Many parents find their social world much reduced by this process. They feel constantly at risk that the ill member of the family will disturb things and that their energies are not sufficient to deal with anything else. The emotional tension is such that it brings on psychosomatic disturbances and many have to take sick leave periodically in order to be able to cope. The siblings can react either by getting deeply involved or by withdrawing from the family. Many carry the fear that they might themselves break down if they were to get too involved and are afraid that the mental illness might be hereditary and that it might get passed on to their children. Here they are in need of information to allay their fears. The risk of having a child who inherits the illness is only slightly elevated in someone who has a parent or sibling with a schizophrenic disorder and it is not a reason for advising against having children.

The over-involved parent

A common development within families with a child who has a schizophrenic disability is that one or both parents (and occasionally a sibling) becomes more and more identified with the sufferer. The value of ordinary life has now ceased to be of interest. It is only the life of the ill member of the family that matters. The person himself becomes slowly deflated and his or her relationship with others in the family circle loses its vitality and meaning. Time can be taken up with cleaning for the ill person, washing, cooking or planning outings. In the long run this kind of involvement is of little help. Even and perhaps especially a person diagnosed with schizophrenia has a need for independence in order to maintain his integrity. Is it not, after all, necessary for a visitor to call in advance before visiting? A certain disorganised freedom must be tolerated. Setting boundaries might be something that can be agreed upon together.

The problem with the 'over-involved' parent is that, paradoxically, the son's or daughter's condition can, as has been shown scientifically, become clinically worsened because of the level of emotional arousal that this over-involvement generates. It can also mean that the involvement offered by other members of the family dwindles or that the attempts made by the authorities to provide assistance become difficult. The parent always knows best what is needed and can assume an overly critical attitude, which irritates and annoys.

What can be done about this? Relatives' support groups have begun to take note of this kind of situation. They can support the members singly or in groups in order to help them to let go of their over-involvement and to let professionals help instead. The family member who has been so completely occupied with the ill person must find other outlets. It is important to accept that it is not possible to maintain complete control over the disabled person's life. Often it can be very helpful to go on a course to find out how better to understand and work with a relative's mental disabilities. These kinds of courses are usually run by a local organisation.

On being the child of a mentally ill parent

The problem of being the child of a psychotic parent has attracted more interest in recent years. Although the attention paid to this situation is insufficient in psychiatry, thinking about the family and work with the family are now expected in adult psychiatry as well as child psychiatry.

One in three patients with first-episode psychosis has children. An unknown number of children under the age of 18 have a parent with long-term psychosis. This will have an even greater effect on a child with a lone parent, the kind of child for whom it is difficult to meet up with friends in their free time because the parent is estranged from society. They are also at risk of being drawn into the parent's system of delusions and sometimes they can become physically neglected. A worse experience for the child occurs when the parent is hard to make emotional contact with and is preoccupied with their own inner thoughts. The child's sense of aloneness is often powerful. At the same time these children maintain a deep loyalty to the parent and find it hard to talk about problems with someone whom they do not trust completely. The problems can lead to truancy from school, which might be hard to understand if one is unaware of the parent's illness. Depression can be a consequence of neglect. The parent's lack of involvement in school activities is a non-specific warning sign for teachers.

It is important that schools' healthcare professionals need to be aware that these problems are not unusual. Supportive activities found in many places today are also very important. The children are given the opportunity, together with other children in the same situation, to talk about how things are at home. Their increased need for support must be identified. They need to be given information to help them understand and cope with their parent's illness, but in such a way that they do not feel disloyal to their parent. Such child support resources need to be available in all large cities. Furthermore, there is a need to work more closely between child and adult psychiatry in order to give the children adequate support in the acute stages of a parent's psychosis. The risk for a child who has a psychotic parent of developing psychosis in adulthood is usually thought to be around 10 per cent, but I would argue that this amount can be significantly reduced if their psychosocial environment is attended to.

When it is a question of a psychotically ill mother who is breastfeeding her child, the decision regarding how to help support her and how she co-operates with the maternity clinic's staff and psychiatry is vital. During the post-natal period the breastfeeding mother with a psychotic illness poses many challenges for both the maternity ward staff and the psychiatric team. Are there any relatives who can help? Are the symptoms under control and has the mother herself any insight regarding her need for support and help? Most can manage their mothering satisfactorily but do often need extra containment. A careful balance has to be maintained: doses of antipsychotic medication should not be so high that the psychological and neurological side effects become marked, while an acceptable protection against relapse needs to be provided. If the dose is too high the mother will find it difficult to respond adequately and sensitively to her baby. Also the presence in breast milk may sedate the baby further reducing interaction. The risk of using lower doses can be offset by close supervision of the mother's symptoms and behaviour by family and mental health professionals. Both mother and family also require a high level of psychological and social support from these professionals. This means that in certain cases one can allow a very low maintenance dose, which can be increased if necessary. The emotional needs of the baby must not be forgotten. Taking the baby into care should be resorted to only if all other attempts to help the mother have failed and the other supportive resources are inadequate.

Epilogue

My brother Erland, who is three years older than me, developed schizo-phrenia in the mid-1950s while studying painting at the Royal Academy of Arts. For many years he struggled with insulin comas, ECT treatment and exclusion from ordinary human life. Professional care ruled and I recall the consultant's irritated dismissal of my parents' complaint that Erland had been physically ill-treated. Eventually he was transferred to another hospital that dispensed with the ECT and insulin treatment in favour of medication.

In these environments there were some enlightened elements. Mr Härsing, head of the insulin department and a serious and attentive person, made people feel respected. The art therapist, Johanne Grieg-Cederblad, managed to give Erland the opportunity to paint. Dr Segnestam, consultant at Sundby Hospital, found time to talk to us, the relatives, whenever we asked. Eventu-ally Erland was discharged 'at his own risk'. He suffered and still suffers from his illness and his hospital experiences but has managed, more or less, to live in the outside world since then. With an incredible strength of mind, he has also been creative and successful as an artist.

I recount my brother's story because this book would not have happened without Erland, who taught me so much about what it means to have a schizophrenic disorder. At the same time, I can see how the conditions for psychiatry have changed as I have closely followed its development – as a relative and a psychiatrist – for almost half a century. As Erland's brother, I have experienced the sense of impotence that comes from observing the humiliating effects of a system of care that is not attuned to the patient's needs. But I must also admit that, as a doctor, I have committed much the same kinds of misjudgement for which I, as a relative, have criticised my colleagues.

Working in medical care has an almost irresistible tendency to numb prac-titioners to the realisation that they are treating and tending individuals who are just like themselves. Many claim that they have to dissociate themselves from their feelings in order to function in the wards; this is plainly not the case. There is more to good care than ethical principles and staff training. It also requires an organisation that accords priority to and accordingly finds room for empathy and humanity without any loss of professional standards. I have seen many places where this has been achieved. It is very much a matter of wanting and being sufficiently courageous to break away from ingrained attitudes. An organisation in which truly humane care is not feasible is a bad organisation. In other words, this has to do with the politics of care in the widest sense.

Classification

ICD-10 and DSM-IV

There are two diagnostic systems in use in psychiatry today. One is the ICD-10 (*International Classification of Mental and Behavioural Disorders*, 10th edn.), published by the World Health Organisation in 1994. The other is DSM-IV (*Diagnostic and Statistical Manual of Mental Disorders*, 4th edn.), published in 1995 by the American Psychiatric Association. The two systems conform in most of their essential features.

Both ICD-10 and DSM-IV detail a number of criteria for the diagnosis of each disorder and in each case a research manual has been published. The classifications are intentionally atheoretical: that is to say, they do not commit themselves to any specific viewpoint in relation to the aetiology of psychiatric disorders. The classification is confined to that which is directly observable and does not concern that which might be interpretable according to a specific theory – at least, such is the intention. Hence, different symptoms and signs can be operationalised: that is, they may be expressed in quantifiable terms and can then be 'measured' by means of rating scales of different kinds.

This implies that *reliability*, that is to say, agreement between what different judges arrive at, is high. The *validity* is lower, that is, whether it is clinically possible or useful to precisely delineate or separate out different psychiatric disorders is much debated. The psychiatrist who is interested in dynamics is going to find the system lacking and will need to add a diagnostic system that includes developmental and intentional aspects (i.e. the background circumstances, the psychological meaning of the symptom). Furthermore, behavioural disorders, anxiety disorders, affective disorders, psychotic disorders and personality disorders connect and influence each other in the face of different outer and inner conditions. These systems give a mistaken impression that types of disorders are distinctly delineated from each other. In actuality, transitional forms are more commonly found than are 'typical' forms.

This does not exclude phenomenological thinking from being useful for a scientifically orientated psychiatry. Operationalised systems of classification are indispensable especially with respect to research development.

Psychoses in relation to other mental disorders

Many mental disorders can usefully be thought of in terms of reactions to inner or outer conditions or as unsuccessful strategies for adjusting to the difficulties of life. The notion of 'illness' is a term that distracts from the possibility of phenomena being adaptive or biologically 'natural' ways of reacting, emphasising instead the deviant and 'pathological' in the form of abstracted symptoms. In this way, any interest in understanding the underlying psychodynamic and intentional factors is easily reduced. Any attempt to engage with these underlying processes to allow or facilitate natural recovery or healing is then undermined. The notion of 'disorder' is used both in ICD-10 and in DSM-IV. The use of the term 'illness' in psychiatry is easily associated with cause–effect conditions and with a medicalised culture. In fact, psychiatric reality is far more complex and humanistic theories of understanding and psychosocial methodologies are indispensable. The notion of a 'syndrome', by which we mean groups of symptoms tending to occur together, is more flexible for clinical practice in this area.

On the one hand it has become evident that the attention centred on psychodynamic factors in the middle of the twentieth century resulted in a decreased interest in studying and researching biological factors related to mental illness. However, on the other hand, in the last decades progress made within the neuro-psychiatric and bio-medical areas reversed this situation. The immense economic support that the bio-medically concerned clinical researchers get from the pharmaceutical industry has tended to marginalise the interest in humanistic research and psychosocial attitudes. In some places they may be given an honorary status, but evidently as second-rank phenomena.

Therefore, we sometimes speak about psychic problems, sometimes about disorders, illnesses, disabilities or handicap. In this book I use the term that I deem most relevant for what I am describing. Usually this means that I talk about *disorders* or a *syndrome*. In cases where the circumstances demand chiefly biological treatment or where we know the pathology of the brain to be dominant, I use the notion of *illness*. Psychological *disability* refers to the behavioural disturbance or thought disorders that lead to the person having difficulty in living up to basic psychosocial requirements. Where a disability can no longer be compensated for by the person themselves or by means of social support, it is referred to as *handicap*. (A somatic analogy might be a visual disability, which should not be termed handicap if it can be corrected by means of glasses.)

The psychiatric diagnostic groups

Figure A.1 shows the psychiatric diagnostic groups according to ICD-10. The first group consists of disorders that are due to organic central nervous system (CNS) damage (that is, the brain and the spinal cord) or developmental disorders that give different forms of *dementia* (a permanent and progressive reduction of the brain's capacity for thought from an earlier greater capacity) and cognitive disorders of other kinds. Also included are *disorders from brain damage* causing hallucinations (for example, certain forms of epilepsy) or delusions (for example, the early stages of dementia).

There are many psychotic disorders that are due to psychoactive substances (including alcohol) during both states of intoxication and as a result of withdrawal.

The group that includes other psychotic and schizophrenic disorders is singled out by the fact that we do not yet have knowledge of their possible organic causes. Sometimes they are called functional psychoses as opposed to organic psychoses. Research over the coming decades is expected to produce findings that describe the essential and characteristic organic features of many disorders which are currently included in the group of functional psychoses.

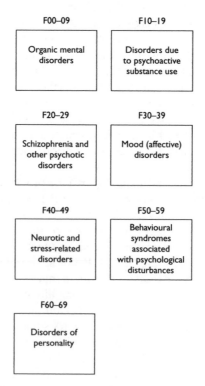

Figure A.1 Psychiatric diagnostic groups according to ICD-10.

Affective syndromes or disorders of mood include different degrees of depressive or manic states. Many of these patients can also suffer from transitory psychotic symptoms of a varying severity. It is essential to identify the underlying affective trait in these cases, so that opportunities for treatment are not missed. In addition many non-affective psychoses have secondary depressive disorders, which are in fact a consequence of the psychotic illness.

A large group consists of different anxiety disorders or syndromes. They include neurotic and stress-related *difficulties in adjustment, somatoform* (which means expressed through the body) and *dissociative disorders.*

Eating disorders, sexual problems, etc. are included in the group related to behavioural disorders connected with physiological disturbances.

Personality disorders imply a maintained behaviour and pattern of experience, which deviates from what might be expected within the cultural environment. For diagnosis there should be suffering to a clinically significant degree for the person or for those around them (see further Chapter 7 regarding the connection between psychosis and personality).

An overview and comparison between the classification systems for psychosis in DSM-IV and ICD-10

It is important to point out that these systems will not be of much use to those engaged in work with patients in the early stages of psychosis. The content and form of acute psychosis can change rapidly and surprise even the most experienced diagnostician (see Chapter 5 for a fuller picture of the evolution of acute psychosis).

The diagnostic systems described in this book are used whilst we await a clearer and more comprehensive system. I am certain that within a few years they will be replaced or completed by other systems which build on a deeper biological and psychological knowledge.

Definitions

To be psychotic is defined in DSM-IV as to be suffering from delusions and hallucinations without accompanying insight into their pathological nature. A broader definition is also suggested where those hallucinatory conditions are included when the person is aware of (has insight into) the hallucinatory nature of the sensations. An additional dimension to the definition also includes confused speech and acutely disorientated or catatonic behaviour. Along with this, a more dynamically orientated definition is suggested in the DSM-IV that includes a loss of ego boundaries and a deeply ingrained deterioration of the capacity for reality testing.

ICD-10 uses a broad definition of the concept of psychosis including hallucinations, delusions or other marked disorders of behaviour such as excitation and hyperactivity, marked psychomotor slowness and catatonic behaviour.

In this book I agree with a combination of descriptive and dynamic definitions, where a greater or lesser loss of the ego's (actually that of the self!) boundaries against the world becomes expressed in delusions and hallucinations without insight into their real nature. It means that reality testing is clearly limited and insight is reduced. A hallucinatory experience accompanied by the full recognition of its hallucinatory nature, something which for example certain schizophrenics can experience after many years, cannot be called psychosis. Rather, it is a disorder of perception. The ego would then be intact and the patient would have reached a paradigm shift in relation to his hallucinations and dependence on his illness.

Although the criteria for schizophrenia are somewhat different between the two systems, both depend on symptoms and on the duration of illness. ICD-10 leans towards Schneider's 'first range symptoms' (see Chapter 11) as it includes manifestations of thought withdrawal, thought insertion and thought broadcasting (others can hear one's thoughts on the radio), etc. DSM-IV emphasises the concurrence of several psychotic symptoms together with a bizarre component to the symptoms.

Both demand at least a month's active phase of illness while DSM-IV also demands that the whole course of events should have endured for at least six months if both prodromal (Chapter 5, p. 50) and residual symptoms (Chapter 11, p. 138) are included. This means that according to DSM-IV it would not be possible to make a diagnosis before six months, at the earliest. Furthermore, DSM-IV demands that there should be a reduction in functioning capacity in important aspects of living. In spite of its expressed atheoretical inception, DSM-IV, more than ICD–10, leans towards a point of view which assumes that there is a basic degenerative process. Hence, the schizophrenia diagnosis according to the American DSM-IV classification is more serious, which suggests that there will be a tendency to see individuals with a good prognosis as wrongly diagnosed. This difference will have consequences in attitudes towards patients and is further discussed in Chapter 11.

ICD-10 also includes as a specific subtype an unusual condition called *schizophrenia simplex* or *simple schizophrenia*. It describes a slow personality change with diminishing ability in functioning, together with a strange affectless and passive behaviour without any obvious psychotic symptoms. DSM-IV considers this disorder to be a variant of the *schizotypal personality disorder*.

Both systems have a subtype called *schizo-affective disorders*, a condition which at the same time has an affective (depressive or manic) disorder and schizophrenic symptoms. The schizophrenic symptoms must occur without affective symptoms during a period of at least two weeks – otherwise the condition must be attributed to the *affective psychoses*.

Psychoses which are schizophrenia-like (that is, psychoses which fulfil the criteria for schizophrenia's symptoms but which last a short term), according to DSM-IV, are called *schizophreniform psychoses* if they last at least one and not more than six months. Psychoses which last less than a month are called *brief psychoses*.

ICD-10 mentions *acute or transient psychotic disorders* if the period does not last more than a month. It should, moreover, be noted if symptoms of a schizophrenic nature occur. An example of acute, transient psychosis is *acute polymorphic psychosis* (also known as 'cycloid psychosis' and in large part these overlap with the schizo-affective psychoses) that is characterised by very variable and changing affective symptoms.

Delusional disorder, according to ICD-10, should continue beyond three months, otherwise it is known as *other acute delusional disorder*. According to DSM-IV the delusions should be present for at least one month and should not have any bizarre content: that is to say, things, which would be completely impossible according to the individual's culture. Examples of bizarre ideas include (in mainstream European culture) thought broadcast, the belief that one can control the weather with one's mind.

Final comments

A system of classification should have a practical value. It should be able to assist us in marking out those conditions that have a good or bad prognosis and which patients will respond most favourably to this or that form of treatment. It is not clear if ICD-10 and DSM-IV have such validity. Perhaps all these subgroupings hide more than they reveal? There is a simple way of grouping early psychoses that is clinically useful – see Chapter 10 for further details. Hopefully, the future will supply us with completely new classifications based on new research into clinical, neuropsychological, psychodynamic, receptor physiological and morphological (anatomical) factors.

Psychotic syndromes

Table A.1 Criteria for psychosis (somewhat simplified) according to DSM-IV and ICD-10 (see further Chapters 10 and 11)

	DSM-IV	ICD-10
DSM-IV: Brief psychotic disorders **ICD-10: Acute transient psychosis**	**Symptoms:** Delusions/ hallucinations/disorganisation. **Duration:** Over one day, under one month, with or without evident stressor.	As for DSM-IV.

	DSM-IV	ICD-10
DSM-1V: Schizophreniform psychotic disorder ICD-10: Acute (or polymorphic) schizophrenia-like psychotic disorder	**Symptoms:** Same as for schizophrenia. **Duration:** Over one month, under six months.	Under one month.
DSM-IV: Schizo-affective disorders ICD-10: Schizo-affective syndrome	**Symptoms and duration:** Unbroken illness with simultaneous schizophrenic and affective symptoms during some period. Also hallucinations or delusions of at least two weeks duration without affective symptoms. Affective symptoms during a considerable part of the illness.	As for DSM-IV.
Schizophrenia	**Symptoms:** Two or more psychotic symptoms (only one if bizarre). Social functions lowered (performance at work, relationships, or self-care). **Duration:** Continuous symptoms over six months one of which containing active symptoms.	At least 1 Schneider symptom (bizarre) or at least two non-bizarre psychotic symptoms. Over one month.
Delusional disorder	**Symptoms:** Non-bizarre delusions. No noticeable lowering of function. **Duration:** Over one month. Under three months for 'acute delusional disorder'. Over three months for 'chronic delusional disorder'.	As for DSM-IV.
DSM-IV: Psychosis UNS (unspecified psychotic disorder) ICD-10: Unspecified non-organic psychosis	Psychotic symptoms and behaviour without sufficient information or which is not referable to another specific group.	As for DSM-IV.

Notes

1 Reason – a thin veil over chaos

1 Many suggest that the experience of being in love, where psychic and physical intimacies unite, is a psychotic-like reality, a denial with minimal reality testing. It is built on the fact that idealised inner representations of our selves and the other can be projected out onto a recipient who may or may not reciprocate the desire. It is our own idealised inner world more than the other person's which we see realised in the representation of this person. Sometimes it becomes clear that fantasy and reality can adapt to each other under the aegis of the reality principle.

3 The concept of psychosis, delusions and hallucinations

1 The so-called balance of terror between east and west during the latter half of the twentieth century contained a steady occurrence of incidents of this kind: the difference being that the fear concerned atomic weapons on both sides. The threat was increased by problems of perceiving activities with a barely dependable radar and air supervision. Naturally the problems of interpretation become much more difficult for someone with a narcissistic-paranoid personality problem with a tendency to quick reactions and seeing events in terms of black and white, good and bad.

2 A similar assumption of ideas and delusions lying far from a rational self can also occur in an extreme religious or political sect where the leader is a charismatic and narcissistic personality who wants to form everyone into his own mould and is unable to accept dissident thought. In the democratic atmosphere of today we underestimate many people's need to radically submit to authoritative personalities or ideologies. These people prefer to obey a strict and demanding leader rather than live with a lonely and uncertain self with little recognition from other people.

3 The difference between this kind of delusion and, for example, the Christian missionary vocation, is that eventually it is usually experienced as an invitation – a calling – which does not contain the grandiose belief that God is closer to you than to anyone else. This is well described in depth by Selma Lagerlöf in her book *Jerusalem* (1901–1902). The story is about a revivalist movement in a country district in Southern Dalecarlia at the end of the nineteenth century, which, under the leadership of a revivalist preacher, persuaded all the people living there to sell their farms and to move to Jerusalem.

4 The ego, the self and psychosis

1 The word 'object' refers to internal representations of important people in the environment. This term is used in order to differentiate between object and subject where the latter stands for the individual himself.

5 Phases of acute psychosis: A crisis model

1 A friend of the author August Strindberg asked him six months after his paranoid psychosis in 1895 how he now thought about his paranoid experiences. He answered, 'With three quarters of my being I believe in the reality of these constellations, but with a quarter of my being I ask myself if all this is not in the end, my own thoughts, all the same.'

6 Neurobiological vulnerability factors

1 For Tienari (1991) the notion of schizophrenic borderline states includes non–schizophrenic psychoses as well as borderline personality disorders.

2 That the children from the mother's and not the father's illness have been sought out is wholly a practical fact. It does not mean that the father's genes are less important.

3 It is possible that the early developmental disorders in the form of autism spectrum disorders which occur in 4 out of 1000 children may have an increased vulnerability factor for psychosis. There is still no clear evidence for this in the literature (see further Chapter 12).

4 One can, somewhat polemically, compare the notion of psychosis with fainting. It is easy to find a diagnostic agreement between different clinicians regarding fainting (the reliability is high) but everyone agrees that the explanatory value – (the validity) of the notion of fainting is low. Behind the symptom, a brain tumour, a lack of blood sugar, low blood pressure, emotional instability and much else can lie. It is a matter of a clear, yet non-specific propensity to react in a certain way. If one were to give a recommendation as to how 'fainting' should be treated, the result would be unacceptably rough and of little use. Has psychosis research advanced any further? Psychosis, like fainting is a final common pathway for a range of diverse pathological genetic, developmental and psychosocial factors, all of which appear to have the potential to interact.

5 Positron emissions tomography (PET) is a method by which radioactivity marks certain molecules, for example, glucose, which is included in the brain's metabolism and bound to the receptor for the signal substance. Variations in metabolic function can later be graphically illustrated by detecting the precise point of emission of this radiation in the brain. This method allows us to study how the different areas of the brain work under different conditions.

6 A meta-analysis means that findings from several researches, which have been carried out by certain scientific centres, are put together according to specific scientific criteria. By this means it is possible to make use of a greater number of subjects giving the statistical analysis a higher power.

7 Magnetic resonance imaging (MRI) refers to the fact that the brain is subject to a magnetic field which induces detectable changes in different structures of the brain. These changes can be computerised and displayed as high resolution pictures of different brain structures. Computerised tomographic (CT) scanning is a cheaper method of imaging which gives a less clear differentiation of the structures in the brain.

8 Pre-eclampsia is diagnosed when the blood pressure is high and there is protein in

the urine during pregnancy. A less well-functioning placenta is evident in these cases, which is thought to influence the child's nutrition.

7 Psychodynamic vulnerability factors

1 Recently the pendulum has swung in the other direction so that it has been difficult to have a scientific discussion about the possibility of experiences in childhood and family relationships as important for a psychotic development. Researchers who take an interest in this area find it difficult to get noticed or to get published and are a priori treated as being unscientific. This reaction, which is not hard to understand, has been strongly supported by influential organisations of relatives of schizophrenic patients.

2 DSM-III, which was used during the 1980s, shows no decisive diagnostic differences in relation to schizophrenia compared with the present DSM-IV.

3 There is a growing body of knowledge about how a serious deficiency in the lives of infant monkeys causes underdevelopment in certain brain centres. This underdevelopment relates to the unavailability of a mother to function as stimulus during a critical period of infancy. Negative effects can later be seen in the monkey, when it becomes adult, in the form of behaviour disorders, aggression or inwardness. A psychotic state is triggered with low doses of amphetamine, which suggests that the dopamine system has been sensitised through the early deprivation (Kraemer et al. 1984). If the important nurturing stimuli necessary to build up the brain's dopamine 'reward system' are lacking in the earliest stage of childhood, then essential brain functions become imbalanced or do not develop sufficiently. This is also discussed later in this chapter in connection with schizoid personality characteristics.

4 In the different myths about Faust, he enters into a pact with the Devil whereby he may have all his wishes come true in exchange for the Devil taking his soul.

5 To speak about choice here may seem unrealistic. Of course, it has not much to do with the kind of choice that older children or adults can make. The infant has no freedom to reflect upon different alternatives. The use of the word here is to do with a specific process where the rudimentary self plays a part and which will constitute the centre for the adult self.

6 The occurrence of alexithymic traits has been studied by the psychoanalyst Aaron Karush (1969), who concluded that it is a contraindication to treatment with dynamic psychotherapy. He divided up a group of 30 people with ulcerative colitis in order to find out if insight orientated psychotherapy was appropriate. Six patients were considered to be possible candidates for this kind of therapy but most cases were not considered appropriate. All these cases were described as having a marked degree of alexithymia. They were considered to be better off with supportive treatment or behaviour therapy.

8 Factors that trigger psychosis

1 Naturally, even a physiological stress can be measured (rated) in terms of experience. In this case it is the subjective experience of the stress that is rated. This can be correlated to a larger or lesser extent with biological markers measuring the organism's physiological reactions.

2 The design of post-operative wards may well have contributed to these psychoses. They were, for practical reasons, unintentionally arranged in such a way that the risk of sensory deprivation became heightened. The patients were left motionless, listening to a monotonous sound, lights were kept low and did not

vary with the time of day as natural light would. When attempts were made to make the post-operative ward more psychologically stimulating, the duration of the psychosis diminished markedly. (See Chapter 13 for further discussion.)

3   The term transition is used in anthropological literature when discussing ritualised initiations that mark the big changes in life and give support to the individual and his or her environment during these changes.

4   The American anthropologist and psychoanalyst Erik H. Erikson introduced the term moratorium in *Childhood and Society* (1950) and *Identity: Youth and Crisis* (1968). He developed ideas concerning psychosocial maturation. He argues that divergent behaviour and illness may have a developmental role in some sensitive individuals: they may allow maturation by an indirect route. Psychiatry's fixation on symptoms can easily lead to a dismissal of the creative contents in these events. Consequently, the moratorium represents a period when something which appears to be an unhealthy activity turns out to be psychically meaningful (see Chapter 14).

5   As we saw in Chapter 4, the primary process refers to thinking which is not dependent on ordinary logical consistency, time or place. This is the case in the tiny infant, in dreams and in psychosis. In contrast, the normal secondary process thinking in essence consists in logical reflection.

6   Strindberg himself has dramatised his experience in 'Inferno' (1897) which gives a more schizophrenic picture than that of his letters, diary notes and contemporary comments by eyewitnesses.

9 Protective factors

1   For more evidence, look at Tienari's (1991) research into families of adopted high-risk children (p. 61).

10 Psychotic disorders I

1   Such a diagnostic rationale can appear academic. However, it has a certain value in relation to the treatment as psychotic symptoms in schizophrenia often respond to medication. In the case of delusional disorder, medication is seldom effective.

11 Psychotic disorders II: Schizophrenia – the sickness of the self

1   In spite of the spectrum concept's clear clinical relevance, there is a risk that it might be used all too lightly. People whom one does not understand are without careful consideration labelled schizotypal, that is to say, pre-schizophrenic. Thus a wide concept of schizophrenia may be misused by including those introverted people who simply oppose mainstream thinking. We have seen situations of this kind in Soviet psychiatry which, by using a very wide concept of schizophrenia (that did not follow the above described fundamental symptoms), allowed for the inclusion and treatment by force of many people for their dissident thoughts.

2   In order to simulate this kind of experience, healthy people have been invited to listen to their own voices through earphones with a few seconds delay. They describe their actions to the researcher and themselves through a microphone. They usually give up after a short period because of feelings of impotence or they lose the will to speak.

12 Autism spectrum disorders and childhood psychoses

1 The neurologist and author Oliver Sacks has provided a sensitive description of many highly gifted people with Asperger's syndrome in *An Anthropologist on Mars* (1995).

14 The two critical periods in acute psychosis and the potential for recovery

1 Of course, 'toxic' could be seen as a metaphor for a slowly advancing damaging influence. However, the risk is great that the word 'toxic' will rule and the concept will remain entrenched in its concrete meaning. It is worth spelling out the alternative process here as it is such an important point: a less concrete, more psychosocial conception of 'toxic psychosis' allows for dynamic (and hence modifiable) negative reinforcing effects such as stigma and understimulation which impair recovery, sometimes irretrievably.

15 Cognitive disorders and the psychotic thought process

1 Metaphoric and symbolic ideas often overlap in their use. A metaphor implies that associative similarities or inner agreements (correspondences) mean that an object or a piece of behaviour is exchanged for another idea or some other form of behaviour. A question that no one wishes to 'hold on to' becomes 'a hot potato'; the poet talks about 'the red pan of the autumn moon' or of the camel as 'the desert ship'. Metaphors are normally used in our culture in order to make ideas surrounding time, concrete and spatial: for example, before Christmas, within three days, etc. People in certain cultures, just like small children, live concretely with this spatial view of time where, for example, yesterday lies on the other side of the forest.

The notion of a symbol is comprehensive and implies that signs, an icon or concentrated picture stand for a complex content: for example, computer icons for different functions. The symbol can have an aesthetic-metaphysical aspect which is absent in the metaphor: for example, 'the way of the cross' and 'Eve's apple'. A condition for its ability to function in language is that the person who uses it is conscious of its double meaning. In this way, it is possible to connect the function of symbolisation with the pretence aspect of children's play (see Chapter 1).

17 Towards a bio-psycho-social model of psychoses

1 I mean that the ego does not 'exist in reality' other than as a mode of thought. It has a significant usefulness as a means for expressing the existence of an organising bio-psycho-social principle.
2 The expression 'gestalt' in its psychological meaning refers to when the whole is more than simply the sum of the parts.

18 Traditions of thought in the history of psychiatric ideas

1 See, for example, Antonio Damasio's *Descartes' Error* (1996) and Oliver Sacks (1998) *The Man Who Mistook His Wife for a Hat*. Another example is the new *International Journal of Neuro-Psychoanalysis* (Karnac).

19 Attitudes in the twentieth-century treatment of psychosis

1   A stark, autobiographical account of the unprotected and angst-ridden suffering that a patient undergoes in this kind of electro-convulsive treatment is given by the New Zealand writer Janet Frame (1961) in *Faces in the Water*.

2   The term 'social psychiatry' is used here in its original context, to convey the development of a 'therapeutic community' and working in groups. It gradually gained a more theoretical meaning as an explanatory system for psychic ill health in addition to those of biological and dynamic psychiatric theory. Psychic health is dependent on containing relationships and a functioning social network. Social psychiatry became the branch of psychiatry that examined the relationship between the occurrence of psychiatric illness in the population (epidemiology) and different factors in the social environment.

20 The requirements, demands and organisation of treatment for psychosis

1   *Compliance* actually means being amenable or obedient. The expression has been introduced into psychiatry as a remnant of a more authoritarian attitude. Since amenability is not considered a particularly desirable state of mind in today's world, the word co-operation is more applicable.

21 The assessment and treatment of patients with an acute psychotic episode

1   The WAIS-R (Wechsler Adult Intelligence Scale, revised version) has been used to investigate cognitive functioning. It contains 11 subtests, divided into verbal and performance subscales.

23 People with long-term psychosis in the community

1   The word 'client' is used instead of 'patient' in the Wisconsin project since it implies a more assertive and active role.

24 Pharmacological treatment of psychosis

1   Currently, such an attitude is common within psychiatry. It is grounded in the idea that mental processes are products of and hence are secondary to the bio-logical and molecular context. This way of thinking is countered by most modern scientific theorists and neurophysiologists who claim instead that mental phe-nomena imply a perception (conscious and unconscious) of processes within and between our inner and outer worlds. The mental system will ensure survival by means of optimising our adjustment to the exigencies of life. The psychological processes influence and alter the neuropsychological processes. In other words, the mental is neither primary nor secondary to the molecular, rather it occurs simultaneously and expresses another aspect of biological activity. Psychology in its exact meaning is just as much biology (theory of life) as neurophysiology.

References

Alanen, Y. O. (1968) From the mothers of schizophrenic patients to interactional family dynamics, *Journal of Psychiatric Research, 6*, suppl 1, 202–212.

—— (1997) *Schizophrenia – Its origins and need-adapted treatment.* London: Karnac.

Alanen, Y., Lehtinen, K., Räkkökäinen, V. *et al.* (1991) Need-adapted treatment of new schizophrenic patients. Experiences and results of the Turku project, *Acta Psychiatrica Scandinavica, 83*, 363–372.

Allebeck, P., Adamsson, C., Engström, A. *et al.* (1993) Cannabis and schizophrenia: A longitudinal study of cases treated in Stockholm County, *Acta Psychiatrica Scandinavica 88*, 21–24.

American Psychiatric Association (APA) (1995) *DSM-IV, Diagnostic and Statistical Manual of Mental Disorders* (4th ed.). Washington, DC: American Psychiatric Association.

Andersen, T. (1990) *The reflecting team.* Broadstairs: Borgmann.

Antonovsky, A. (1987) *Unravelling the mystery of health.* San Francisco: Jossey-Bass.

Arnold, S. E., Hyman, B. T., Van Hoesen, G. W. *et al.* (1991) Some cytoarchitectural abnormalities of the enthorinal cortex in schizophrenia, *Archives of General Psychiatry, 48*, 625–632.

Balint, M. (1972) *The doctor, his patient and the illness.* New York: International Universities Press.

Baron, M., Gruen, R., Asnis, L. and Kane, J. (1983) Age-of-onset in schizophrenia and schizotypal disorders: Clinical and genetic implications, *Neuropsychobiology, 10*, 199–204.

Basaglia, F. (1964) *The doctrine of the mental hospital as a place of institutionalism.* Paper presented at the First International Congress of Social Psychiatry, London.

Bebbington, P., Wilkins, S., Jones, P. *et al.* (1993) Life events and psychosis. Initial results from the Camberwell Collaborative Psychosis Study, *British Journal of Psychiatry, 162*, 72–79.

Beck, J. C. and van der Kolk, B. (1987) Reports of childhood incest and current behaviour of chronically hospitalized psychotic women, *American Journal of Psychiatry, 144*, 1474–1476.

Beckman, V. (1984) *Sinnesjukhuset. Bilder ur psykiatrins historia.* Stockholm: Norstedts.

Bion, W. (1967) *Second thoughts.* London: Heinemann.

Birchwood, M. (1999) Psychological and social treatments: Course and outcome, *Current Opinion in Psychiatry, 12*, 61–66.

Bleuler, E. (1950/1911) *Dementia praecox or the group of schizophrenias*. New York: International Universities Press.

Bleuler, M. (1972) *Die schizophrenen Geistesstörungen in Lichte lang-jähriger Kranken-und Familiengeschichten*. Stuttgart: Georg Thieme Verlag.

—— (1974) The long-term course of schizophrenic psychoses, *Psychological Medicine, 4*, 244–254.

—— (1979) *Lehrbuch der Psychiatrie* (14th ed.). Berlin: Springer Verlag.

—— (1984) Das alte und das neue Bild des Schizophrenen, *Scheizer Archiv für Neurologie, Neurochirurgie und Psychiatrie, 135*, 143–149.

Bowlby, J. (1969–1980) *Attachment and loss* (Vols 1–3). London: Hogarth Press.

Buber, M. (1962) *Ich und Du*. Leipzig: Inselverlag.

Cannon, M., Jones, P., Huttunen, M. O. *et al.* (1999) School performance in Finnish children and later development in schizophrenia, *Archives of General Psychiatry, 56*, 457–563.

Cannon, T. D. and Mednick, S. A. (1993) The schizophrenia high-risk project in Copenhagen: Three decades of progress, *Acta Psychiatrica Scandinavica*, suppl 370, 33–47.

Cappelen-Smith, C. Tunström, G. and Öhnell, A. (1994) *Inge Schiöler*. Uddevalla: Bohusläns Museum.

Castle, D. J. and Murray, R. M. (1991) The neuro-developmental basis of sex differences in schizophrenia, editorial, *Psychological Medicine, 21*, 565–575.

Chapman, J. (1966) The early symptoms of schizophrenia, *British Journal of Psychiatry, 112*, 225–251.

Ciompi, L. (1980) The natural history of schizophrenia in the long term, *British Journal of Psychiatry, 136*, 413–420.

—— (1997) The concept of affect-logic: An integrative psycho-social-biological approach to understanding and treatment of schizophrenia, *Psychiatry, 60*, 158–170.

Ciompi, L. and Hoffman, H. (2004) Soteria Berne: An innovative milieu therapeutic approach to acute schizophrenia based on the concept of affect-logic, *World Psychiatry, 3*, 140–146.

Ciompi, L., Dauwalder, H.-P., Aebi, E., *et al.* (1992) A new approach of acute schizophrenia. Further results of the pilot project Soteria Bern. In A. Werbart and J. Cullberg (Eds.), *Psychotherapy of schizophrenia: Facilitating and obstructive factors* (pp. 95–109). Oslo: Scandinavian University Press.

Conrad, C. (1958) *Die beginnende Schizophrenie*. Stuttgart: Georg Thieme Verlag.

Coryell, W., Endicott, J., Keller, M. *et al.* (1989) Bipolar affective disorder and high achievement. A familiar association, *American Journal of Psychiatry, 146*, 983–988.

Crow, T. J. (1980) Molecular pathology of schizophrenia: More than one disease process?, *British Medical Journal, 280*, 66–68.

Cullberg, J. (1997) Effekten av psykodynamisk terapi på neuroleptikaanvändningen vid psykoser [The effect of psychodynamic therapy on the use of neuroleptics], *Behandling med neuroleptika*. Report 133/1 from the Swedish Council on Technology Assessments in Health Care, 181–192.

—— (2002) Stressful life events preceding the first onset of psychosis, An explorative study, *Nordic Journal of Psychiatry, 57*, 209–214.

Cullberg, J. and Levander, S. (1991) Fully recovered schizophrenic patients who received intensive psychotherapy. A Swedish case-finding study, *Nordic Journal of Psychiatry, 45*, 253–262.

Cullberg, J. and Nybäck, H. (1992) Persistent auditory hallucinations correlate with the size of the third ventricle in schizophrenic patients, *Acta Psychiatrica Scandinavica, 86*, 469–472.

Cullberg, J., Stefansson, C. G. and Wennersten, E. (1981) Psychiatry in low status dwelling areas, *Psychiatry and Social Science, 1*, 118–123.

Cullberg, J., Thorén, G., Åbb, S. *et al.* (2000) Integrating intense psychosocial and low dose neuroleptic treatment. A three year follow-up. In B. Martindale (Ed.), *Psychosis – Psychological approaches and their effectiveness* (pp. 200–209). London: Gaskell.

Cullberg, J., Levander, S. and Holmqvist, R. (2002) One-year results in first episode patients in the Swedish Parachute project, *Acta Psychiatrica Scandinavica, 106*, 276–285.

Cullberg. J., Mattsson, M., Levander, S. *et al.* (2005) *Three-year outcome for the Swedish Parachute Project.* Manuscript submitted for publication.

Dahl, M. L. and Sjöqvist, F. (1997) Faktorer som påverkar neuroleptikas omsättning I kroppen [Factors influencing the metabolism of neuroleptics], *Behandling med neuroleptika.* Report 133/2 from the Swedish Council on Technology Assessments in Health Care, 103–128.

Dalén, P. (1978) *Season of birth. A study of schizophrenia and other mental disorders.* Amsterdam: Elsevier,.

Dalgaard, O. S. (1980) *Bomiljø og psykisk helse.* Oslo: Universitetsforlaget.

Dalman, C. and Cullberg, J. (1999) Neonatal hyperbilirubinaemia – a vulnerability factor for mental disorder?, *Acta Psychiatrica Scandinavica, 100*, 469–471.

Dalman, C., Allebeck, P., Cullberg, J. *et al.* (1999) Obstetric complications and the risk of schizophrenia. A longitudinal study of a national birth cohort, *Archives of General Psychiatry, 56*, 234–240.

Damasio, A. (1996) *Descartes' error.* London: Papermac.

Der, G., Gupta, S. and Murray, R. M. (1990) Is schizophrenia disappearing?, *Lancet, 335*, 513–516.

Drury, V., Birchwood, M., Cochrane, R. and Macmillan, F. (1996) Cognitive therapy and recovery from acute psychosis: A controlled trial. I. Impact on symptoms. II. Impact on recovery time, *British Journal of Psychiatry, 169*, 593–607.

Eggers, C. (1978) Course and prognosis of childhood schizophrenia, *Journal of Autism and Childhood Schizophrenia, 8*, 21–36.

—— (1989) Schizo-affective psychoses in childhood: A follow-up study, *Journal of Autism and Developmental Disorders, 19*, 327–342.

Eivergård, M. and Jönsson, L. E. (1993) *Sidsjöns sjukhus 1943–1993. From Den moderna sinnesjukvårdens historuia.* Sundsvalls: Sundsvalls Museum.

Elkis, H., Friedman, L., Wise, A. and Meltzer, H. (1995) Metaanalyses of studies of ventricular enlargement and cortical sulcal prominence in mood disorders. Comparisons with controls or patients with schizophrenia, *Archives of General Psychiatry, 52*, 735–746.

Erikson, E.H. (1950) *Childhood and society.* New York: WW Norton.

—— (1968) *Identity: Youth and crisis.* New York: WW Norton.

Falloon, I. R. H., Boyd, J. L., McGill, C. W. *et al.* (1985) Family management in the prevention of morbidity of schizophrenia. Clinical outcome of a two-year longitudinal study, *Archives of General Psychiatry, 42,* 887–896.

Farde, L. (1997) Brain imaging of schizophrenia – the dopamine hypothesis, *Schizophrenia Research, 8,* 157–162.

Farde, L., Wiesel, F-A., Stone-Elander, S. *et al.* (1990) D2-Dopamine receptors in neuroleptic-naïve schizophrenic patients, *Archives of General Psychiatry, 47,* 213–219.

Farde, L., Nordström, A.-L., Wiesel, F.-A. *et al.* (1992) Positron emission tomographic analysis of central D1-and D2-dopamine receptor occupancy in patients treated with classical neuroleptics and clozapine – relation to extrapyramidal side effects, *Archives of General Psychiatry, 49,* 538–544.

Farde, L., Gustavsson, J.P. and Jönsson, E. (1997) D2-Dopamine receptors and personality traits, *Nature, 590.*

Fish, B., Marcus, J., Sydney, H. L. *et al.* (1992) Infants at risk for schizophrenia: Sequelae of a genetic neurointegrative defect, *Archives of General Psychiatry, 49,* 221–235.

Foucault, M. (1961) *Histoire de la folie à l'age classique.* Paris : PUF.

Fowler, D., Garety, P. and Kuipers, E. (1995) *Cognitive behaviour therapy for psychoses. Theory and practice.* New York: Wiley.

—— (1998) Cognitive therapy for psychosis: Formulation, treatment, effects and service implications, *Journal of Mental Health, 7,* 123–133.

Frame, J. (1961) *Faces in the water.* New York: Georges Braziller.

Freud, S. (1923) *The Ego and the Id.* London: Hogarth Press.

—— (1940 [1938]) *Abriss der Psychoanalyse*, SE. London:Hogarth Press,

Friis, S. (1986) Characteristics of a good ward atmosphere, *Acta Psychiatrica Scandinavica, 74,* 469–473.

Frith, C.D. (1995) *The cognitive neuropsychology of schizophrenia.* Hove, UK: Lawrence Erlbaum Associates Ltd.

Geijer, E. G. (1856) *Föreläsningar öfver menniskans historia* [Lectures on the history of man]. Upsala: P A Norstedt & Söner.

Glass, L. L., Katz, H. M., Schnitzer, R. D. *et al.* (1989) Psychotherapy of schizophrenia: An empirical investigation of the relationship of process to outcome, *American Journal of Psychiatry, 146,* 603–608.

Goffman, E. (1990) *Asylums.* New York: Doubleday.

Goldstein, K. (1943) The significance of psychological research in schizophrenia, *Journal of Nervous and Mental Disease, 97,* 261–279.

Goldstein, M. (1992) The family in schizophrenia – some current issues. In A. Werbart and J. Cullberg (Eds.), *Psychotherapy of schizophrenia: Facilitating and obstructing factors.* Oslo: Scandinavian Universities Press.

Green, H. (1964) *I never promised you a rose garden.* New York: Holt.

Green, J. F. (1988) *Schizophrenia from a neurocognitive perspective – Probing the impenetrable darkness.* Boston: Allyn and Bacon.

Grotstein, J. S. (1995) Orphans of the 'real': I. Some modern and postmodern perspectives on the neurobiological and psychosocial dimensions of psychosis and other primitive mental disorders, *Bulletin of the Menninger Clinic, 50,* 287–311.

Gunderson, J. G., Frank, A. F. and Katz, H. M. (1984) Effects of psychotherapy in schizophrenia: II. Comparative outcome of two forms of treatment, *Schizophrenia Bulletin, 10*, 564–598.

Häfner, H., der Heiden, W. and Behrens, S (1998) Causes and consequences of the gender differences in age at onset of schizophrenia, *Schizophrenia Bulletin, 24*, 99–113.

Harding, C. M., Brooks, C. W., Ashikaga, T. *et al.* (1987) The Vermont longitudinal study of persons with severe mental illness. II: Long term outcome of subjects who retrospectively met DSM-III criteria for schizophrenia, *American Journal of Psychiatry, 144*, 727–735.

Healy, D. (1989) Neuroleptics and psychic indifference: A review, *Journal of the Royal Society of Medicine, 82*, 615–619.

—— (1990) Schizophrenia: Basic, release reactive and defect processes, *Human Psychopharmacology, 5*, 105–121.

Healy, D. and Farquhar, G. (1998) Immediate effects of Droperidol, *Human Psychopharmacology, 13*, 113–120.

Hegarty, J. D. *et al.* (1994) One hundred years of schizophrenia: A meta-analysis of the outcome literature, *American Journal of Psychiatry, 151*, 1409–1416.

Hoek, H. W., Brown, A. S. and Susser, E. (1998) The Dutch famine and schizophrenia spectrum disorders, *Social Psychiatry and Psychiatric Epidemiology, 33*, 373–379.

Hogarty, G. E., Anderson, C. M., Reiss, D. J. *et al.* (1991) Family psychoeducation, social skills training and maintenance chemotherapy in the aftercare treatment of schizophrenia: II. Two-year effects of a controlled study on relapse and adjustment, *Archives of General Psychiatry, 48*, 340–347.

Hogarty, G. E., Kornblith, S. J., Greenwald, D. *et al.* (1995) Personal therapy: A disorder-relevant psychotherapy for schizophrenia, *Schizophrenia Bulletin, 21*, 379–393.

Hogarty, G., Greenwald, D., Ulrich, R. *et al.* (1997) Three-year trials of personal therapy among schizophrenic patients living with or independent of family. II: Effects on adjustment of patients, *American Journal of Psychiatry, 154*, 1514–1524.

Horrobin, D. F. (1999) The phospholipid concept of psychiatric disorders and its relationship to the neuro-developmental concept of schizophrenia. In M. Peet, I. Glen and D. Horrobin (Eds.), *Phospholipid spectrum disorder in psychiatry*. Carnforth: Marius Press.

Huber, G., Gross, G., Schüttler, R. *et al.* (1980) Longitudinal studies of schizophrenic patients, *Schizophrenia Bulletin, 6*, 592–605.

Hughlings-Jackson, J. (1958/1894) *The factors of insanities. Selected writings. Vol 2: Evolution and Dissolution of the Nervous System*, James Taylor (Ed.). London: Staples Press

Huttunen, M. O. and Niskanen, P. (1978) Prenatal loss of father and psychiatric disorders, *Archives of General Psychiatry, 35*, 429–431.

Huxley, A. (1954) *The doors of perception*. London: Chatto & Windus.

—— (1956) *Heaven and hell*. London: Chatto & Windus.

Ingvar, D. H. and Franzén, G. (1974) Abnormalities of blood flow distribution in patients with chronic schizophrenia, *Acta Psychiatrica Scandinavica, 50*, 425–462.

Isohanni, M., Isohanni, I., Jones, P., Järvelin, M.-R. *et al.* (1999) School predictors of schizophrenia in the 1966 Northern Finland birth cohort study. Paper presented at the Conference for Schizophrenia Research, Santa Fé.

Jackson, H., Edwards, J., Hulbert, C. and McGorry, P. (1999) Recovery from psychosis: Psychological interventions. In P. McGorry and H. Jackson (Eds.), *The recognition and management of early psychosis.* Cambridge: Cambridge University Press.

Jackson, M. (1994) *Unimaginable storms.* London: Karnac.

Jakob, H. and Beckmann, H. (1986) Prenatal developmental disturbances in the limbic allo-cortex in schizophrenics, *Journal of Neural Transmission, 65,* 303–326.

Jaskiw, G. E., Juliano, D. M., Goldberg, T. E. *et al.* (1994) Cerebral ventricular enlargement in schizophreniform disorder does not progress. A seven year follow-up study, *Schizophrenia Research, 14,* 23–28.

Johnson, E. (1968) *The days of his grace.* (E. Harley Schubert, Trans.). London: Chatto & Windus.

Jones, M. (1970) *The therapeutic community.* New York: Basic Books.

Jones, P., Rodgers, B., Murray, R. and Marmot, M. (1994) Child developmental risk factors for schizophrenia in the British 1946 birth cohort, *Lancet, 344,* 1398–1402.

Jonsson, E. (1986) *Tokfursten.* Stockholm: Rabén and Sjögren.

Kapur, S. (2003) Psychosis as a state of aberrant salience: A framework linking biology, phenomenology, and pharmacology in schizophrenia, *American Journal of Psychiatry, 160,* 13–23.

Karon, B. and VandenBos, G. (1972) The consequences of psychotherapy for schizophrenic patients, *Psychotherapy: Theory, Research and Practice, 9,* 11–19.

Karush, A. (1969) The response to psychotherapy in chronic ulcerative colitis, *Psychosomatic Medicine, 31,* 201–207.

Keenan, B. (1992) *An evil cradling.* London: Vintage.

Kernberg, O. (1980) *Internal world and external reality. Object relations theory applied.* New York: Jason Aronson.

—— (1984) *Severe personality disorders.* Cambridge, MA: Yale University Press.

Kety, S. S., Wender, P. H., Jacobsen, B., Ingraham, L. J., Jansson, L., Faber, B. and Kinney, D.K. (1994) Mental illness in the biological and adoptive relatives of schizophrenic adoptees, *Archives of General Psychiatry, 51,* 442–455.

Kinney, D. K., Holzman, P. S., Jacobsen, B., Jansson, L. *et al.* (1997) Thought disorder in schizophrenic and control adoptees and their relatives, *Archives of General Psychiatry, 54,* 475–479.

Klein, M. (1988) *Love, guilt and reparation. Envy and gratitude.* London: Virago.

Knoll, J. L., Garver, D. L., Ramberg, J. E. *et al.* (1998) Heterogeneity of the psychoses: Is there a neurodegenerative psychosis?, *Schizophrenia Bulletin, 24,* 365–379.

Kopala, L. C., Fredrikson, D., Good, K. P. *et al.* (1996) Symptoms in neuroleptic naïve first episode schizophrenia: Response to risperidone, *Biological Psychiatry, 39,* 296–298.

Kopala, L. C., Kimberley, P. G. and Honer, W. G. (1997) Extrapyramidal signs and clinical symptoms in first-episode schizophrenia: Response to low dose Risperidone, *Journal of Clinical Psychopharmacology, 17,* 308–313.

Kraemer, G. W., Ebert, M. H., Lake, C. R. *et al.* (1984) Hypersensitivity to d-amphetamine several years after early social deprivation in rhesus monkeys, *Psychopharmacology, 82*, 266–271.

Kraepelin, E. (1971/1919) *Dementia praecox and paraphrenia.* New York: Huntington.

Kretschmer, E. (1966) *Der sensitive Beziehungswahn* (4th ed.). Berlin: Springer-Verlag.

Kuipers, E., Fowler, D., Garety, P. *et al.* (1998) London-East Anglia randomised controlled trial of cognitive-behavioural therapy for psychosis. III. Follow-up and economic evaluation at 18 months, *British Journal of Psychiatry, 173*, 61–68.

Kuipers, L., Leff, J. and Lam, D. (1992) *Family work for schizophrenia. A practical guide.* London: Gaskell.

Lagerlöf, S. (1901–1902) *Jerusalem.* Stockholm: Bonnier.

Laing, R. D. (1960) *The divided self.* London: Tavistock.

Laing, R. D. and Esterson, A. (1964) *Sanity, madness and the family.* London: Tavistock.

Larsen, T. K., Johannesen, J. O. and Opjordsmoen, S. (1998) First-episode schizophrenia with long duration of untreated psychosis, *British Journal of Psychiatry, 172*, suppl 1, 45–52.

Lawrie, S. M. and Abukmeil, S. S. (1998) Brain abnormality in schizophrenia – a systematic and quantitative review of volumetric magnetic resonance imaging studies, *British Journal of Psychiatry, 172*, 110–120.

Leff, J. P., Kuipers, L., Berkowitz, R. *et al.* (1985) A controlled trial of social intervention in the families of schizophrenic patients: A two-year follow-up, *British Journal of Psychiatry, 146*, 594–600.

Lehtinen, K. (1993) Need-adapted treatment of schizophrenia: A five-year follow-up study from the Turku project, *Acta Psychiatrica Scandinavica, 87*, 96–101.

Lehtinen, K. and Cullberg, J. (1999) Neonatal hyperbilirubinaemia – a vulnerability factor for mental disorder?, *Acta Psychiatrica Scandinavica, 100*, 469–471.

Leighton, A. (1963) *The character of danger.* New York: Basic Books.

Levander, S. and Cullberg, J. (1993) Sandra: Successful psychotherapeutic work with a schizophrenic woman, *Psychiatry, 56*, 284–293.

Lewander, T. (1994) Neuroleptics and the neuroleptic-induced deficit syndrome, *Acta Psychiatrica Scandinavica, 89*, suppl 380, 8–13.

Liberman, R., Wallace, C. J., Blackwell, G. *et al.* (1998) Social skills training versus psychosocial occupational therapy for persons with persistent schizophrenia, *American Journal of Psychiatry, 155*, 1087–1091.

Loebel, A. D., Lieberman, J. A., Alvir, J. M. J. *et al.* (1992) Duration of psychosis and outcome in first episode schizophrenia, *American Journal of Psychiatry, 149*, 1183–1188.

Luborsky, L., Singer, B. and Luborsky, L. (1975) Comparative studies of psychotherapies. Is it true that everyone has won and all must have prizes?, *Archives of General Psychiatry, 32*, 995–1008.

Luborsky, L., Barber, J. P. and Beutler, L. (1993) Introduction to special section: A briefing on curative factors in dynamic psychotherapy, *Journal of Consulting and Clinical Psychology, 61*, 539–541.

Lundquist, G. (1949) *Modern svensk sinnessjukvård.* Stockholm: Modern Litteratur.

McEvoy, J. P., Hogarty, G. E. and Steingard, S. (1991) Optimal dose of neuroleptic in acute schizophrenia. A controlled study of the neuroleptic threshold and higher haloperidol dose, *Archives of General Psychiatry, 48*, 739–745.

McGlashan, T. H. (1984) The Chestnut Lodge follow-up study: II. Long-term outcome of schizophrenia and the affective disorders, *Archives of General Psychiatry, 41*, 141–144.

McGlashan, T. H. and Johannessen, J. O. (1996) Early detection and intervention with schizophrenia: Rationale, *Schizophrenia Bulletin, 22*, 201–222.

McGlashan, T. H. and Keats, C. J. (1989) *Schizophrenia – treatment process and outcome*. Washington, DC: American Psychiatric Press.

McGorry, O. P. K. and Jackson, H. J. (Eds.) (1999) *The recognition and management of early psychosis. A preventive approach.* Cambridge: Cambridge University Press.

McGorry, P. D. (1994) The influence of illness duration on syndrome clarity and stability in functional psychosis: Does the diagnosis emerge and stabilize with time?, *Australia and New Zealand Journal of Psychiatry, 28*, 607–619.

McGorry, P. D., Chanen, A., McCarty, E. *et al.* (1991) Post traumatic stress disorder following recent-onset psychosis; an unrecognized post-psychotic syndrome, *Journal of Nervous and Mental Disorders, 179*, 251–258.

McGorry, P. D., Edwards, J., Mihalopoulos, C. *et al.* (1996) EPPIC: An evolving system of early detection and optimal management, *Schizophrenia Bulletin, 22*, 305–326.

McGuire, P. K., Shah G. M. S. and Murray, R. M. (1994) Increased blood flow in Broca's area during auditory hallucinations in schizophrenia, *Lancet, 342*, 703–706.

Masterman, D. L. and Cummings, J. L. (1997) Frontal-subcortical corciots: The anatomical basis of executive, social and motivated behaviours, *Journal of Psychopharmacology, 11*, 107–114.

May, R. A., Tuma, A. H. and Dixon, W. J. (1968) *Treatment of schizophrenia. A comparative study of five treatment methods.* New York: Science House.

Mednick, S. A., Machon, R. A., Huttunen, M. O. *et al.* (1988) Adult schizophrenia following prenatal exposure to an influenza epidemic, *Archives of General Psychiatry, 45*, 189–192.

Meltzer, D. (1992) *The claustrum*. Worchester: Clunie Press.

Merwin, W. S. (1970) A Garden. In W. S. Merwin, *The Miner's Pale Children* (pp. 213–214). New York: Atheneum.

Meuser, K. T., Rosenberg, S. D., Goodman, L. A. and Trumbetta, S. L. (2002) Trauma, PTSD, and the course of severe mental illness: An interactive model, *Schizophrenia Research, 53*, 123–143.

Milgram, S. (1958) Some conditions of obedience and disobedience to authority, *International Journal of Psychiatry, 6*, 259–276.

Mill, J. S. (1859) *On liberty*. London.

Miller, R. (1987) The time course of neuroleptic therapy for psychosis; role of learning processes and implications for concepts of psychotic illness, *Psychopharmacology, 92*, 405–415.

Mortensen, P. B., Pedersen, C. B., Westergaard, T. *et al.* (1999) Effects of family history and place and season of birth on the risk of schizophrenia, *New England Journal of Medicine, 340*, 603–608.

Mosher, L. R., Vallone, R. and Menn, A. (1995) The treatment of acute psychosis without neuroleptics: Six-week psychopathology data from the Soteria project, *International Journal of Social Psychiatry, 41,* 157–173.

Munk-Jørgensen, P. and Mortensen, P. B. (1992) Incidence and other aspects of the epidemiology of schizophrenia in Denmark, 1971–1987, *British Journal of Psychiatry.*

Nordentoft, M., Jeppesen, P., Petersen, L. *et al.* (2004) *The Opus trial: A randomised multi-center trial of integrated versus standard treatment for 547 first-episode patients.* Poster presentation, Davos.

Nyberg S., Eriksson, O. Oxenstierna, B. *et al.* (1999) Suggested minimal effective dose of risperidone based on PET measured D2-and 5-HT2A-receptor occupancy in schizophrenic patients, *American Journal of Psychiatry, 156,* 869–875.

Ödegard, Ö. (1964) Pattern of discharge from Norwegian psychiatric hospitals before and after the introduction of psychotropic drugs, *American Journal of Psychiatry, 120,* 772–778.

Palmblad, E. and Cullberg, J. (1990) Grannars reaktioner på ett psykoterapeutiskt behandlingshem [Neighbours' reactions to a psychotherapeutic residence for treatment], *Nord Psykiatrika Tidsskrift, 44,* 551–558.

Pao, P. N. (1979) *Schizophrenic disorders.* Madison, CT: International Universities Press.

Paulesu, E., Frith, C. D. and Frackowiak, R.S.J. (1993) The neural correlates of the verbal components of working memory, *Nature, 362,* 342–344.

Perris, C. (1988) *Kognitiv psychoterapi vid schizofrena störningar.* Stockholm: Pilgrim Press.

Rabkin, J. G. (1980) Stressful life events and schizophrenia: A review of recent literature, *Psychological Bulletin, 87,* 408–425.

Räkköläinen, V. (1977) *Onset of psychosis. A clinical study of 68 cases.* Unpublished PhD thesis, University of Turku.

Rang, H. P., Dale, M. M. and Ritter, J. M. (1999) *Pharmacology.* Edinburgh: Churchill Livingstone.

Read, J. (1997) Child abuse and psychosis: A literature review and implications for professional practice, *Professional Psychology: Research and Practice, 28,* 448–456.

Robbins, M. (1993) *Experiences of schizophrenia. An integration of the personal, scientific and therapeutic.* New York: Guilford Press.

Romme, M. and Escher, S. (1989) Hearing voices, *Schizophrenia Bulletin, 15,* 209–216.

—— (2000) *Making sense of voices – a guide for mental health professionals working with voice-hearers.* London: MIND Publications.

Rosenbaum, B. (2000) *Tankeformer og talemåder* [Kinds of thinking and talking]. Copenhagen: Multivers forlag.

Rosenbaum, B. and Sonne, H. (1986) *The language of psychosis.* New York: New York University Press.

Sacks, O. (1995) *An anthropologist on Mars.* New York: Knopf.

—— (1998) *The man who mistook his wife for a hat.* New York: Simon and Schuster.

Sandin, B. (1986) *Den Zebrarandiga pudelkärnan.* Stockholm: Rabén and Sjögren.

Schneider, K. (1967) *Klinische Psychopathologie* (8th ed.). Stutttgart: Georg Thieme Verlag.

Schwartz, M. L. and Goldman-Rakic, P. (1990) Development and plasticity of the primate cerebra cortex, *Clinics in Perinatology, 17*, 83–102.

Searles, H. (1965) *Collected papers on schizophrenia and related subjects.* London: Hogarth Press.

Sechehaye, M. (1947) *La réalisation symbolique.* Bern: Huber.

Sedvall, G. and Farde, L. (1995) Chemical brain anatomy in schizophrenia, *Lancet, 346,* 743–749.

Shepherd, M., Watt, D., Falloon, I. and Smeeton, N. (1989) The natural history of schizophrenia: A five year follow-up study of outcome and prediction in a representative sample of schizophrenics, *Psychological Medicine,* suppl 15.

Siegel, D. J. (1999) *The developing mind: Toward a neurobiology of interpersonal experience.* London: Guilford Press.

Sifneos, P. E. (1973) The prevalence of 'alexithymnic' characteristics in psychosomatic patients, *Psychotherapy and Psychosomatics, 22,* 255–262.

Sjöström, R. (1985) Effects of psychotherapy in schizophrenia. A retrospective study, *Acta Psychiatrica Scandinavica, 71,* 513–522.

Slade, P. D. (1984) Sensory deprivation and clinical psychiatry, *British Journal of Hospital Medicine, 32,* 256–260.

Solomon, G. S. (1987) Psycho-neuroimmunology. Interactions between central nervous system and immune system, *Journal of Neuroscience Research, 18,* 1–9.

SOU (1958) Mentalsjukvården – Planering och organisation, 38.

SOU (1992) Välfärd och valfrihet service, stöd och vård för psykiskt störda, 73.

Stefenson, A. and Cullberg, J. (1995) Committed suicide in a total schizophrenic cohort: In the search of the suicidal process, *Nordic Journal of Psychiatry, 49,* 429–437.

Stefenson, A. and Cullberg, J. (2005) *Suicidality in persons with schizophrenia – subjective perspectives.* Manuscript submitted for publication.

Stein, L. I. and Test, M. A. (1980) Alternative to mental hospital treatment. I. Conceptual model, treatment program and clinical evaluation, *Archives of General Psychiatry, 37,* 392–397.

Stern, D. (1985) *The interpersonal world of the infant.* New York: Basic Books.

Stone, M. H. (1986) Explorative psychotherapy in schizophrenia-spectrum patients: A reevaluation in the light of long-term follow up of schizophrenic and borderline patients, *Bulletin of the Menninger Clinic, 50,* 287–306.

Strauss, J. S. (1989) Mediating processes in schizophrenia – towards a new dynamic psychiatry, *British Journal of Psychiatry, 55,* suppl 5, 22–28.

Strauss, J., Carpenter, W. T. and Bartko, J. J. (1974) An approach to the diagnosis and understanding of schizophrenia. III: Speculations on the processes that underlie schizophrenia symptoms and signs, *Schizophrenia Bulletin, 2,* 61–69.

Suddath, R. L., Christison, G. W., Torrey, E. F. *et al.* (1990) Anatomical abnormalities in the brains of monozygotic twins discordant for schizophrenia, *New England Journal of Medicine, 322,* 789–794.

Svedberg, B., Mesterton, A. and Cullberg, J. (2001) First episode non-affective psychosis in a total urban population: A five year follow-up, *Social Psychiatry and Psychiatric Epidemiology, 36,* 332–337.

Svensson, B. (1999) *Treatment process and outcome for long-term mentally ill patients in a comprehensive treatment program based on cognitive therapy.* Academic dissertation, Lunds University.

Tarrier, N., Wittkowski, A., Kinney, C. *et al.* (1999) Durability of the effects of cognitive behavioural therapy in the treatment of chronic schizophrenia: 12-month follow-up, *British Journal of Psychiatry, 174,* 500–504.

Tienari, P. (1991) Interactions between genetic vulnerability and family environment: The Finnish adoptive family study of schizophrenia, *Acta Psychiatrica Scandinavica, 84,* 460–465.

Torrey, E. F., Taylor, E. H., Bracha, H. S. *et al.* (1994) Prenatal origin of schizophrenia in a subgroup of discordant monozygotic twins, *Schizophrenia Bulletin, 20,* 423–432.

Tranströmer, T. (1983) Carillon. In T. Tranströmer, *Det vilda torget.* Stockholm: Bonnier; trans. R. Fulton, *New Collected Poems,* Newcastle, Bloodaxe Books (2002).

Tsuang, M. T., Woolson, R., Fleming, J. A. (1979) Long-term outcome of major psychoses: I. Schizophrenia and affective disorders compared with psychiatrically symptom-free surgical conditions, *Archives of General Psychiatry, 39,* 1295–1301.

Van Os, J. and Selten, J. P. (1998) Prenatal exposure to maternal stress and subsequent schizophrenia, *British Journal of Psychiatry, 172,* 324–326.

Vaughn, C. E. and Leff, J. P. (1976) The influence of family and social factors on the course of psychiatric illness. A comparison of schizophrenic and depressed neurotic patients, *British Journal of Psychiatry, 129,* 125–137.

Verdoux, H. and Cougnard, A. (2003) The early detection and treatment controversy in schizophrenia research, *Current Opinion in Psychiatry, 16,* 175–179.

Wahlberg, K. E., Wynne, L. C., Oja, H., Keskitalo, P. *et al.* (1997) Gene-environment interation in vulnerability to schizophrenia: Findings from the Finnish adoptive family study of schizophrenia, *American Journal of Psychiatry, 154,* 355–362.

Warner, R. (1994) *Recovery from schizophrenia. Psychiatry and political economy* (2nd ed.). London: Routledge.

Weinberger, D. (1995) From neuropathology to neurodevelopment, *Lancet, 346,* 552–557.

Werbart, A. (1997) Separation, termination-process, and long-term outcome in psychotherapy with severely disturbed patients, *Bulletin of the Menninger Clinic, 61,* 16–43.

Widerlöv, B., Borgå, P. and Cullberg, J. (1989) Epidemiology of long-term functional psychosis in three different areas in Stockholm county, *Acta Psychiatrica Scandinavica, 80,* 40–46.

Wing, J. (1960) A pilot experiment of long hospitalized male schizophrenic patients, *British Journal of Preventive and Social Medicine, 14,* 173–180.

Winnicott, D. W. (1971) *Playing and reality.* London: Tavistock.

World Health Organization (WHO) (1994) *ICD-10, International statistical classification of diseases and related health problems* (10th ed.). Genève: World Health Organization.

Yung, A. R. and McGorry, P. D. (1996) The prodromal phase of first episode psychosis: Past and current conceptualisations, *Schizophrenia Bulletin, 22,* 353–370.

Yung, A. R., McGorry, P. D., McFarlane, C. A. *et al.* (1996) Monitoring and care of young people at incipient risk of psychosis, *Schizophrenia Bulletin, 22*, 283–303.

Zubin, J. and Spring, B. (1977) Vulnerability – a new view of schizophrenia, *Journal of Abnormal Psychology, 86*, 103–126.

Index

Page entries for main headings which have subheadings refer to general aspects of that topic.

Page entries in **bold** refer to tables/figures/diagrams.